Obstetric Clinical Algorithms

Obstetric Clinical Algorithms

Second Edition

Errol R. Norwitz, M.D., Ph.D., M.B.A.
Louis E. Phaneuf Professor of Obstetrics & Gynecology
Tufts University School of Medicine
Chairman., Department of Obstetrics & Gynecology
Tufts Medical Center
Boston, USA

George R. Saade, M.D.
University of Texas Medical Branch
Galveston, TX, USA

Hugh Miller, M.D.
Department of Obstetrics and Gynecology
University of Arizona
Tuscon, AZ, USA

Christina M. Davidson, M.D.
Baylor College of Medicine
Ben Taub Hospital
Houston, TX, USA

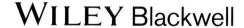

Registered Office
John Wiley & Sons, Ltd, The Atrium, Southern Gate, Chichester, West Sussex, PO19 8SQ, UK

Editorial Offices
9600 Garsington Road, Oxford, OX4 2DQ, UK
The Atrium, Southern Gate, Chichester, West Sussex, PO19 8SQ, UK
111 River Street, Hoboken, NJ 07030-5774, USA

For details of our global editorial offices, for customer services and for information about how to apply for permission to reuse the copyright material in this book please see our website at www.wiley.com/wiley-blackwell.

Library of Congress Cataloging-in-Publication Data

Names: Norwitz, Errol R., author. | Saade, George R., 1960– author. |
    Miller, Hugh S. (Hugh Stephen), author. | Davidson, Christina (Christina Marie) author.
Title: Obstetric clinical algorithms / Errol R. Norwitz, George R. Saade, Hugh Miller, Christina M. Davidson.
Description: 2nd edition. | Chichester, West Sussex, UK ; Hoboken, NJ : John Wiley & Sons, Inc., 2017. |
    Preceded by: Obstetric clinical algorithms : management and evidence / Errol R. Norwitz ... [et al.]. 2010. |
    Includes bibliographical references and index.
Identifiers: LCCN 2016024815 (print) | LCCN 2016026085 (ebook) | ISBN 9781118849903 (pbk.) | ISBN
    9781118849873 (pdf) | ISBN 9781118849880 (epub)
Subjects: | MESH: Pregnancy Complications–diagnosis | Pregnancy Complications–therapy | Algorithms |
    Decision Support Techniques
Classification: LCC RG571 (print) | LCC RG571 (ebook) | NLM WQ 240 | DDC 618.3–dc23
LC record available at https://lccn.loc.gov/2016024815

A catalogue record for this book is available from the British Library.

Wiley also publishes its books in a variety of electronic formats. Some content that appears in print may not be available in electronic books.

Cover image: Jasmina/Gettyimages

Set in 8.5/12pt Meridien by SPi Global, Pondicherry, India
Printed and bound in Malaysia by Vivar Printing Sdn Bhd

1   2017

Contents

Preface

Recent advances in obstetrical practice and research have resulted in significant improvements in maternal and perinatal outcome. Such improvements carry with them added responsibility for the obstetric care provider. The decision to embark on a particular course of management simply because *"that's the way we did it when I was in training"* or because *"it worked the last time I tried it"* is no longer acceptable. Clinical decisions should, wherever possible, be evidence-based. Evidence-based medicine can be defined as *"the conscientious, explicit, and judicious use of current best evidence in making decisions about the care of individual patients"* [1]. In practice, evidence-based medicine requires expertise in retrieving, interpreting, and applying the results of scientific studies and in effectively communicating the risks and benefits of different courses of action to patients. This daunting task is compounded by the fact that the volume of medical literature is doubling every 10–15 years. Even within the relatively narrow field of Obstetrics & Gynecology, there are more than five major publications each month containing an excess of 100 original articles and 35 editorials. How then does a busy practitioner maintain a solid foundation of up-to-date knowledge and synthesize these data into individual management plans? New information can be gleaned from a variety of sources: the advice of colleagues and consultants, textbooks, lectures and continuing medical education courses, original research and review articles, and from published clinical guidelines and consensus statements. The internet has created an additional virtual dimension by allowing instant access to the medical literature to both providers and patients. It is with this background in mind that we have written *Obstetric Clinical Algorithms: Management and Evidence, 2nd edition.*

Standardization of management reduces medical errors and improves patient safety and obstetrical outcomes [2,3]. In this text, we have developed a series of obstetric algorithms based on best practice to mimic the decision-making processes that go on in our brains when faced with a vexing clinical problem. To further facilitate decision-making, we have superimposed "levels of evidence" as defined by the report of the US Preventive Services Task Force (USPSTF) of the Agency for Healthcare Research Quality, an independent panel of experts appointed and funded by the US government to systematically review evidence of effectiveness and develop recommendations for clinical preventive services [4]. The table below summarizes the 'levels of evidence' used in this text.

'Levels of Evidence' used in *Obstetric Clinical Algorithms: Management and Evidence, 2nd edition:*

Color key	Levels of evidence available on which to base recommendations*	Recommendation/ suggestions for practice
Red bold	Level I/II-1	Definitely offer or provide this service
Red regular	Level II-1/II-2	Consider offering or providing this service
Red italics	*Level II-2/II-3/III*	*Discuss this service, but insufficient evidence to strongly recommend it*
Black regular	Level II-3/III	Insufficient evidence to recommend this service, but may be a reasonable option

*Levels of evidence are based on the 'hierarchy of research design' used in the report of the 2nd US Preventive Services Task Force:

Level I: Evidence obtained from at least one properly powered and conducted randomized controlled trial (RCT); also includes well-conducted systematic review or meta-analysis of homogeneous RCTs.

Level II-1: Evidence obtained from well-designed controlled trials without randomization.

Level II-2: Evidence obtained from well-designed cohort or case-control analytic studies, preferably from more than one center or research group.

Level II-3: Evidence obtained from multiple time series with or without the intervention; dramatic results from uncontrolled trials might also be regarded as this type of evidence.

Level III: Opinions of respected authorities, based on clinical experience; descriptive studies or case reports; or reports of expert committees.

Obstetric care providers can be broadly divided into two philosophical camps: those who believe that everything possible should be offered in a given clinical setting in the hope that something may help (also called the *"we don't have all the information we need"* or *"might as well give it, it won't do any harm"* group) and those who hold out until there is consistent and compelling scientific evidence that an individual course of action is beneficial and has a favorable risk-to-benefit ratio (sometimes referred to as *"therapeutic nihilists"*). As protagonists of the latter camp, we argue that substantial harm can be done—both to individual patients and to society as a whole—by implementing management plans that have not been the subject of rigorous scientific investigation followed by thoughtful introduction into clinical practice. In *Obstetric Clinical Algorithms: Management and Evidence,* 2nd edition, we provide evidence-based management recommendations for common obstetrical conditions. It is the sincere hope of the authors that the reader will find this book both practical and informative. However, individual clinical decisions should not be based on medical algorithms alone, but should be guided also by provider experience and judgment.

Errol R. Norwitz
George R. Saade
Hugh Miller
Christina M. Davidson

1. Sackett DL, Rosenberg WM, Gray JA *et al.* Evidence based medicine: what it is and what it isn't. *BMJ* 1996;**312**:71–72.
2. Pettker CM, Thung SF, Norwitz ER *et al.* Impact of a comprehensive patient safety strategy on obstetric adverse events. *Am J Obstet Gynecol* 2009;**200**:492 (e1-8).
3. Clark SL, Belfort MA, Byrum SL *et al.* Improved outcomes, fewer cesarean deliveries, and reduced litigation: results of a new paradigm in patient safety. *Am J Obstet Gynecol* 2008;**199**:105 (e1-7).
4. Report of the US Preventive Services Task Force (USPSTF). Available at http://www.ahrq.gov/clinic/uspstfix.htm (last accessed on 19 February 2016).

List of Abbreviations

ABG	arterial blood gas	BV	bacterial vaginosis
AC	abdominal circumference	CAOS	chronic abruption-oligohydramnios sequence
ACA	anticardiolipin antibody		
ACE	angiotensin-converting enzyme	CBC	complete blood count
ACIP	Advisory Committee on Immunization Practices	CDC	Centers for Disease Control and Prevention in the U.S.
ACOG	American College of Obstetricians and Gynecologists	CFU	colony-forming units
		CI	cervical insufficiency
AED	antiepileptic drug	CL	cervical length
AED	automated external defibrillator	CMV	cytomegalovirus
AFE	amniotic fluid embolism	CO	cardiac output
AFI	Amniotic Fluid Index	CPD	cephalopelvic disproportion
AGA	appropriate for gestational age	CST	contraction stress test
AGC	atypical glandular cells	CT	computed tomography
AHA	American Heart Association	CTG	cardiotocography
AIDS	acquired immune deficiency syndrome	CVS	chorionic villous sampling
		CXR	chest radiograph
AIS	adenocarcinoma in situ	DCIS	ductal carcinoma in situ
AMA	advanced maternal age	DES	diethylstilbestrol
ANA	antinuclear antibodies	DIC	disseminated intravascular coagulopathy
APLAS	antiphospholipid antibody syndrome		
ARB	angiotensin receptor blockers	DKA	diabetic ketoacidosis
ARDS	acute respiratory distress syndrome	DVT	deep vein thrombosis
ART	assisted reproductive technology	ECC	endocervical curettage
ART	antiretroviral therapy	ECG	electrocardiography
ARV	antiretroviral	ECT	electroconvulsant therapy
ASCUS	atypical squamous cells of undetermined significance	ECV	external cephalic version
		EDD	estimated date of delivery
ATP	alloimmune thrombocytopenia	EFM	electronic fetal monitoring
AZT	azidothymidine	EFW	estimated fetal weight
BCG	Bacillus Calmette-Guérin	ELISA	enzyme-linked immunosorbant assay
BMI	body mass index	EMB	endometrial biopsy
BP	blood pressure	FEV1	forced expiratory volume in one second
BPD	biparietal diameter		
BPP	biophysical profile	fFN	fetal fibronectin
BUN	blood urea nitrogen	FFP	fresh frozen plasma

FL	femur length		LFT	liver function test
FSE	fetal scalp electrode		LGA	large-for-gestational age
FTA-ABS	fluorescent treponemal antibody absorption		LGSIL	low-grade squamous intraepithelial lesions
FVC	forced vital capacity		LMP	last menstrual period
GBS	Group B β-hemolytic streptococcus		LMWH	low molecular weight heparin
GCT	glucose challenge test		LTL	laparoscopic tubal ligation
GDM	gestational diabetes mellitus		MCA	middle cerebral artery
GFR	glomerular filtration rate		MDI	metered dose inhaler
GLT	glucose load test		MFM	maternal-fetal medicine
GTT	glucose tolerance test		MFPR	multifetal pregnancy reduction
HBsAb	anti-hepatitis B surface antibodies		MHA-TP	microhemagglutination assay for antibodies to *T. pallidum*
HBsAg	hepatitis B surface antigen			
HBIg	hepatitis B immunoglobulin		MoM	multiples of the median
HBV	hepatitis B virus		MRCP MR	cholangiopancreatography
HC	head circumference		MRI	magnetic resonance imaging
hCG	human chorionic gonadotropin		MS-AFP	maternal serum α-fetoprotein
HEG	hyperemesis gravidarum		MTX	methotrexate
HELLP	hemolysis, elevated liver enzymes, low platelets		NIDDM	non-insulin-dependent diabetes mellitus
HGSIL	high-grade squamous intraepithelial lesions		NIPT	noninvasive prenatal testing
			NR-NST	non-reactive NST
HIE	hypoxic ischemic encephalopathy		NSAIDs	non-steroidal anti-inflammatory drugs
HIV	human immunodeficiency virus			
HPV	human papilloma virus		NST	non-stress testing
HSV	herpes simplex virus		NT	nuchal translucency
IAI	intraamniotic infection		NTD	neural tube defect
ICP	intrahepatic cholestasis of pregnancy		NVP	nausea and vomiting in pregnancy
ICU	intensive care unit		OCT	oxytocin challenge test
IgA	immunoglobulin A		OST	oxytocin stimulation test
IgG	immunoglobulin G		PCOS	polycystic ovarian syndrome
IGRA	interferon gamma release assay		PCP	*pneumocystis carinii* pneumonia
INH	isoniazid		PCR	polymerase chain reaction
IOL	induction of labor		PE	pulmonary embolism
IOM	Institute of Medicine		PEFR	peak expiratory flow rate
ITP	immune thrombocytopenic purpura		PKU	phenylketonuria
			po	per os (orally)
IUFD	intrauterine fetal demise		POC	products of conception
IUGR	intrauterine growth restriction		PPD	purified protein derivative
IUPC	intrauterine pressure catheter		PPH	postpartum hemorrhage
IV	intravenous		pPROM	preterm PROM
IVIG	intravenous immune globulin		PRBC	packed red blood cell
LAC	lupus anticoagulant		PROM	premature rupture of membranes
LEEP	loop electrosurgical excision procedure		PTT	partial thromboplastin time
			PTU	propylthiouracil

PUBS	percutaneous umbilical blood sampling	**TPPA**	*T. pallidum* particle agglutination assay
q	every	**TRAP**	twin reverse arterial perfusion
QFT-GIT	QuantiFERON®-TB Gold In-Tube test	**TST**	tuberculin skin testing
RhoGAM	anti-Rh[D]-immunoglobulin	**TTP/HUS**	thrombotic thrombocytopenic purpura/hemolytic uremic syndrome
R-NST	reactive NST		
RPL	recurrent pregnancy loss	**TTTS**	twin-to-twin transfusion syndrome
RPR	rapid plasma reagin		
SC	subcuticular	**UA C&S**	urine culture and sensitivity
SGA	small for gestational age	**UDCA**	ursodeoxycholic acid
SIADH	syndrome of inappropriate ADH secretion	**UFH**	unfractionated heparin
		UTI	urinary tract infection
SLE	systemic lupus erythematosus	**VAS**	vibroacoustic stimulation
SMA	spinal muscular atrophy	**VBAC**	vaginal birth after cesarean
SSI	surgical site infection	**VDRL**	Venereal Disease Research Laboratory
STI	sexually transmitted infection		
TB	tuberculosis	**VL**	viral load
TBG	thyroxine-binding globulin	**V/Q**	ventilation-perfusion
TFT	thyroid function test	**VTE**	venous thromboembolism
TORCH	toxoplasmosis, rubella, cytomegalovirus, herpes	**ZDV**	zidovudine

SECTION 1

Preventative Health

1 Abnormal Pap Smear in Pregnancy

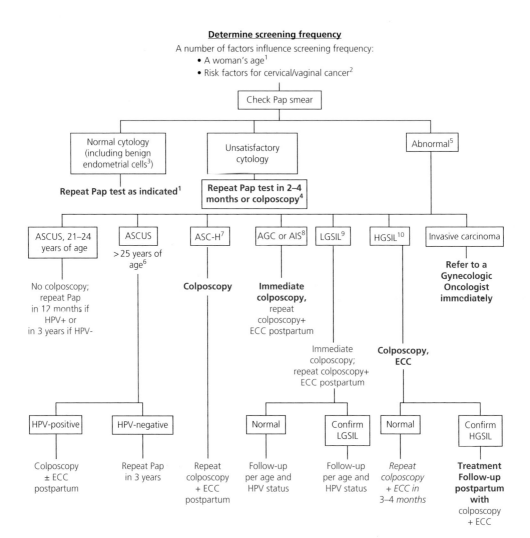

1. Recommendations for screening and management of abnormal cervical cytology in pregnancy follow from the general guidelines for screening onset and frequency that were updated in 2012 to reflect the recommendations of the American Cancer Society ACOG, and U.S. Preventive Services Task Force for detection of cervical cancer. Routine pap screening should **not** be collected until age 21 regardless of first vaginal intercourse. The risk of severe dysplasia or cancer

Obstetric Clinical Algorithms, Second Edition. Errol R. Norwitz, George R. Saade, Hugh Miller and Christina M. Davidson.
© 2017 John Wiley & Sons, Ltd. Published 2017 by John Wiley & Sons, Ltd.

is very low among adolescents, but they should be encouraged to receive human papilloma virus (HPV) vaccination and counseled about safe sex practices to limit exposure to sexually transmitted infections. Women between the age of 21–29 years should be screened with cervical cytology alone. Women >30 years of age should be screened with cytology and HPV testing every 5 years (or with cytology alone every 3 years). Women with a history of cervical cancer, HIV or other risk factors (such as immunocompromise) should continue annual screening. These guidelines and the associated algorithm are based on a large database of patients including adolescents who were managed using former criteria in the Kaiser Healthcare system. The American Society of Colposcopy and Cervical Pathology (ASCCP) has developed an updated free App that can assist with the current recommendations.

2. Women who have risk factors for cervical/vaginal cancer (such as a history of *in utero* diethylstilbestrol (DES) exposure, HIV, women who are immunocompromised, or those on chronic steroids) should be screened annually.

3. Women aged 21–29 with normal cytology but absent or insufficient endocervical–transformation zone elements can continue regular screening, which should not include HPV testing. In women ≥30 years with a similar cytology result, HPV testing is recommended. Positive HPV results should prompt repeat co-testing in one year, unless the HPV genotype is known to be 16 or 18, in which case, immediate colposcopy is recommended. A negative HPV result in a woman ≥30 years means that she can go back to routine screening.

4. Unsatisfactory cytology is less common in current practice with the use of liquid-based media for cervical screening. Insufficient squamous cells to detect epithelial abnormalities generally arise from blood or inflammation that obscures the result. Repeat cytology is recommended in 2–4 months. Colposcopy can be considered in

women >30 years with positive HPV, and is recommended in those women who have had two consecutive unsatisfactory cytology test results.

5. Women should always be informed of an abnormal Pap result by her physician or another healthcare professional who can answer basic questions and allay anxiety. Verbal notification should be followed with written information and clear recommendations for follow-up. Additionally, if there is evidence of infection along with cellular abnormalities, the infection should be treated.

6. The 2012 criteria substantially clarify the management of ASCUS, which is guided by HPV test results whether obtained reflexively or as a co-test. The management in pregnancy differs only in that colposcopy and endocervical curettage (ECC) should be deferred until 6 weeks postpartum unless a CIN 2+ lesion is suspected. Women ≥25 years old with a negative HPV test should be returned to a regular three-year follow-up cycle. Following pregnancy colposcopy is recommended in women who are HPV+ with annual co-test follow-up. Similarly, an endocervical curettage (ECC) should be obtained whenever possible and excisional procedures should be avoided to prevent over-treatment. In women 21–24 years old, cytology should be repeated in one year. A positive HPV result does not change the recommended follow-up, but a negative result should return the woman to a three-year follow-up cycle.

7. Atypical squamous cells cannot exclude high-grade squamous intraepithelial lesions (HSIL) (ASC-H), which is associated with a higher risk of CIN 3+ regardless of patient age and a five-year invasive cancer risk of 2% regardless of HPV status. That said, HPV is highly correlated with ASC-H, but the cancer risk demands that all women receive immediate colposcopy, including those 21–24 years of age. Colposcopy with directed biopsies of any area that might be concerning for micro invasion

should be done by a highly trained clinician. Treatment should be dictated by histologic evaluation of the biopsied lesions.

8. Atypical glandular cells (AGC) or adenocarcinoma in situ (AIS) warrant aggressive investigation and close follow-up. Although the risk of cancer is lower in younger age groups, women ≥30 years have a 9% risk of CIN3+ and 2% risk of invasive cancer. All such women of all ages should have antenatal colposcopy with 6-weeks postpartum follow-up to include colposcopy, ECC and endometrial biopsy (EMB). Subsequent treatment and follow-up are dictated by the biopsy results, maternal age, and the histologic evaluation of the glandular elements.

9. Approximately 60% of low-grade squamous intraepithelial lesions (LGSIL) will regress spontaneously without treatment depending on the age of the patient, HPV status, and HPV genotype. For women ≥25 years old in whom HPV testing is negative, repeat co-testing in ome year is preferred but colposcopy is acceptable. However, if the HPV is positive, then colposcopy is preferred. If colposcopy is not part of the initial evaluation, subsequent co-testing needs to be entirely normal to allow patients to return to three-year follow-up. Any abnormality at the one-year follow-up visit should result in colposcopy. In women 21–24 years old, annual repeat cytology without HPV testing is preferred and colposcopy should be avoided unless the results recur for two consecutive years or if one of the following lesions is detected: ASC-H, AGC, or HSIL. Pregnant women ≥25 years old with low-grade squamous intraepithelial lesions should undergo immediate colposcopy without ECC, while those 21–24 years old should be evaluated postpartum.

10. High-grade squamous intraepithelial lesions (HGSIL) are associated with a 60% risk of CIN2+ and a 2% risk of invasive cervical cancer. Immediate colposcopy with directed biopsies of any area that might be concerning for micro invasion is recommended, regardless of maternal age. The antepartum diagnosed of HGSIL should prompt a 6-weeks postpartum follow-up colposcopy with ECC and treatment as dictated by the biopsy results. If diagnosed early in pregnancy, colposcopy can be repeated every 12 weeks. Treatment during pregnancy should be reserved for invasive carcinoma and should be managed in concert with a gynecologic oncologist.

2 Immunization

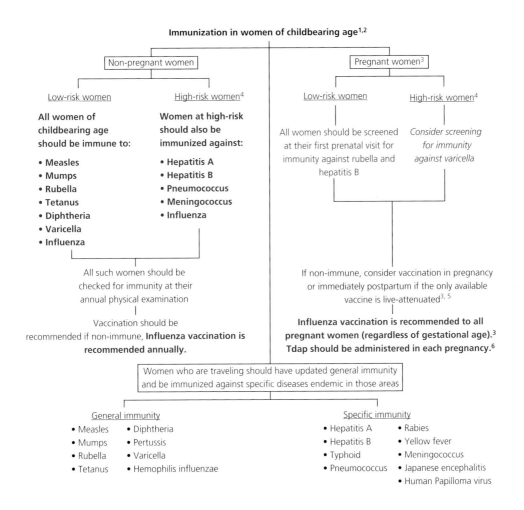

Immunization in women of childbearing age[1,2]

Non-pregnant women | **Pregnant women[3]**

Non-pregnant women

Low-risk women

All women of childbearing age should be immune to:

- Measles
- Mumps
- Rubella
- Tetanus
- Diphtheria
- Varicella
- Influenza

High-risk women[4]

Women at high-risk should also be immunized against:

- Hepatitis A
- Hepatitis B
- Pneumococcus
- Meningococcus
- Influenza

All such women should be checked for immunity at their annual physical examination

Vaccination should be recommended if non-immune, **Influenza vaccination is recommended annually.**

Pregnant women[3]

Low-risk women

All women should be screened at their first prenatal visit for immunity against rubella and hepatitis B

High-risk women[4]

Consider screening for immunity against varicella

If non-immune, consider vaccination in pregnancy or immediately postpartum if the only available vaccine is live-attenuated[3, 5]

Influenza vaccination is recommended to all pregnant women (regardless of gestational age).[3] Tdap should be administered in each pregnancy.[6]

Women who are traveling should have updated general immunity and be immunized against specific diseases endemic in those areas

General immunity
- Measles   • Diphtheria
- Mumps   • Pertussis
- Rubella   • Varicella
- Tetanus   • Hemophilis influenzae

Specific immunity
- Hepatitis A   • Rabies
- Hepatitis B   • Yellow fever
- Typhoid   • Meningococcus
- Pneumococcus   • Japanese encephalitis
- Human Papilloma virus

1. Immunization can be active (vaccines, toxoid) or passive (immunoglobulin, antiserum/antitoxin). In *active immunity*, the immune response is induced by wild infection or vaccination, which is generally robust and long-lasting. As such, subsequent exposure to the vaccine-preventable infection will result in the release of antibodies and the prevention of illness. In *passive immunity*, antibodies are acquired passively through maternal transfer across the placenta or breast milk or through the receipt of exogenous immunoglobulins. Protection is temporary and fades within a few weeks to months. The immune system of the recipient is

Obstetric Clinical Algorithms, Second Edition. Errol R. Norwitz, George R. Saade, Hugh Miller and Christina M. Davidson.
© 2017 John Wiley & Sons, Ltd. Published 2017 by John Wiley & Sons, Ltd.

therefore not programmed, and subsequent exposure to vaccine-preventable infections can lead to active infection.

2. *Vaccination* works by inducing antibodies in recipients that protects them against infection after future exposure to specific disease-causing microbes. The level of protection varies according to the strength and durability of the immune response induced by the vaccine as well as the virulence, prevalence, and ease of transmission of the infection itself. Vaccination programs may have different goals: (i) to protect at-risk individuals (e.g., meningococcal disease); (ii) to establish control by minimizing the overall prevalence of the infection (e.g., measles, varicella); or (iii) to attain global elimination of an infection (e.g., neonatal tetanus, polio).

3. Vaccination in pregnancy is of benefit and at times poses concern relative to the increased vulnerability of the mother and fetus. Inactivated vaccines are approved for use in pregnancy. The inactivated influenza vaccine should be given to **all pregnant women** during the influenza season (October through May in the northern hemisphere), regardless of gestational age. It is clear that there are significant maternal benefits including fewer cases of fever and respiratory illness and substantial neonatal protection through the transplacental passage of antibodies that provide months of protection at a time when the infant is vulnerable and could not be directly vaccinated. However, live-attenuated vaccines (including rubella, MMR, varicella) are not recommended for pregnant women despite the fact that no cases of congenital anomalies have been documented. Exceptions include yellow fever and polio, which can be given to pregnant women when traveling to high prevalence areas. In addition, women should be advised not to get pregnant within 1 month of receiving a live-attenuated vaccine. The live-attenuated influenza vaccine is available as an intranasal spray, which is considered safe in the postpartum period. Vaccines

considered safe in pregnancy include tetanus, diphtheria, hepatitis B, and influenza. Tetanus immunization during pregnancy is a common strategy used in the developing world to combat neonatal tetanus

4. Risk factors for specific vaccine-preventable illnesses include:
- illicit drug users (hepatitis A and B, tetanus)
- men who have sex with men (hepatitis A) or >1 sexual partner in the past 6 months (hepatitis A, human papilloma virus)
- travel to or immigration from areas where infection is endemic (hepatitis A and B, measles, meningococcus, rubella, tetanus, varicella)
- healthcare workers (hepatitis B, influenza, varicella)
- nursing home residents (meningococcus, pneumococcus, varicella) or ≥50 years of age (influenza)
- chronic medical diseases: diabetes, asthma, HIV, liver disease and/or renal disease (hepatitis A, influenza, pneumococcus)
- adults who have had their spleens removed (meningococcus, pneumococcus)
- accidental or intentional puncture wounds (tetanus)

5. One of the ongoing controversies about vaccination in pregnancy is whether vaccines containing thimerosal pose a risk to the fetus. Thimerosal is a mercury-containing preservative that has been used in multidose vaccines since the 1930s. Although there has been concern about the cumulative levels of mercury, the current scientific evidence does not consider thimerosal to be associated with adverse outcomes in children exposed in utero. The Centers for Disease Control and Prevention's Advisory Committee on Immunization Practices (ACIP) does not recommend avoiding thimerosal containing vaccines. Although the ACIP does not recommend any specific formulation, there are newer trivalent and quadrivalent influenza vaccines (containing two A and two B influenza strains) that are available for use. The following

adult vaccines are thimerosal-free: Tdap (but not Td), Recombivax hepatitis B vaccine (but not Engerix-B), and some influenza vaccines (Fluzone with no thimerosal).

6. Tetanus toxoid, reduced diphtheria toxoid and acellular pertussis vaccine (Tdap) may be given at any time of pregnancy or the postpartum period but ideally is administered between 27–36 weeks to confer the best passive immunity through the transfer of antibodies to the fetus. This recommendation has developed to address the significant impact of pertussis disease in the newborn.

3 Preconception Care

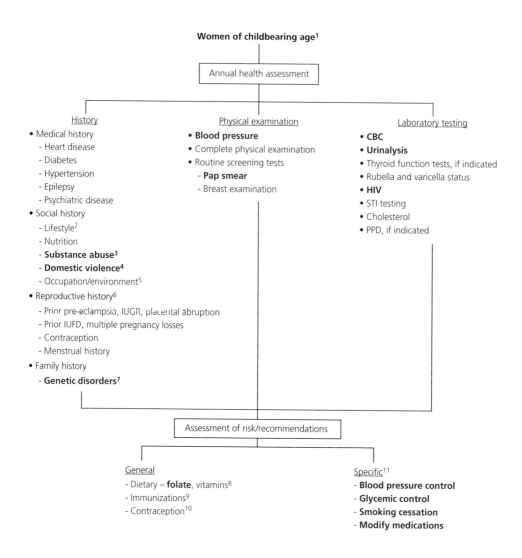

Women of childbearing age[1]

Annual health assessment

History
- Medical history
  - Heart disease
  - Diabetes
  - Hypertension
  - Epilepsy
  - Psychiatric disease
- Social history
  - Lifestyle[2]
  - Nutrition
  - **Substance abuse[3]**
  - **Domestic violence[4]**
  - Occupation/environment[5]
- Reproductive history[6]
  - Prior pre-eclampsia, IUGR, placental abruption
  - Prior IUFD, multiple pregnancy losses
  - Contraception
  - Menstrual history
- Family history
  - **Genetic disorders[7]**

Physical examination
- **Blood pressure**
- Complete physical examination
- Routine screening tests
  - **Pap smear**
  - Breast examination

Laboratory testing
- **CBC**
- **Urinalysis**
- Thyroid function tests, if indicated
- Rubella and varicella status
- **HIV**
- STI testing
- Cholesterol
- PPD, if indicated

Assessment of risk/recommendations

General
- Dietary – **folate**, vitamins[8]
- Immunizations[9]
- Contraception[10]

Specific[11]
- **Blood pressure control**
- **Glycemic control**
- **Smoking cessation**
- **Modify medications**

1. Fetal organogenesis occurs before most women are aware that they are pregnant. As such, the ideal time for addressing primary prevention of reproductive health risks is in the preconception period. Since approximately half of all pregnancies in the United States are unplanned, all women of reproductive age should be considered candidates for discussion of these issues.

Obstetric Clinical Algorithms, Second Edition. Errol R. Norwitz, George R. Saade, Hugh Miller and Christina M. Davidson.
© 2017 John Wiley & Sons, Ltd. Published 2017 by John Wiley & Sons, Ltd.

2. Discuss social, financial, and psychological issues in preparation for pregnancy.

3. Maternal alcohol use is the leading known cause of congenital mental retardation and is the leading preventable cause of birth defects in the Western world. An accurate drinking history is best elicited using a tool that employs standardized screening questions (such as the CAGE questionnaire). The adverse effects of alcohol may be compounded with abuse of other drugs. Cigarette smoking, cocaine, and other drug use should be included in the history. Patients at risk should be provided education, contraceptive counselling, and referral for treatment as necessary.

4. Screen for domestic violence. Be aware of available state and local resources and state laws regarding mandatory reporting. Risk increases with pregnancy. Domestic violence is not isolated to any particular risk group in pregnancy; it cuts across socio-economic and ethnic lines.

5. Take an occupational history that will allow assessment of workplace risks to the pregnancy. Elicit information about any exposures to hazardous materials or biologic hazards (HIV, cytomegalovirus (CMV), toxoplasmosis) and review the use of safety equipment. Talk to patients about the appropriate and correct use of seat belts while in a moving vehicle.

6. Counsel patients with a history of preeclampsia, placental abruption, unexplained fetal death, or severe intrauterine growth restriction (IUGR) about the risks of recurrence. Low-dose aspirin starting at the end of the first trimester is recommended to prevent recurrent preeclampsia. The use of low-dose aspirin, calcium supplementation, and/or anticoagulation for women with documented inherited thrombophilias to prevent adverse pregnancy outcome is controversial, and cannot be routinely recommended.

7. Personal and family histories should be examined for evidence of genetic diseases. Genetic testing is available to determine a patient's carrier status for some autosomal recessive conditions such as Tay–Sachs, Canavan disease, sickle cell disease, and the thalassemias. Consider referral for further genetic counselling if patients are at high risk. ACOG currently recommends that all couples be offered prenatal testing for cystic fibrosis. ACMG (but not ACOG) recommends that all couples also be offered genetic testing for spinal muscular atrophy (SMA).

8. Emphasize the importance of nutrition. Assess appropriateness of patient's weight for height, special diets and nutrition patterns such as vegetarianism, fasting, pica, bulimia, and vitamin supplementation. Recommend folic acid supplementation as necessary: 0.4 mg per day for all pregnant women or women considering pregnancy, 4.0 mg per day if the woman has a personal/family history of a child with a neural tube defect or is on anticonvulsant medications (especially valproic acid). Counsel to avoid oversupplementation (such as vitamin A). Review the recommendations on dietary fish ingestion (<12 ounces per week of cooked fish) to minimize mercury intake, and steps for prevention of listeriosis (avoiding raw or undercooked meat/fish, unpasteurized milk and soft cheeses, unwashed fruit and vegetables) and toxoplasmosis (exposure to cat feces).

9. A thorough immunization history should be obtained that addresses vaccination. Women should be tested for immunity to rubella and vaccinated prior to pregnancy if not immune. Women without a history of chickenpox (varicella) should be tested and offered vaccination prior to pregnancy. Hepatitis B vaccination should be offered to all women at high risk, and screening for other sexually transmitted infections should be offered as needed. The U.S. Centers for Disease Control and Prevention (CDC) recommends that pregnancy be delayed for at least 1 month after receiving a live-attenuated vaccine

(such as MMR, varicella, live-attenuated influenza, BCG).

10. Discuss birth spacing and the options available for postpartum contraception.

11. Effects of the pregnancy on any medical conditions for both mother and fetus should be discussed. Pregnancy outcomes can be improved by optimizing control of chronic medical conditions prior to pregnancy (such as glycemic control in patients with diabetes and blood pressure control in patients with hypertension). Medications should be reviewed, and patients counselled regarding alternatives that may be safer in pregnancy. Close communication with the patient's primary care and subspecialty physicians should always be maintained.

4 Prenatal Care[1]

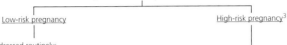

Initial prenatal visit

- Take a detailed history and physical examination
- Send routine prenatal laboratory tests[2]

Low-risk pregnancy

Issues that should be addressed routinely:

- **Folic acid supplementation** (1 mg daily for all reproductive age women) to prevent neural tube defect
- Identify and treat existing sexually transmitted infections, diabetes, thyroid disease, obesity, HIV, hepatitis B
- Identify maternal phenylketonuria (PKU)
- **Discontinue teratogenic drugs (such as coumadin, vitamin A)**
- **Counsel on risks of smoking, alcohol, and illicit drug use**
- Counsel about appropriate use of seatbelts and airbags
- *Reassure about safety of sexual intercourse, moderate exercise*
- **Screen for domestic violence and depression**
- Review symptoms/signs of complications (e.g. preterm birth)
- **Check rubella immunity status**
- Ask about chickenpox ($\sqrt{}$ varicella immunity status if unknown)
- Counsel about toxoplasmosis prevention
- **Counsel about influenza vaccination in pregnancy**
- Counsel about food safety, multivitamins
- Encourage breastfeeding

Regular follow-up prenatal visits[4]

Routine testing for all low-risk pregnancies
- Weight/Body Mass Index (BMI in kg/m^2) at each prenatal visit
- **BP and urine dipstix at each prenatal visit[5]**
- **UA C&S** q trimester to exclude asymptomatic bacteriuria and urinary tract infection (UTI)
- 1st trimester risk assessment for fetal aneuploidy[6]
- *Serum analyte ("quad") screen for fetal aneuploidy at 15–20 weeks[6]*
- MS-AFP for neural tube defect at 15–20 weeks[6]
- PPD (to screen for TB exposure) in 2nd trimester
- **1-hour GLT screening for gestational diabetes (GDM) at 24–28 weeks[7]**
- **GBS perineal culture at 35–36 weeks[8]**

High-risk pregnancy[3]

- Address issues as for low-risk pregnancies (opposite)
- Schedule follow-up visits based on individual risk factors
- Individualize prenatal testing based on risk factors

Maternal tests

- Hemoglobin electrophoresis (for sickle cell trait in African-Americans; for β-thalassemia in Mediterranean/Italians)
- Genetics testing for α-thalassemia in Mediterranean/Italians (esp. if anemia unresponsive to iron supplementation)
- **Urine toxicology screen** (for women with a history of illicit drug use)
- Chest x-ray if PPD positive
- Smoking cessation counseling
- Baseline renal/liver function tests, 24-hour urinalysis in high-risk patients[5]
- Early GLT screening for GDM at first prenatal visit in high-risk patients[7]
- **3-hour GTT to confirm diagnosis of**
- **GDM in women with a positive GLT[7]**
- Cervical length and fetal fibronectin in women at risk of preterm birth[9]
- **UA C&S** q month in women at high risk for UTI (diabetes, sickle cell trait, history of recurrent UTI, HIV)
- Maternal EKG, echo, cardiology consultation in women at risk

Fetal tests

- Early dating ultrasound to confirm gestational age, exclude multiple pregnancy
- Genetic counseling in high-risk women (e.g. AMA, personal or family history of an inherited disorder, abnormal aneuploidy screening test, CF carrier)
- **Genetic amniocentesis/CVS to exclude fetal aneuploidy[6]**
- Fetal anatomic survey (level II ultrasound) at 18–20 weeks
- Fetal echo at 20–22 weeks to diagnose cardiac anomaly in women at high risk
- **Serial ultrasounds** for fetal growth q 3–4 weeks after 24 weeks in pregnancies at risk for IUGR or macrosomia
- Fetal testing q week after 32–36 weeks in high-risk women (e.g. diabetes, AMA, chronic hypertension)
- **Amniocentesis at 36–39 weeks for fetal lung maturity testing**

Obstetric Clinical Algorithms, Second Edition. Errol R. Norwitz, George R. Saade, Hugh Miller and Christina M. Davidson.
© 2017 John Wiley & Sons, Ltd. Published 2017 by John Wiley & Sons, Ltd.

1. The goal of prenatal care is to promote the health and well-being of the pregnant woman, fetus, infant, and family up to 1 year after birth. To achieve these aims, prenatal care must be available and accessible. The three major components are: (i) early and continuing risk assessment, including preconception assessment (see Chapter 3, Preconception Care); (ii) continued health promotion; and (iii) both medical and psychosocial assessment and intervention.

2. Routine prenatal tests that should be completed for all pregnant women include complete blood count (CBC), blood group type and screen (Rh status), rubella serology, HIV, hepatitis B, syphilis serology (VDRL/RPR), Pap smear, cystic fibrosis (CF) carrier status, chlamydia/gonorrhea cultures, and urine culture and sensitivity (UA C&S).

3. Approximately 20% (1 in 5) of pregnancies are considered high risk. Risk factors for adverse pregnancy outcome may exist prior to pregnancy or develop during pregnancy or even during labor (examples are listed below, although this list should not be regarded as comprehensive).

4. The frequency and timing of prenatal visits will vary depending on the risk status of the pregnant woman and her fetus. In low-risk women, prenatal visits are typically recommended q 4 weeks to 28 weeks, q 2 weeks to 36 weeks, and then weekly until delivery.

5. See Chapter 12 (Preeclampsia).

6. See Chapter 53 (Prenatal diagnosis).

7. See Chapter 10 (Gestational diabetes mellitus)

8. See Chapter 24 (GBS)

9. See Chapter 55 (Screening for preterm birth)

High-Risk Pregnancies

Maternal factors

- Pre-existing medical conditions (diabetes, chronic hypertension, cardiac disease, renal disease, pulmonary disease)
- Preeclampsia
- Gestational diabetes
- Morbid obesity
- Extremes of maternal age
- Active venous thromboembolic disease
- Poor obstetric history (prior preterm birth, preterm PROM, stillbirth, IUGR, placental abruption, preeclampsia, recurrent miscarriage)

Fetal factors

- Fetal structural or chromosomal anomaly
- History of a prior baby with a structural or chromosomal anomaly
- Family or personal history of a genetic syndrome
- Toxic exposure (to environmental toxins, medications, illicit drugs)
- IUGR
- Fetal macrosomia
- Multiple pregnancy (esp. if monochorionic)
- Isoimmunization
- Intra-amniotic infection (chorioamnionitis)
- Nonreassuring fetal testing

Uteroplacental factors

- Preterm premature rupture of membranes
- Unexplained oligohydramnios
- Large uterine fibroids (esp. if submucosal)
- Prior cervical insufficiency
- Prior uterine surgery (especially prior "classic" hysterotomy)
- Placental abruption
- Placenta previa
- Uterine anomaly (didelphys, septate)
- Abnormal placentation (placenta accreta, increta or percreta)
- Vasa previa

SECTION 2
Maternal Disorders

5 Antiphospholipid Antibody Syndrome

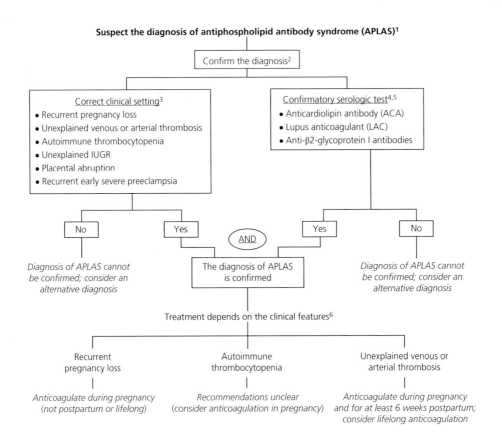

Suspect the diagnosis of antiphospholipid antibody syndrome (APLAS)[1]

Confirm the diagnosis[2]

Correct clinical setting[3]
- Recurrent pregnancy loss
- Unexplained venous or arterial thrombosis
- Autoimmune thrombocytopenia
- Unexplained IUGR
- Placental abruption
- Recurrent early severe preeclampsia

Confirmatory serologic test[4,5]
- Anticardiolipin antibody (ACA)
- Lupus anticoagulant (LAC)
- Anti-β2-glycoprotein I antibodies

No — Yes — AND — Yes — No

Diagnosis of APLAS cannot be confirmed; consider an alternative diagnosis

The diagnosis of APLAS is confirmed

Diagnosis of APLAS cannot be confirmed; consider an alternative diagnosis

Treatment depends on the clinical features[6]

Recurrent pregnancy loss	Autoimmune thrombocytopenia	Unexplained venous or arterial thrombosis
Anticoagulate during pregnancy (not postpartum or lifelong)	*Recommendations unclear (consider anticoagulation in pregnancy)*	*Anticoagulate during pregnancy and for at least 6 weeks postpartum; consider lifelong anticoagulation*

1. Antiphospholipid antibody syndrome (APLAS) is an autoimmune disease characterized by the presence in the maternal circulation of one or more autoantibodies against membrane phospholipid as well as one or more specific clinical syndromes. It is an acquired rather than an inherited condition. As such, it cannot explain a family history of venous thromboembolism (VTE). A significant family history of VTE should prompt testing to exclude inherited thrombophilias, including factor V Leiden mutation, prothrombin gene mutation, and protein S, protein C, and antithrombin deficiency.

2. The diagnosis of APLAS requires two distinct elements: (i) the correct clinical setting; and (ii) confirmatory serologic testing. Approximately 2–4% of healthy pregnant women will have circulating antiphospholipid antibodies in the absence of any clinical symptoms. As such, routine screening for these antibodies in all pregnant women is strongly discouraged.

Obstetric Clinical Algorithms, Second Edition. Errol R. Norwitz, George R. Saade, Hugh Miller and Christina M. Davidson.
© 2017 John Wiley & Sons, Ltd. Published 2017 by John Wiley & Sons, Ltd.

3. Clinical manifestations of APLAS include: (i) recurrent pregnancy loss (defined as ≥ 3 unexplained first-trimester pregnancy losses or ≥ 1 unexplained second-trimester pregnancy loss); (ii) unexplained thrombosis (venous, arterial, cerebrovascular accident or myocardial infarction); and/or (iii) autoimmune thrombocytopenia (platelets <100,000/mm³). Recent consensus opinions suggest that such clinical conditions as unexplained intrauterine growth restriction (IUGR), massive placental abruption, and recurrent early-onset severe pre-eclampsia be included.

4. At least one of three serologic tests confirming the presence of circulating antiphospholipid antibodies (below) is required to make the diagnosis of APLAS. Moreover, the diagnosis requires the persistence of such antibodies as confirmed by two or more positive tests at least 12 weeks apart.

- Lupus anticoagulant (LAC) is an unidentified antiphospholipid antibody (or antibodies) that causes prolongation of phospholipid-dependent coagulation tests *in vitro* by binding to the prothrombin–activator complex. Examples of tests that can confirm the presence of LAC include the activated PTT test, dilute Russel viper venom test, kaolin clotting time, and recalcification time. *In vivo*, however, LAC causes thrombosis. LAC results are reported as present or absent (no titers are given). The term LAC is a misnomer: it is not specific to lupus (SLE) and it acts *in vivo* as a procoagulant and not an anticoagulant.
- Antibodies against specific phospholipids as measured by enzyme-linked immunosorbant assay (ELISA). These high-avidity IgG antibodies have anticoagulant activity *in vitro*, but procoagulant activity *in vivo*. The most commonly used ELISA test is the anticardiolipin antibody (ACA). Cardiolipin is a negatively charged phospholipid isolated from ox heart. ACA ELISA is at best semi-quantitative. Results have traditionally been reported as low, medium or high titers. More recently, standardization of the phospholipid extract

has allowed for standard units to be developed (GPL units for IgG, MPL units for IgM). ACA IgM alone, IgA alone, and/or low-positive IgG may be a nonspecific (incidental) finding since they are present in 2–4% of asymptomatic pregnant women. As such, moderate-to-high levels of ACA IgG (>40 GPL units) are required to make the diagnosis of APLAS.

- The presence of anti-β2-glycoprotein I antibodies.

5. A number of additional antiphospholipid antibodies are described, including antiphosphatidylserine, antiphosphatidylethanolamine, antiphosphatidylcholine, anti-Ro, and anti-La, but these are not sufficient to make the diagnosis. A false-positive test for syphilis (defined as a positive rapid plasma reagin (RPR) or Venereal Disease Research Laboratory (VDRL) test, but negative definitive test for syphilis) is another common finding in women with APLAS, but is nonspecific and is not sufficient to confirm the diagnosis. Antinuclear antibodies (ANA) are not antiphospholipid antibodies, and may suggest the diagnosis of SLE but not APLAS.

6. Treatment for APLAS depends on the clinical features:
- For women with thrombosis (such as stroke or pulmonary embolism), *therapeutic* anticoagulation is indicated with either unfractionated heparin (UFH) or low molecular weight heparin (LMWH) during pregnancy followed by oral anticoagulation (coumadin) postpartum because of a 5–15% risk of recurrence. In pregnancy, regular blood tests are required 4 hours after administration of the drug to ensure that anticoagulation is therapeutic: the PTT should be 1.5- to 2.5-fold normal and anti-Xa activity levels should be 0.6–1.0 U/mL. Side-effects include hemorrhage, thrombocytopenia, and osteopenia and fractures. Such women may need lifelong treatment.

  For women with recurrent pregnancy loss, treatment should include *prophylactic* UFH

(5000–10,000 units sc bid) or LMWH (enoxa-parin (Lovenox) 30–40 mg sc daily or daltepa-rin (Fragmin) 2500–5000 U sc daily) starting in the first trimester of pregnancy. Although pro-phylactic dosing does not change PTT, it will increase anti-Xa activity to 0.1–0.2 U/mL. However, it is not necessary to follow serial anti-Xa activity in such patients. The goal of this treatment is to prevent pregnancy loss and to prevent VTE, which is possible in women with APLAS in pregnancy even if they have not had a VTE in the past. Therefore, anticoagulation should be administered throughout pregnancy and typically for 6–12 weeks after delivery.

- For women with <u>autoimmune thrombocyto-penia or a history of severe pre-eclampsia, IUGR or placental abruption</u>, the optimal treatment is unknown. Consider treating as for recurrent pregnancy loss. Postpartum anticoagulation is probably not necessary.

6 Asthma

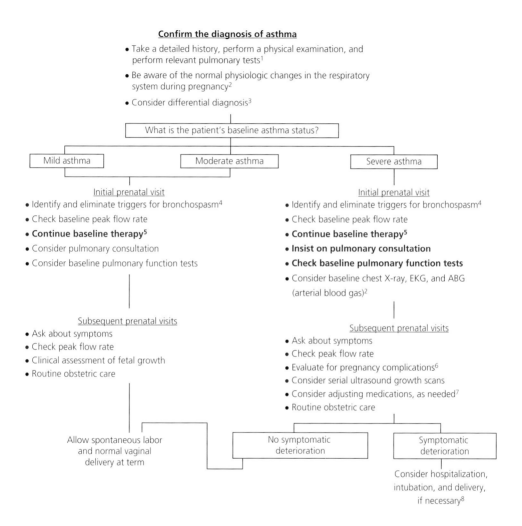

Confirm the diagnosis of asthma
- Take a detailed history, perform a physical examination, and perform relevant pulmonary tests[1]
- Be aware of the normal physiologic changes in the respiratory system during pregnancy[2]
- Consider differential diagnosis[3]

What is the patient's baseline asthma status?

| Mild asthma | Moderate asthma | Severe asthma |

Mild / Moderate asthma

Initial prenatal visit
- Identify and eliminate triggers for bronchospasm[4]
- Check baseline peak flow rate
- **Continue baseline therapy[5]**
- Consider pulmonary consultation
- Consider baseline pulmonary function tests

Subsequent prenatal visits
- Ask about symptoms
- Check peak flow rate
- Clinical assessment of fetal growth
- Routine obstetric care

Severe asthma

Initial prenatal visit
- Identify and eliminate triggers for bronchospasm[4]
- Check baseline peak flow rate
- **Continue baseline therapy[5]**
- **Insist on pulmonary consultation**
- **Check baseline pulmonary function tests**
- Consider baseline chest X-ray, EKG, and ABG (arterial blood gas)[2]

Subsequent prenatal visits
- Ask about symptoms
- Check peak flow rate
- Evaluate for pregnancy complications[6]
- Consider serial ultrasound growth scans
- Consider adjusting medications, as needed[7]
- Routine obstetric care

Allow spontaneous labor and normal vaginal delivery at term

No symptomatic deterioration

Symptomatic deterioration

Consider hospitalization, intubation, and delivery, if necessary[8]

1. Asthma is a chronic inflammatory disorder of the airways characterized by intermittent episodes of reversible bronchospasm. The "classic" signs and symptoms of asthma are intermittent dyspnea, cough, and wheezing. Pulmonary function tests that are most helpful in diagnosing asthma are peak expiratory flow rate (PEFR), spirometry (which includes measurement of forced expiratory volume in one second [FEV1] and forced vital capacity [FVC]), and bronchoprovocation testing (such as with a metacholine or exercise challenge). PEFR,

Obstetric Clinical Algorithms, Second Edition. Errol R. Norwitz, George R. Saade, Hugh Miller and Christina M. Davidson.
© 2017 John Wiley & Sons, Ltd. Published 2017 by John Wiley & Sons, Ltd.

which correlates well with FEV1, can be measured using a hand-held peak flow meter and is a useful measure in the clinic or home setting. PEFR is determined for each patient (personal best) or by using charts adjusted for age, height, gender, and race. PEFR results are categorized into green (80–100% of normal or personal best), yellow (50–80%), and red (less than 50%). Usually, the green zone means that the asthma is well controlled, yellow means that adjustments to medications and/or environment are needed, and red is a medical alert that needs immediate attention. Findings consistent with asthma include a variability of >20% in PEFR, a reduction in FEV1 and FEV1/FVC ratio on spirometry, an increase in FEV1 of more than 15% from the baseline following administration of 2–4 puffs of a bronchodilator, and heightened sensitivity to bronchoprovocation. Asthma complicates 1–4% of all pregnancies. Pregnancy has a variable effect on asthma (25% improve, 25% worsen, 50% are unchanged). In general, women with mild, well-controlled asthma tolerate pregnancy well. Women with severe asthma are at risk of symptomatic deterioration.

2. Respiratory adaptations during pregnancy are designed to optimize maternal and fetal oxygenation, and to facilitate transfer of CO_2 waste from the fetus to the mother. The mechanics of respiration change with pregnancy. The ribs flare outward and the level of the diaphragm rises 4 cm. During pregnancy, tidal volume increases by 200 mL (40%) resulting in a 100–200 mL (5%) increase in vital capacity and a 200 mL (20%) decrease in the residual volume, thereby leaving less air in the lungs at the end of expiration. The respiratory rate remains unchanged or increases slightly. The end result is an increase in minute ventilation and a drop in arterial PCO_2. Arterial PO_2 is essentially unchanged. A compensatory decrease in bicarbonate enables the pH to remain unchanged. Pregnancy thus represents a state of *compensated respiratory alkalosis*.

	pH	PO_2 (mmHg)	PCO_2 (mmHg)
Non-pregnant	7.40	93–100	35–40
Pregnant	7.40	100–105	28–30

3. The differential diagnosis of asthma includes pneumonia, pulmonary embolism, pneumothorax, congestive cardiac failure, pericarditis, pulmonary edema, and rib fracture.

4. Characteristic triggers for asthma include exercise, cold air, and exposure to allergens. Exercise-triggered symptoms typically develop 10–15 minutes after exertion and are more intense when the inhaled air is cold. Allergens that typically trigger asthma symptoms include dust, molds, furred animals, cockroaches, pollens, and other irritant-type exposures (cigarette smoke, strong fumes, airborne chemicals). Viral infections can also trigger asthma symptoms. Influenza vaccination is recommended (see Chapter 2 on Immunization).

5. The principal goals of treatment are to minimize symptoms, normalize pulmonary function, prevent exacerbations, and improve health-related quality of life. Initial treatment for relief of symptoms should be an inhaled short-acting beta-agonist used on an as-needed basis rather than at regularly scheduled intervals. The most commonly used agent is an albuterol inhaler at a dose of 2–4 puffs as needed every 4–6 hours. If this is not adequate to control symptoms, inhaled glucocorticoids (such as beclomethasone dipropionate) should be given by metered dose inhaler (MDI) and should be taken at regular intervals two to three times daily.

6. Pregnancy-related complications of severe asthma include intrauterine growth restriction (IUGR), stillbirth, and maternal mortality.

7. A number of alternative therapies are available on an outpatient basis. These include a

short course of oral glucocorticoids. A typical regimen is prednisone 0.5 mg per kg body weight given orally each day and tapered over a period of one to two weeks. This can be given alone or in combination with a leukotriene modifying agent—such as the leukotriene D4 receptor antagonists zafirlukast (Accolate) and montelukast (Singulair) or the 5-lipoxygenase inhibitor zileuton (Zyflo)—or a slow-release theophylline.

8. See Chapter 75 (Acute Asthma Exacerbation).

7 Cholestasis of Pregnancy

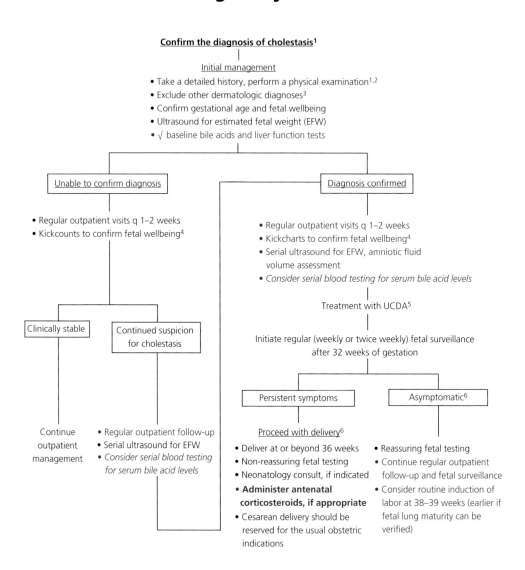

Confirm the diagnosis of cholestasis[1]

Initial management
- Take a detailed history, perform a physical examination[1,2]
- Exclude other dermatologic diagnoses[3]
- Confirm gestational age and fetal wellbeing
- Ultrasound for estimated fetal weight (EFW)
- √ baseline bile acids and liver function tests

Unable to confirm diagnosis
- Regular outpatient visits q 1–2 weeks
- Kickcounts to confirm fetal wellbeing[4]

Diagnosis confirmed
- Regular outpatient visits q 1–2 weeks
- Kickcharts to confirm fetal wellbeing[4]
- Serial ultrasound for EFW, amniotic fluid volume assessment
- *Consider serial blood testing for serum bile acid levels*

Treatment with UCDA[5]

Initiate regular (weekly or twice weekly) fetal surveillance after 32 weeks of gestation

Clinically stable

Continued suspicion for cholestasis

Persistent symptoms

Asymptomatic[6]

Continue outpatient management

- Regular outpatient follow-up
- Serial ultrasound for EFW
- *Consider serial blood testing for serum bile acid levels*

Proceed with delivery[6]
- Deliver at or beyond 36 weeks
- Non-reassuring fetal testing
- Neonatology consult, if indicated
- **Administer antenatal corticosteroids, if appropriate**
- Cesarean delivery should be reserved for the usual obstetric indications

- Reassuring fetal testing
- Continue regular outpatient follow-up and fetal surveillance
- Consider routine induction of labor at 38–39 weeks (earlier if fetal lung maturity can be verified)

1. Cholestasis of pregnancy (also referred to as intrahepatic cholestasis of pregnancy (ICP)) represents a clinical syndrome that results from a complex interplay between reproductive hormones, biliary transport proteins, and genetic factors that contribute to an inability to adequately metabolize and excrete bile acids during pregnancy. Risk factors for cholestasis

Obstetric Clinical Algorithms, Second Edition. Errol R. Norwitz, George R. Saade, Hugh Miller and Christina M. Davidson.
© 2017 John Wiley & Sons, Ltd. Published 2017 by John Wiley & Sons, Ltd.

include cholestasis in a prior pregnancy (recurrence rate is >90%), multiple gestation, pregnancies conceived through IVF, and underlying liver, renal, and/or bowel disease.

2. Cholestasis of pregnancy is a clinical/biochemical diagnosis. Patients typically present with complaints of acute onset of severe pruritus in the latter half of pregnancy, usually >30 weeks' gestation. Physical examination may reveal jaundice and/or skin excoriations, but is often unremarkable. Bile acids will usually be elevated at values >10–14 micromoles/L (6–10 micromoles/L in the fasting state). Bile acids are derived from hepatic cholesterol metabolism. Cholic and chenodeoxycholic acid are the dominant fractionated constituents. Liver function tests, specifically serum transaminases, will frequently be elevated.

3. The differential diagnosis of cholestasis includes skin allergy, parasitic infections, systemic lupus erythematosis (SLE), syphilis, viral/drug-induced hepatitis, preeclampsia, metabolic disorders, and gall bladder diseases.

4. Cholestasis of pregnancy is associated with adverse perinatal outcome, including increase perinatal mortality (unexplained stillbirth), premature birth, and meconium passage and aspiration. Many of these adverse outcomes are directly associated with elevated bile acids, particularly with values ≥40 micromol/L. The association with IUGR is less clear. For these reasons, regular (weekly or twice weekly) fetal surveillance is recommended after 32 weeks of gestation. However, it is not clear whether fetal testing is associated with an improvement in perinatal outcome.

5. Ursodeoxycholic acid (ursodiol (UDCA)) has become the preferred therapeutic intervention for ICP. Although treatment with UDCA has not been conclusively shown to improve perinatal outcome, it does significantly reduce pruritis and normalize LFTs. The recommended initial dose of 300 mg TID can be upward adjusted as needed to a maximum of 2 gms/day in divided doses. Other agents that have been used for symptomatic relief include hydroxyzine (25–50 mg/day, which may have significant somnolent side effects) and cholestyramine (a foul-tasting resin that binds bile acids in the gastrointestinal system). Response to such medications may take several weeks and is highly variable. Alternative treatment options that are less well established include ultraviolet light, rifampicin, phenobarbitone, epomediol, or S-adenosyl-L-methionine.

6. In contrast to the effects on the fetus, cholestasis of pregnancy is not associated with adverse maternal outcome. Many patients remain symptomatic despite treatment and live with anxiety relative to the small risk of fetal death, which is seen most commonly >38 weeks. As a consequence, some consensus bodies recommend delivery at 37–38 weeks even with reassuring fetal testing. Earlier delivery is reserved for fetal indications or maternal jaundice despite treatment. Mode of delivery should be governed by routine obstetric indications. Patients should be aware that symptoms generally resolve in the immediate postpartum period, but recurrence in future pregnancies can be as high as 90%.

8 Chronic Hypertension[1]

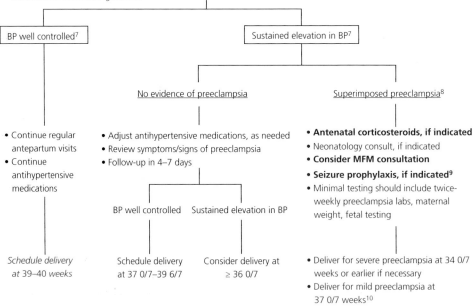

History and/or examination suggestive of chronic hypertension[2]

Initial evaluation
- Consider further evaluation to identify an underlying cause[2]
- Evaluate for target organ damage[3]
- Review the risks to the pregnancy associated with chronic hypertension[4]
- Consider initiating or changing antihypertensive therapy[5,6]
- **Check baseline renal function (creatinine clearance) and preeclampsia lab tests (urinalysis, 24-hour urinary protein, CBC, liver function tests, renal function tests, uric acid)**

Further evaluation
- **Regular antepartum visits including BP checks, urinalysis**
- Fetal testing (weekly biophysical profiles with nonstress tests, serial ultrasound examinations for fetal growth) should be initiated after 32 weeks' gestation

BP well controlled[7]

Sustained elevation in BP[7]

No evidence of preeclampsia

Superimposed preeclampsia[8]

- Continue regular antepartum visits
- Continue antihypertensive medications

- Adjust antihypertensive medications, as needed
- Review symptoms/signs of preeclampsia
- Follow-up in 4–7 days

- **Antenatal corticosteroids, if indicated**
- Neonatology consult, if indicated
- **Consider MFM consultation**
- **Seizure prophylaxis, if indicated[9]**
- Minimal testing should include twice-weekly preeclampsia labs, maternal weight, fetal testing

BP well controlled

Sustained elevation in BP

Schedule delivery at 39–40 weeks

Schedule delivery at 37 0/7–39 6/7

Consider delivery at ≥ 36 0/7

- Deliver for severe preeclampsia at 34 0/7 weeks or earlier if necessary
- Deliver for mild preeclampsia at 37 0/7 weeks[10]

1. Hypertension is defined as systolic BP ≥140 mmHg and/or diastolic BP ≥90 mm Hg on two occasions at least 4 hours (but not more than 7 days) apart. Chronic hypertension refers to the presence of hypertension prior to pregnancy, whether or not the patient was on pharmacologic treatment. Given that BP normally decreases in the first and early second trimester of pregnancy,

---

Obstetric Clinical Algorithms, Second Edition. Errol R. Norwitz, George R. Saade, Hugh Miller and Christina M. Davidson.
© 2017 John Wiley & Sons, Ltd. Published 2017 by John Wiley & Sons, Ltd.

the diagnosis should also be suspected in women with a sustained elevation in BP prior to 20 weeks of gestation. However, if BP was normal in the first trimester and then increases before 20 weeks of gestation, early preeclampsia should also be considered.

2. All women with pre-existing hypertension should be assessed either before pregnancy or early in pregnancy to rule out secondary (and potentially curable) hypertension, and to evaluate for evidence of target organ damage. Most women with chronic hypertension have essential (primary) hypertension. Up to 10% of women have secondary hypertension, due most commonly to chronic kidney disease. Other causes may include renal artery stenosis and an underlying endocrinopathy (such as primary hyperaldosteronism, pheochromocytoma, and Cushing syndrome).

3. Baseline evaluation should include serum analysis for creatinine, electrolytes, uric acid, liver enzymes, and platelet count as well as urinary protein estimation. These values can be used for comparison if superimposed preeclampsia is suspected later in pregnancy. Left ventricular function should be assessed in women with severe hypertension of more than 4 years duration either by electrocardiography (ECG) or echocardiography.

4. Chronic hypertension is associated with an increased risk of superimposed preeclampsia and higher rates of adverse maternal-fetal outcome, such as severe hypertension, cerebrovascular accident (stroke), uteroplacental insufficiency leading to fetal growth restriction, placental abruption, and stillbirth.

5. Pharmacologic treatment of mild hypertension has not been shown to improve pregnancy outcome. The goals of treatment during pregnancy are to minimize acute maternal and fetal risks of severe hypertension. As such, it is rarely necessary to initiate antihypertensive therapy in early pregnancy. If a patient is well controlled

on medications prior to pregnancy, it is usual to leave her medications unchanged. The exceptions are the angiotensin-converting enzyme (ACE) inhibitors and angiotensin receptor blockers (ARB), which should be discontinued as soon as a positive pregnancy test is attained. First trimester exposure has been associated with cardiac and central nervous system anomalies, and use in the second and third trimester can result in progressive and irreversible renal injury as well as oligohydramnios and fetal growth restriction. Drugs of choice include α-methyldopa, β-blockers (labetalol) or calcium channel blockers (nifedipine). Diuretic therapy is generally discouraged in pregnancy.

6. In the absence of maternal end organ damage, treatment is not recommended if the systolic BP remains <160 mmHg and the diastolic BP <105 mmHg. If end organ damage is present, BP goals are more strict (systolic BP <140 mmHg and diastolic BP <90 mmHg) to avoid progression of disease and its associated complications during pregnancy.

7. When antihypertensive therapy is initiated during pregnancy, it is suggested that BP be maintained between 120–160 mmHg systolic and 80–105 mmHg diastolic. Acute-onset, severe systolic hypertension (>160 mmHg) and/or severe diastolic hypertension (>110 mmHg) should be treated with antihypertensive therapy with the aim to achieve BP of 140–150/90–100 mmHg. First-line treatment for the management of acute-onset, severe hypertension includes intravenous labetalol, intravenous hydralazine, or oral nifedipine.

8. Preeclampsia is superimposed on chronic hypertension when there is a sudden increase in BP that was previously well controlled or an escalation of antihypertensive medications needed to control BP; or new onset of proteinuria or a sudden increase in proteinuria in pregnancy. Superimposed preeclampsia can be further classified into with or without severe

features. The diagnosis of superimposed preeclampsia with severe features is established when any of the following are present: (i) severe-range BP despite escalation of antihypertensive therapy; (ii) thrombocytopenia (platelet count <100,000/microliter); (iii) elevated liver transaminases to twice normal concentrations; (iv) new-onset/worsening renal insufficiency (serum creatinine >1.1 mg/dL or a doubling of the creatinine in the absence of other renal disease); (v) pulmonary edema; or (vi) persistent cerebral or visual disturbances.

9. Intravenous magnesium sulfate is the drug of choice for seizure prophylaxis and should be given intrapartum and for at least 24 hours postpartum to prevent eclampsia. An IV loading dose of 4–6 g should be followed by a maintenance dose of 1–2 g/h. The use of magnesium sulfate therapy in superimposed preeclampsia without severe features is not recommended, but should be initiated if there is progression to severe disease either intrapartum or postpartum.

10. Delivery is the only effective treatment for superimposed preeclampsia. It is recommended in women with superimposed preeclampsia without severe features at or beyond 37–0/7 weeks. It is recommended in women with superimposed preeclampsia with severe features if the gestational age is at least 34–0/7 weeks. If the gestational age is <34–0/7 weeks and the diagnosis is superimposed preeclampsia by BP criteria alone, expectant management can be considered (see Chapter 12). There is no proven benefit to routine delivery by cesarean; however, the probability of vaginal delivery decreases with decreasing gestational age. With labor induction, the likelihood of cesarean delivery is 93–97% at <28 weeks, 53–65% at 28–32 weeks, and 31–38% at 32–34 weeks. Preeclampsia and its complications always resolve following delivery (with the exception of stroke). Diuresis (>4 L/day) is the most accurate clinical indicator of resolution. Fetal prognosis is dependent largely on gestational age at delivery.

9 Deep Vein Thrombosis

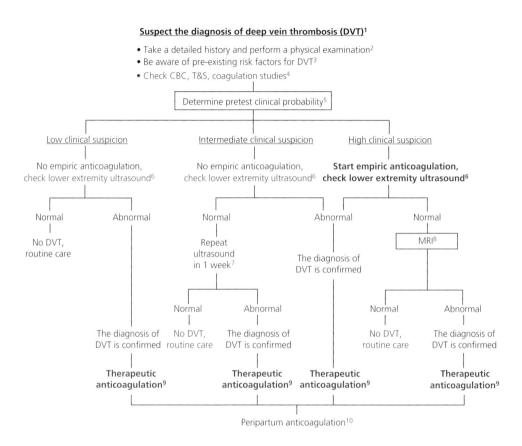

Suspect the diagnosis of deep vein thrombosis (DVT)[1]

- Take a detailed history and perform a physical examination[2]
- Be aware of pre-existing risk factors for DVT[3]
- Check CBC, T&S, coagulation studies[4]

Determine pretest clinical probability[5]

Low clinical suspicion

No empiric anticoagulation, check lower extremity ultrasound[6]

Normal — No DVT, routine care

Abnormal — The diagnosis of DVT is confirmed — **Therapeutic anticoagulation[9]**

Intermediate clinical suspicion

No empiric anticoagulation, check lower extremity ultrasound[6]

Normal — Repeat ultrasound in 1 week[7]

Normal — No DVT, routine care

Abnormal — The diagnosis of DVT is confirmed — **Therapeutic anticoagulation[9]**

Abnormal — The diagnosis of DVT is confirmed — **Therapeutic anticoagulation[9]**

High clinical suspicion

Start empiric anticoagulation, check lower extremity ultrasound[6]

Normal — MRI[8]

Normal — No DVT, routine care

Abnormal — The diagnosis of DVT is confirmed — **Therapeutic anticoagulation[9]**

Peripartum anticoagulation[10]

1. Venous thromboembolic events (VTE), which include both deep vein thrombosis (DVT) and pulmonary embolism (PE), complicate 0.5–2.0 per 1000 pregnancies. VTE is one of the leading causes of maternal mortality in developed nations, accounting for 10–20% of pregnancy-related maternal deaths in the United States. DVTs account for 75–80% of VTEs during pregnancy, with PE comprising the remaining 20–25%.

2. Symptoms suggestive of DVT include pain, swelling, and/or redness in the calf or thigh. Physical findings include objective evidence of calf swelling (a difference in calf circumference of ≥2 cm), localized redness, and calf tenderness with or without a palpable thrombotic "cord." Homan's sign refers to pain in the calf in response to active dorsiflexion of the foot. Pain in the calf is regarded as a "positive" Homan's sign and is taken to be suggestive of acute DVT.

Obstetric Clinical Algorithms, Second Edition. Errol R. Norwitz, George R. Saade, Hugh Miller and Christina M. Davidson.
© 2017 John Wiley & Sons, Ltd. Published 2017 by John Wiley & Sons, Ltd.

However, a "positive" Homan's sign is only around 30–40% sensitive, and a "negative" Homan's sign does not exclude the diagnosis. Isolated iliac-vein thrombosis may present with abdominal pain, back pain, and swelling of the entire leg.

3. A personal history of VTE is the single most important risk factor for VTE during pregnancy. The risk of recurrent VTE during pregnancy is increased three–fourfold, and 15–25% of all cases of VTE in pregnancy are recurrent events. The second most important individual risk factor for VTE in pregnancy is the presence of an inherited thrombophilia (such as factor V Leiden mutation, prothrombin gene mutation, protein S/protein C/antithrombin deficiency) or acquired thrombophilia (antiphospholipid antibody syndrome, see Chapter 5), which is present in 20–50% of women who experience VTE during pregnancy and the puerperium. Other risk factors for VTE include advanced maternal age, black race, heart disease, sickle cell disease, diabetes, lupus, hypertension, hemoglobinopathies, smoking, multiple pregnancy, obesity, prolonged immobility (bedrest), trauma, pregnancy (due to its hypercoagulable state), and cesarean delivery (especially an intrapartum emergency cesarean). VTE is fourfold more common in pregnancy than in nonpregnant women. Two-thirds of DVTs occur antepartum, with these events distributed throughout all three trimesters.

4. Laboratory tests (including circulating D-dimer levels) are generally unhelpful in confirming the diagnosis of DVT, but baseline coagulation studies should be sent if the patient requires anticoagulation.

5. If the clinical suspicion of DVT is high, consider starting anticoagulation immediately to avoid DVT propagation and possible PE.

6. The diagnosis of DVT is usually confirmed noninvasively by compression ultrasonography of the proximal veins, including Doppler duplex. Compression ultrasonography is reliable at detecting proximal lower extremity DVT with a sensitivity of 97%, specificity of 94%, using contrast venography as the gold standard, but is less effective at diagnosing isolated calf and iliac vein thrombosis.

7. If compression ultrasonography is negative, future management depends in large part on the clinical suspicion for DVT. The minimal requirement in a symptomatic patient with a negative lower extremity compression ultrasound examination is to repeat the test in 1 week.

8. If the clinical setting is highly suspicious but compression ultrasound is negative or equivocal, an MRI should be performed. Contrast venography, once the standard technique for DVT diagnosis, has now been replaced by compression ultrasound and an MRI due to the less invasive nature and lack of radiation exposure.

9. Deep vein thrombosis in pregnancy should be treated to prevent propagation of the thrombus and PE. If untreated, 25% of patients with DVT will have a PE as compared with 5% of treated patients. Admission is generally warranted for initiation of treatment in pregnancy. Therapeutic subcutaneous low molecular weight-heparin (LMWH) is now the treatment of choice for DVT in pregnancy. The advantages of LMWH over unfractionated heparin (UFH) include a reduced risk of bleeding, predictable pharmacokinetics allowing weight-based dosing without the need for monitoring, and a reduced risk of heparin-induced thrombocytopenia and heparin-induced osteoporotic fractures. A twice-daily weight-adjusted dosing regimen should be used, such as enoxaparin (Lovenox) 1 mg/kg sc q12h. LMWH does not significantly alter PTT, but serum anti-factor Xa activity can be measured. Therapeutic anticoagulation is achieved with a circulating anti-Xa activity of 0.6–1.0 U/mL, however, routine

monitoring of anti-Xa activity may not be justi-fied due to the absence of large studies using clinical end points that demonstrate an optimal therapeutic anti-Xa LMWH range or that dose adjustments increase the safety or efficacy of therapy, the lack of accuracy and reliability of the measurement, the lack of correlation with risk of bleeding and recurrence, and the cost of the assay. The management of isolated calf vein thrombosis is controversial, with no established guidelines. Since most iliofemoral thromboses originate from calf vein thromboses, full antico-agulation with LMWH is suggested for sympto-matic patients.

- When LMWH cannot be used or when UFH is preferred (e.g., in patients with renal dys-function and when delivery or surgery may be necessary), UFH can be administered as an initial IV therapy followed by subcutaneous UFH. IV treatment should be initiated with a loading dose of 80 U/kg followed by an initial infusion of 18 U/kg/h. Serum PTT should be checked every 4–6 hours, and the infusion adjusted to maintain PTT at 1.5–2.5 times control. Once a steady state has been achieved, PTT levels should be measured daily. After 5–10 days, IV heparin can be changed to SC injection (not IM injection because of the risk of hematoma) as follows: begin with 10,000 U SC three times daily and titrate dosage upward depending on the results of the mid-interval PTT; aim for PTT 1.5–2.5 times control. When subcutaneous UFH is used during pregnancy, higher doses and three times daily dosing are usually required to maintain adequate anticoagulation.
- Alternative therapies (fibrinolytic agents, surgical intervention) are associated with a high incidence of complications in pregnancy and, as such, are best avoided. The use of vena caval filters should be considered only for patients in whom anticoagulation is con-traindicated or in whom extensive venous thromboembolism develops within 2 weeks before delivery.

- Treatment for acute DVT should be continued throughout pregnancy and for at least 6 weeks postpartum (for a minimum total duration of therapy of 3 months).

10. Women receiving therapeutic LMWH may be switched to therapeutic UFH in the last month of pregnancy or if delivery appears imminent due to the shorter half-life of UFH, although the benefit of this approach has not been validated by clinical studies. Alternately, therapeutic LMWH can be discontinued 24 hours prior to induction of labor. The purpose of conversion to UFH is primarily to reduce the risk of an epidural or spinal hematoma with regional anesthesia. The pharmacokinetics of subcutaneous UFH and LMWH are quite simi-lar, though, which may limit the benefit of this approach. The American Society of Regional Anesthesia and Pain Medicine guidelines recommend withholding neuraxial blockade for 24 hours after the last therapeutic dose of LMWH. These guidelines support the use of neuraxial anesthesia in patients receiving dos-ages of 5,000 units of UFH twice daily, but the safety in patients receiving 10,000 units twice daily or more is unknown. Pregnant women at the highest risk of recurrence (e.g., proximal DVT or PE within 2 weeks) can be switched to therapeutic IV UFH, which is then discontinued 4–6 h prior to the expected time of delivery or epidural insertion.

According to the American Society of Regional Anesthesia and Pain Medicine, resumption of therapeutic UFH or LMWH should be delayed for 24 hours after delivery, vaginal or cesarean, in women who have received neuraxial anesthesia. Otherwise, it can be restarted no sooner than 4–6 hours after a vaginal delivery or 6–12 hours after cesarean delivery. Women who require more than 6 weeks of postpartum therapeutic anticoagula-tion may be bridged to warfarin. Warfarin, UFH and LMWH are all compatible with breastfeeding.

10 Gestational Diabetes Mellitus[1,2]

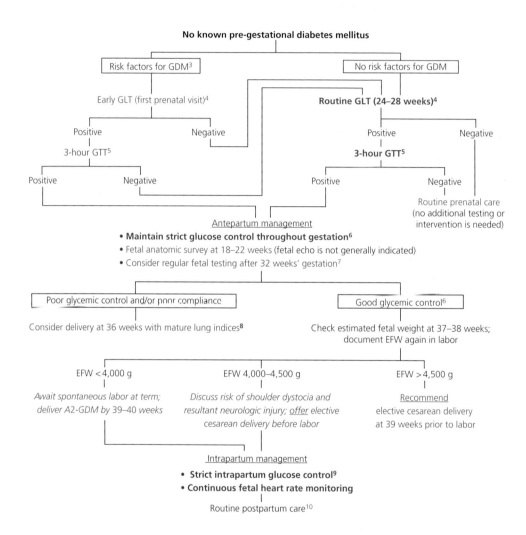

No known pre-gestational diabetes mellitus

Risk factors for GDM[3] — No risk factors for GDM

Early GLT (first prenatal visit)[4] — **Routine GLT (24–28 weeks)[4]**

Positive — Negative — Positive — Negative

3-hour GTT[5] — **3-hour GTT[5]**

Positive — Negative — Positive — Negative

Routine prenatal care
(no additional testing or
intervention is needed)

Antepartum management
• **Maintain strict glucose control throughout gestation[6]**
  • Fetal anatomic survey at 18–22 weeks (fetal echo is not generally indicated)
  • Consider regular fetal testing after 32 weeks' gestation[7]

Poor glycemic control and/or poor compliance — Good glycemic control[6]

Consider delivery at 36 weeks with mature lung indices[8] — Check estimated fetal weight at 37–38 weeks; document EFW again in labor

EFW < 4,000 g — EFW 4,000–4,500 g — EFW > 4,500 g

Await spontaneous labor at term; deliver A2-GDM by 39–40 weeks — *Discuss risk of shoulder dystocia and resultant neurologic injury; offer elective cesarean delivery before labor* — Recommend elective cesarean delivery at 39 weeks prior to labor

Intrapartum management
• **Strict intrapartum glucose control[9]**
• **Continuous fetal heart rate monitoring**

Routine postpartum care[10]

1. Gestational diabetes mellitus (GDM) refers to glucose intolerance present only during pregnancy. Since many pregnant women have never been tested before the pregnancy, it is likely that some patients diagnosed with GDM actually have unrecognized type II pre-gestational diabetes.

2. Pregnancy is a diabetogenic state with evidence of insulin resistance, maternal hyperinsulinism, and reduced peripheral uptake of glucose. This is due to high circulating levels of placental counter-regulatory (anti-insulin) hormones, including placental growth hormone

Obstetric Clinical Algorithms, Second Edition. Errol R. Norwitz, George R. Saade, Hugh Miller and Christina M. Davidson.
© 2017 John Wiley & Sons, Ltd. Published 2017 by John Wiley & Sons, Ltd.

and human chorionic somatomammotropins (previously known as human placental lacto-gens). These mechanisms ensure a continuous supply of glucose for the fetus. In some women, these changes unmask an underlying predisposition to insulin resistance leading to GDM. Depending on the population and the screening method used, up to 18% of pregnancies may be complicated by GDM. Up to 7% of pregnant women will be diagnosed with GDM using the screening approach recommended above.

3. Risk factors for GDM include: a prior history of GDM, a family history (first degree relative) of diabetes, a prior macrosomic or large-for-gestational age (LGA) infant, sustained glycosuria, a prior unexplained late intrauterine fetal demise (IUFD), hypertension, or obesity. Such patients should have early testing for GDM at 16–20 weeks. If the early testing is negative, this should be repeated at 24–28 weeks.

4. Glucose load test (GLT) – also known as a glucose challenge test (GCT) – is a non-fasting test, but the woman should not eat after her 50-g glucose load until a venous blood sample is drawn one hour later. A plasma value of ≥140 mg/dL is considered positive and should be followed with a 3-hour glucose tolerance test (GTT). <2% of women with a GLT <140 mg/dL will have a positive GTT.

5. A definitive diagnosis of GDM requires a 3-hour GTT. There is no GLT cut-off that is diagnostic of GDM. However, almost all women with a GLT value ≥240 mg/dL will have an abnormal GTT and it is acceptable to manage them as GDM without the GTT. To perform a GTT, a 100-g glucose load is administered after an overnight fast. Venous plasma glucose is measured fasting at 1 hour, 2 hours, and 3 hours. GDM requires two or more abnormal values defined as either ≥95, ≥180, ≥155, and ≥140 mg/dL, respectively (Carpenter & Coustan criteria) or ≥105, ≥190, ≥165, and ≥145 mg/dL,

respectively (NDDG criteria). There is no place for HbA1c to diagnose GDM.

6. The goal of antepartum management is to maintain strict glycemic control throughout gestation, defined as fasting blood glucose <95 mg/dL and 1-hour post-prandial <140 mg/dL (or a 2-hour post-prandial <120 mg/dL). A diabetic diet is recommended (defined as 36 kcal/kg or 15 kcal/lb of ideal body weight + 100 kcal per trimester given as 40–50% carbohydrate, 20% protein, 30–40% fat) but, if diet alone does not maintain blood glucose at the desirable levels, additional treatment may be needed. Insulin remains the gold standard, although oral hypoglycemic agents (glyburide, glipizide) appear to be safe and effective and are being used more commonly as first line agents. If fasting glucose levels are >95 mg/dL, treatment can be started right away because you "can't diet more than fasting."

7. Fetal testing is recommended for insulin-requiring GDM (class A2-GDM) after 32 weeks' gestation because of the risks of abnormal fetal growth (IUGR or macrosomia) and fetal demise. Testing should include daily fetal kickcharts, weekly non-stress testing, and serial ultrasound q 3–4 weeks for fetal growth.

8. If an elective delivery is planned prior to 39-0/7 weeks' gestation, ACOG recommends that fetal lung maturity is documented by amniocentesis prior to delivery using diabetes-specific cut-offs.

9. During labor, patients are typically starved. Glucose should therefore be administered (5% dextrose IV at 75–100 mL/h) and blood glucose checked every 1–2 hours. Regular insulin is given as needed (either by subcutaneous injection or IV infusion) to maintain glucose at 100–120 mg/dL.

10. Delivery of the fetus and placenta removes the source of the anti-insulin hormones that

causes GDM. As such, no further management is required in the immediate postpartum period. GDM likely unmasks an underlying predisposition for insulin resistance, and 40–60% of women with GDM will develop type II diabetes later in life. All women with GDM should therefore have a standard, non-pregnant 75-g, 2-hour oral GTT 6–8 weeks after delivery to exclude diabetes. Since the risk of developing type II diabetes remains elevated even if the 6 weeks GTT is negative, it should be repeated at least every 3 years.

11 Gestational Hypertension[1]

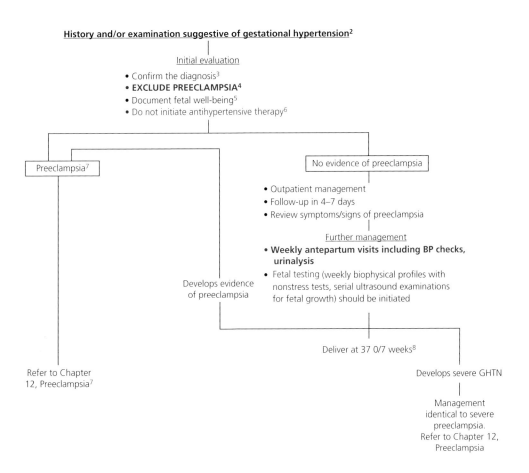

<u>History and/or examination suggestive of gestational hypertension[2]</u>

<u>Initial evaluation</u>
- Confirm the diagnosis[3]
- **EXCLUDE PREECLAMPSIA[4]**
- Document fetal well-being[5]
- Do not initiate antihypertensive therapy[6]

Preeclampsia[7]

No evidence of preeclampsia
- Outpatient management
- Follow-up in 4–7 days
- Review symptoms/signs of preeclampsia

<u>Further management</u>
- **Weekly antepartum visits including BP checks, urinalysis**
- Fetal testing (weekly biophysical profiles with nonstress tests, serial ultrasound examinations for fetal growth) should be initiated

Develops evidence of preeclampsia

Deliver at 37 0/7 weeks[8]

Refer to Chapter 12, Preeclampsia[7]

Develops severe GHTN

Management identical to severe preeclampsia. Refer to Chapter 12, Preeclampsia

1. Characterized by new-onset BP elevation after 20 weeks of gestation, often near term, in the absence of accompanying proteinuria. Hypertension is defined as systolic BP $\geq$140 mmHg and/or diastolic BP $\geq$90 mmHg on two occasions at least 4 hours (but not more than 7 days) apart.

2. Patients with gestational hypertension should be asymptomatic. The diagnosis should

be suspected in a patient who presents with a new-onset sustained elevation in BP without proteinuria in the second or third trimester.

3. Gestational hypertension refers to a sustained elevation in systolic BP $\geq$140 mmHg and/or diastolic BP $\geq$90 mmHg without evidence of preeclampsia in a previously normotensive woman. It is a diagnosis which should only be made after

Obstetric Clinical Algorithms, Second Edition. Errol R. Norwitz, George R. Saade, Hugh Miller and Christina M. Davidson.
© 2017 John Wiley & Sons, Ltd. Published 2017 by John Wiley & Sons, Ltd.

20 weeks of gestation, and likely represents an exaggerated physiologic response of the maternal cardiovascular system to pregnancy.

4. Gestational hypertension may progress to preeclampsia, but preeclampsia can be excluded initially by the absence of maternal symptoms of preeclampsia and laboratory abnormalities. The following tests should be sent: urinalysis, 24-hour urine collection for protein quantitation and creatinine clearance, CBC with platelets, liver and renal function tests, and uric acid. It may be necessary to consider hospitalization for approximately 24 hours to exclude preeclampsia. If the systolic BP is ≥160 mmHg and/or diastolic BP is ≥110 mmHg on two occasions at least 4 hours apart, the diagnosis is severe gestational hypertension. Mild gestational hypertension is rarely associated with adverse maternal or fetal outcome. However, severe gestational hypertension has been associated with outcomes similar to women with preeclampsia. Of note, 14–20% of women with eclampsia (and hence severe preeclampsia) do not have proteinuria prior to their seizure.

5. Such testing should include a nonstress test (looking for evidence of uteroplacental insufficiency), a biophysical profile (BPP) or amniotic fluid estimation, ultrasound for estimated fetal weight (EFW) or a combination of these modalities. Umbilical artery Doppler velocimetry is only useful in the setting of fetal growth restriction.

6. Treatment of mild hypertension has not been shown to improve pregnancy outcome.

Antihypertensive therapy is used to prevent severe gestational hypertension and maternal hemorrhagic stroke. There are only three indications for antihypertensive therapy in the setting of preeclampsia: (i) underlying chronic hypertension; (ii) to achieve BP control to prevent cerebrovascular accident while effecting delivery; and/or (iii) expectant management of severe preeclampsia by BP criteria alone (Sibai protocol).

7. In women with mild gestational hypertension, the progression to severe gestational hypertension or preeclampsia often develops within 1–3 weeks after diagnosis. Elevated concentrations of uric acid (>5.2 mg/dL) might be predictive of progression to preeclampsia and a risk factor for adverse maternal-fetal outcome.

8. Delivery is the only effective treatment for gestational hypertension and preeclampsia. It is recommended in women with mild gestational hypertension and preeclampsia without severe features at or beyond 37-0/7 weeks or at or beyond 34-0/7 weeks of gestation if there is evidence of fetal growth restriction <5th percentile. If severe gestational hypertension develops, management is similar to women with preeclampsia with severe features and delivery is recommended at 34-0/7 weeks of gestation. There is no proven benefit to routine delivery by cesarean; however, the probability of vaginal delivery decreases with decreasing gestational age. With labor induction, the likelihood of cesarean delivery is 93–97% at <28 weeks, 53–65% at 28–32 weeks, and 31–38% at 32–34 weeks.

12 Preeclampsia

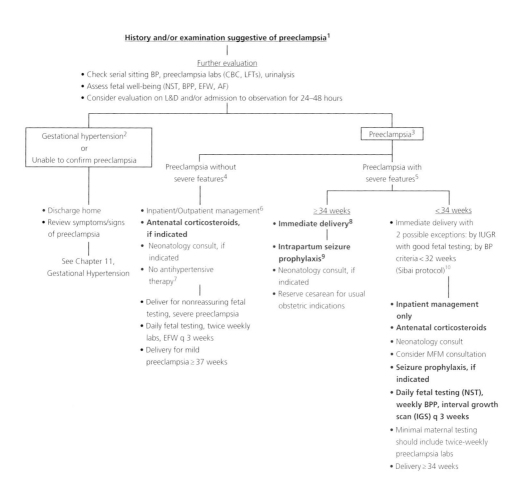

<u>History and/or examination suggestive of preeclampsia[1]</u>

Further evaluation
- Check serial sitting BP, preeclampsia labs (CBC, LFTs), urinalysis
- Assess fetal well-being (NST, BPP, EFW, AF)
- Consider evaluation on L&D and/or admission to observation for 24–48 hours

Gestational hypertension[2]
or
Unable to confirm preeclampsia

Preeclampsia[3]

Preeclampsia without severe features[4]

Preeclampsia with severe features[5]

- Discharge home
- Review symptoms/signs of preeclampsia

See Chapter 11, Gestational Hypertension

- Inpatient/Outpatient management[6]
- **Antenatal corticosteroids, if indicated**
- Neonatology consult, if indicated
- No antihypertensive therapy[7]
- Deliver for nonreassuring fetal testing, severe preeclampsia
- Daily fetal testing, twice weekly labs, EFW q 3 weeks
- Delivery for mild preeclampsia ≥ 37 weeks

≥ 34 weeks
- **Immediate delivery[8]**
- **Intrapartum seizure prophylaxis[9]**
- Neonatology consult, if indicated
- Reserve cesarean for usual obstetric indications

< 34 weeks
- Immediate delivery with 2 possible exceptions: by IUGR with good fetal testing; by BP criteria < 32 weeks (Sibai protocol)[10]

- **Inpatient management only**
- **Antenatal corticosteroids**
- Neonatology consult
- Consider MFM consultation
- **Seizure prophylaxis, if indicated**
- **Daily fetal testing (NST), weekly BPP, interval growth scan (IGS) q 3 weeks**
- Minimal maternal testing should include twice-weekly preeclampsia labs
- Delivery ≥ 34 weeks

1. Most patients are asymptomatic. Symptoms may include headache, visual aberrations, and right upper quadrant or epigastric pain. Signs may include elevated blood pressure (BP), excessive weight gain, brisk deep tendon reflexes or excessive clonus, and right upper quadrant or epigastric tenderness. Hypertension is defined as systolic BP of ≥ 140 mm Hg and/or diastolic BP of ≥ 90 mm Hg on two occasions at least 4 hours (but not more than 7 days) apart.

2. Gestational hypertension refers to a sustained elevation in systolic BP of ≥ 140 mm Hg and/or diastolic BP of ≥ 90 mm Hg without evidence of preeclampsia in a previously normotensive woman. It is a diagnosis which

Obstetric Clinical Algorithms, Second Edition. Errol R. Norwitz, George R. Saade, Hugh Miller and Christina M. Davidson.
© 2017 John Wiley & Sons, Ltd. Published 2017 by John Wiley & Sons, Ltd.

should only be made after 20 weeks of gestation, and likely represents an exaggerated physiologic response of the maternal cardiovascular system to pregnancy.

3. Preeclampsia is a multisystem disorder specific to pregnancy and the puerperium. More precisely, it is a disease of the placenta since it occurs in pregnancies where there is trophoblast but no fetal tissue (complete molar pregnancies). Preeclampsia usually occurs after 20 weeks of gestation, most often near term. Evidence of gestational proteinuric hypertension prior to 20 weeks should raise the possibility of an underlying molar pregnancy, drug withdrawal or (rarely) chromosomal abnormality in the fetus. Diagnostic criteria for preeclampsia include the following: hypertension after 20 weeks of gestation in a woman with a previously normal BP and proteinuria ($\geq$300 mg of protein in a 24-hour urine collection or this amount extrapolated from a timed collection; or protein/creatinine ratio $\geq$0.3; or urine dipstick test of 1+). In the absence of proteinuria, preeclampsia is diagnosed in the setting of new-onset hypertension and any of the following: thrombocytopenia (platelet count <100,000/microliter); renal insufficiency (serum creatinine >1.1 mg/dL or a doubling of the creatinine in the absence of other renal disease); impaired liver function (elevated serum transaminases to twice normal concentration and/or severe, persistent right upper quadrant or epigastric pain); pulmonary edema; cerebral or visual disturbances. Preeclampsia is classified as "mild" or "severe." The terminology has recently undergone revision and "mild" preeclampsia is now referred to as "preeclampsia without severe features," while "severe" preeclampsia is preeclampsia with severe features. Proteinuria is no longer required for the diagnosis of preeclampsia and massive proteinuria (>5 gm) has been eliminated from the consideration of preeclampsia as severe.

4. Refers to all women with only mild hypertension (systolic BP of $\geq$140 mm Hg but <160 mm

Hg and/or diastolic BP of $\geq$90 mmHg but <110 mm Hg) and proteinuria.

5. Refers to all women with severe hypertension (systolic BP of $\geq$160 mm Hg and/or diastolic BP of $\geq$110 mmHg on two occasions at least 4 hours apart, or sooner if antihypertensive medication is administered) and proteinuria or women with new-onset hypertension (mild or severe) and any of the features outlined above.

6. Outpatient management of preeclampsia without severe features is an option for women as long as both patient and physician are comfortable with the plan and understand the risks. The patient will report symptoms of severe preeclampsia immediately, and the patient can comply with regular visits that include all of the following:

- Maternal evaluation: once-weekly clinic visits with assessment for symptoms of preeclampsia and lab evaluation (CBC with platelets, AST, ALT, serum creatinine).
- Fetal evaluation: daily kick counts, once-weekly antenatal testing (i.e., BPP), ultrasound assessment of fetal growth every 3 weeks.

7. Antihypertensive therapy is used to prevent severe gestational hypertension and maternal hemorrhagic strokes. There are only three indications for antihypertensive therapy in the setting of preeclampsia: (i) underlying chronic hypertension; (ii) to achieve BP control to prevent cerebrovascular accident while effecting delivery; and/or (iii) expectant management of severe preeclampsia by BP criteria alone (Sibai protocol). BP control is important to prevent cerebrovascular accident, but does not affect the natural course of preeclampsia. The degree of systolic hypertension (as opposed to the level of diastolic hypertension or relative increase or rate of increase of mean arterial pressure from baseline levels) may be the most important predictor of cerebral injury and infarction. Acute-onset, severe systolic ($\geq$160 mm Hg) hypertension; severe diastolic ($\geq$110 mm Hg)

hypertension, or both should be treated with antihypertensive therapy with the aim of achieving a BP of 140–150/90–100 mm Hg. First line treatment for the management of acute-onset, severe hypertension includes intravenous labetalol and hydralazine and oral nifedipine.

8. Delivery is the only effective treatment. It is recommended in women with mild gestational hypertension and preeclampsia without severe features by 37 0/7 weeks of gestation or at or beyond 34 0/7 weeks of gestation if fetal growth restriction of less than the 5th percentile develops. It is recommended in women with preeclampsia with severe features if the gestational age is at least 34 0/7. There is no proven benefit to routine delivery by cesarean, however, the probability of vaginal delivery is directly related to gestational age. With labor induction, the likelihood of cesarean delivery is 93–97% at <28 weeks of gestation, 53–65% at 28–32 weeks of gestation, and 31–38% at 32–34 weeks of gestation. Preeclampsia and its complications always resolve following delivery (with the exception of stroke). Diuresis (.4 L/day) is the most accurate clinical indicator of resolution. Fetal prognosis is dependent largely on gestational age at delivery.

9. Intravenous magnesium sulfate is the drug of choice and should be given intrapartum and for at least 24 hours postpartum to prevent eclampsia. An IV loading dose of 4–6 gm should be followed by a maintenance dose of 1–2 gm/hr. The use of magnesium sulfate therapy in preeclampsia without severe features is not recommended, but should be initiated if there is progression to severe disease either intrapartum or postpartum.

10. If the gestational age is <34 0/7 weeks and the diagnosis is by BP criteria alone, expectant management can be considered. During the first 24–48 hours of observation and confirmation of diagnosis, the woman should be monitored in labor and delivery with administration of antenatal corticosteroids for fetal maturity, magnesium sulfate for maternal seizure prophylaxis, and antihypertensive medications (as needed for acute-onset, severe hypertension). Expectant management should only be undertaken in facilities with adequate maternal and neonatal intensive care resources and should be abandoned if the BP cannot be controlled, if any other severe features present and persist, and/or if fetal growth restriction (<5th %) develops. Magnesium sulfate should be discontinued during the period of expectant management and re-initiated at the time of induction of labor or immediately postpartum if cesarean delivery is planned.

13 Pregestational Diabetes Mellitus

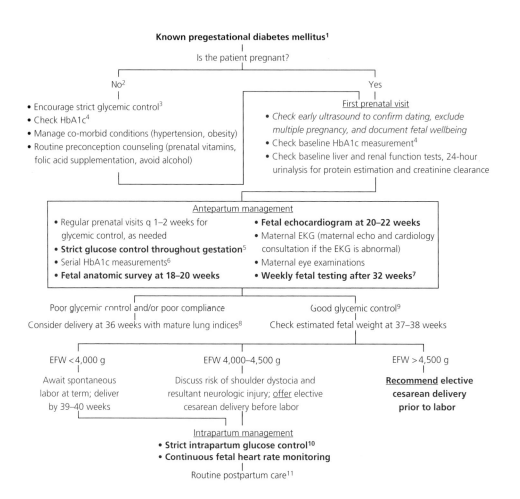

Known pregestational diabetes mellitus[1]

Is the patient pregnant?

No[2]

- Encourage strict glycemic control[3]
- Check HbA1c[4]
- Manage co-morbid conditions (hypertension, obesity)
- Routine preconception counseling (prenatal vitamins, folic acid supplementation, avoid alcohol)

Yes

First prenatal visit
- *Check early ultrasound to confirm dating, exclude multiple pregnancy, and document fetal wellbeing*
- Check baseline HbA1c measurement[4]
- Check baseline liver and renal function tests, 24-hour urinalysis for protein estimation and creatinine clearance

Antepartum management
- Regular prenatal visits q 1–2 weeks for glycemic control, as needed
- **Strict glucose control throughout gestation[5]**
- Serial HbA1c measurements[6]
- **Fetal anatomic survey at 18–20 weeks**
- **Fetal echocardiogram at 20–22 weeks**
- Maternal EKG (maternal echo and cardiology consultation if the EKG is abnormal)
- Maternal eye examinations
- **Weekly fetal testing after 32 weeks[7]**

Poor glycemic control and/or poor compliance
Consider delivery at 36 weeks with mature lung indices[8]

Good glycemic control[9]
Check estimated fetal weight at 37–38 weeks

EFW <4,000 g
Await spontaneous labor at term; deliver by 39–40 weeks

EFW 4,000–4,500 g
Discuss risk of shoulder dystocia and resultant neurologic injury; <u>offer</u> elective cesarean delivery before labor

EFW >4,500 g
<u>**Recommend**</u> **elective cesarean delivery prior to labor**

Intrapartum management
- **Strict intrapartum glucose control[10]**
- **Continuous fetal heart rate monitoring**

Routine postpartum care[11]

1. Pregestational diabetes results from either an absolute deficiency of insulin (type I, insulin-dependent diabetes mellitus) or increased peripheral resistance to insulin (type II, non-insulin-dependent diabetes mellitus (NIDDM)). It occurs in <1% of women of childbearing age. The age of onset and duration of diabetes (White classification) do not correlate with pregnancy outcome. Poor prognostic features include a history of diabetic ketoacidosis (DKA), poor compliance, poorly controlled hypertension, pyelonephritis, and vasculopathy.

2. Pregestational diabetes is associated with significant maternal and perinatal mortality and morbidity. Diabetic women should ideally be

Obstetric Clinical Algorithms, Second Edition. Errol R. Norwitz, George R. Saade, Hugh Miller and Christina M. Davidson.
© 2017 John Wiley & Sons, Ltd. Published 2017 by John Wiley & Sons, Ltd.

seen prior to conception. Pregnancy complications such as fetal congenital anomalies (diabetic embryopathy) and spontaneous abortion correlate directly with the degree of diabetic control around the time of conception.

3. Strict glycemic control is defined as fasting blood glucose <95 mg/dL and 1-hour postprandial <140 mg/dL (or 2-hour postprandial <120 mg/dL).

4. Approximately 5% of maternal hemoglobin is glycosylated (bound to glucose). This fraction is known as hemoglobin A1 (HbA1). HbA1c refers to the 80–85% of HbA1 that is irreversibly glycosylated and, as such, is a more reliable and reproducible measurement. Since red blood cells have a life span of 120 days, HbA1c measurements reflect the degree of glycemic control over the prior 3–4 months. A normal HbA1c is <5.9%.

5. The aim of antepartum management is to maintain strict glycemic control throughout gestation, defined as fasting blood glucose <95 mg/dL and 1-hour post-prandial <140 mg/dL (or 2-hour postprandial <120 mg/dL). A diabetic diet is recommended (defined as 36 kcal/kg or 15 kcal/lb of ideal body weight + 100 kcal per trimester given as 40–50% carbohydrate, 20% protein, 30–40% fat). Almost all patients with pregestational diabetes will also require pharmacologic therapy, particularly those with type I diabetes. Insulin remains the gold standard for women with pregestational diabetes. Although oral hypoglycemic agents (glyburide, glipizide) appear to be safe and effective and are being used more commonly as first line agents, they are not recommended for women with pregestational diabetes, particularly those with type I diabetes. Intense antepartum management and strict glycemic control can reduce perinatal mortality from 20% to 3–5%.

6. HbA1c measurements should be checked prior to conception, at first prenatal visit, and every 4–6 weeks throughout pregnancy.

7. Fetal testing is recommended in all cases of pregestational diabetes after 32 weeks' gestation because of the risks of abnormal fetal growth (intrauterine growth restriction or macrosomia), abnormal amniotic fluid volume, and fetal demise. Testing should include daily fetal kick-charts, weekly non-stress testing (NST) with or without sonographic estimation of amniotic fluid volume, and serial ultrasound q 3–4 weeks for fetal growth.

8. If an elective delivery is planned prior to 39 0/7 weeks' gestation, ACOG recommends that fetal lung maturity be documented by amniocentesis prior to delivery using diabetes-specific cut-offs.

9. If metabolic control is good, spontaneous labor at term can be awaited. Because of the risk of unexplained fetal demise, women with pregestational diabetes should be delivered by 39–40 weeks.

10. During labor, patients are typically starved. Glucose should therefore be administered (5% dextrose IV at 75–100 mL/h) and blood glucose checked every 1–2 hours. Regular insulin is given as needed (either by subcutaneous injection or IV infusion) to maintain glucose at 100–120 mg/dL.

11. During the first 48 hours postpartum, women may have a "honeymoon period" during which their insulin requirement is decreased. Blood glucose levels of 150–200 mg/dL (8.2–11.0 mmol/L) can be tolerated during this period. Once a woman is able to eat, she can be placed back on her regular insulin regimen.

14 Pulmonary Edema

Pulmonary edema[1]
|
Confirm the diagnosis
- Identify risk factors for pulmonary edema[2]
- Take a detailed history and perform a physical examination[3]
- √ chest x-ray
- Consider alternative diagnoses[4]

Initiate treatment immediately	
• **Admit to hospital, manage in an ICU setting**	• **L – Lasix (to promote diuresis)**
• Vital signs and oxygen saturation q 15 min	• **M – Morphine (decreases anxiety and promotes**
• √ EKG	**pulmonary vascular dilatation)**
• Confirm gestational age and fetal wellbeing	• **N – Na^{2+} (sodium) and water restriction**
• *Consider empiric antibiotic therapy and*	• **O – Oxygen supplementation at 4–6 L/min**
ionotropic support, if needed	• **P – Position patient in an upright posture**

Identify the cause
(√ maternal echocardiography)[5]

Non-cardiogenic pulmonary edema[6]
- **Treat the underlying cause (e.g., with antibiotics or anticoagulation)**
- **Suspend tocolysis and excessive fluid management**
- Consider MFM, NICU, anesthesia consultation
- Continuous fetal heart rate monitoring

Does the patient have preeclampsia?

No
- Continue expectant management
- Treat the underlying cause
- Discharge home once stable

Yes[7]
- Stabilize the mother
- Resuscitate the fetus *in utero*
- **Consider antenatal steroids**
|
Proceed with urgent delivery
regardless of gestational age

Cardiogenic pulmonary edema[8]
- **Urgent cardiology consultation**
- Exclude myocardial injury: √ serial EKG and cardiac enzymes (troponin, creatine kinase) q 8 hourly × 3
- Consider MFM, NICU, anesthesia consultation
- √ CBC, renal and liver function
- Consider serial arterial blood gas (ABG) to monitor the extent of hypoxemia
- Continuous fetal heart rate monitoring

- Stabilize the mother
- Resuscitate the fetus *in utero*
- **Consider antenatal steroids, if indicated**
- Reserve delivery for usual obstetric indications

Obstetric Clinical Algorithms, Second Edition. Errol R. Norwitz, George R. Saade, Hugh Miller and Christina M. Davidson.
© 2017 John Wiley & Sons, Ltd. Published 2017 by John Wiley & Sons, Ltd.

1. Pulmonary edema refers to an abnormal and excessive accumulation of fluid in the alveolar and interstitial spaces of the lungs.

2. Risk factors for pulmonary edema include preeclampsia, infection, iatrogenic fluid overload, and tocolytic therapy (such as β-agonist medications).

3. Accumulation of fluid in the alveolar space leads to decreased diffusing capacity, hypoxemia, and shortness of breath (dyspnea). Patients present with worsening dyspnea and orthopnea (inability to lie flat) which may be acute or slowly progressive in onset. Other symptoms may include cough, chest pain, palpitations, fatigue, and low-grade fever. Physical examination may reveal tachycardia, elevated blood pressure, and peripheral edema. Cardiac evaluation may uncover an irregular heart beat, elevated jugular venous pressure (which reflects an elevated right-sided filling pressure), and the presence of a S3 or S4 heart sound or both ("summation gallop") as well as a new or changed heart murmur. Chest examination usually reveals crackles indicative of interstitial pulmonary edema and some patients may have wheezing ("cardiac asthma"). The diagnosis is typically confirmed on chest radiograph. Radiographic findings can range from mild pulmonary vascular redistribution to extensive bilateral interstitial marking and pleural effusions. The presence of bilateral peri-hilar alveolar edema may give the typical "butterfly" appearance. The presence of cardiomegaly suggests a cardiac cause.

4. Consider alternative diagnoses, including pulmonary embolism (see Chapter 15, Pulmonary Embolism), severe asthma exacerbation, and pneumonia.

5. All pregnant women with pulmonary edema should have a maternal echocardiogram (ideally a trans-esophageal echo) to exclude underlying cardiac disease.

6. **Non-cardiogenic pulmonary edema** is defined as radiographic evidence of fluid and protein accumulation in the alveolar space of the lungs without evidence of a cardiogenic cause (i.e., a normal maternal echo and pulmonary capillary wedge pressure <18 mmHg). The major causes of non-cardiogenic pulmonary edema include: the acute respiratory distress syndrome (ARDS) and, less often, high altitude pulmonary edema, neurogenic pulmonary edema, pulmonary embolism, salicylate toxicity, opiate overdose, preeclampsia, amniotic fluid embolism, and reperfusion pulmonary edema. ARDS can develop as a result of a number of insults, including sepsis, acute pulmonary infection, non-thoracic trauma, inhaled toxins, disseminated intravascular coagulation, shock lung, freebase cocaine smoking, post-coronary artery bypass grafting, inhalation of high oxygen concentrations, and acute radiation pneumonia. Frequently overlooked is the common iatrogenic cause associated with tocolytic therapy. The combination of betamimetics, excessive fluid, and corticosteroids can cause significant pulmonary edema. Hypoalbuminemia alone is not a cause of non-cardiogenic pulmonary edema. The primary pathophysiologic mechanism of non-cardiogenic pulmonary edema is an increase in capillary permeability. Treatment is primarily supportive care.

7. If the patient has preeclampsia (gestational proteinuric hypertension), the presence of pulmonary edema puts her in the "severe preeclampsia" category (see Chapter 12, Preeclampsia) and is a contraindication to continued expectant management. Immediate delivery should be recommended regardless of gestational age. Whether delivery can be delayed for 24–48 hours to complete a course of antenatal corticosteroids in women remote from term (<32 weeks) should be individualized.

8. **Cardiogenic pulmonary edema** is characterized by increased transudation of protein-poor fluid into the pulmonary interstitium and

alveolar space. Fluid transudation results from a rise in pulmonary capillary pressure (as measured by pulmonary capillary wedge pressure ≥18mmHg) due to an increase in pulmonary venous and left atrial pressures. This typically occurs in the absence of a change in vascular integrity or permeability. The major causes of cardiogenic pulmonary edema include: myocardial injury or infarction, valvular heart disease, cardiomyopathy, cardiac arrhythmia, poorly controlled systemic hypertension, and, less often, severe anemia, thyroid disease, toxins such as cocaine and alcohol, fever, intercurrent infection (such as pneumonia), and uncontrolled diabetes.

15 Pulmonary Embolism[1]

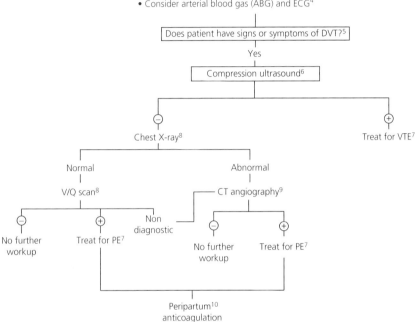

Suspected pulmonary embolism (PE)
- Take a detailed history and perform a physical examination[2]
- Be aware of pre-existing risk factors for DVT/PE[3]
- Check CBC, coagulation studies, oxygen saturation[4]
- Consider arterial blood gas (ABG) and ECG[4]

Does patient have signs or symptoms of DVT?[5]

Yes

Compression ultrasound[6]

Chest X-ray[8]

Treat for VTE[7]

Normal

Abnormal

V/Q scan[8]

CT angiography[9]

Non diagnostic

No further workup

Treat for PE[7]

No further workup

Treat for PE[7]

Peripartum[10] anticoagulation

1. Venous thromboembolic events (VTE) – which includes both deep vein thrombosis (DVT) and pulmonary embolism (PE) – complicate 0.5–2.0 per 1000 pregnancies. VTE is one of the leading cause of maternal mortality in developed nations, accounting for 10–20% of pregnancy-related maternal deaths in the United States. DVTs account for 75–80% of VTEs during pregnancy, with PE comprising the remaining 20–25%.

2. Symptoms of PE include acute-onset shortness of breath (dyspnea), pleuritic chest pain,

cough, and/or hemoptysis. Physical signs suggestive of PE may include low-grade fever, tachypnea, tachycardia, diminished oxygen saturation, diminished breath sounds, audible crackles and/or evidence of pleural effusion on pulmonary examination. In women with confirmed PE, dyspnea (62%), pleuritic chest pain (55%), cough (24%) and sweating (18%) are the four most common features at presentation.

3. Risk factors for VTE are summarized in Chapter 9, Deep Vein Thrombosis. Up to 60% of

Obstetric Clinical Algorithms, Second Edition. Errol R. Norwitz, George R. Saade, Hugh Miller and Christina M. Davidson.
© 2017 John Wiley & Sons, Ltd. Published 2017 by John Wiley & Sons, Ltd.

pregnancy-related PEs occur in the 4–6 weeks after delivery.

4. Laboratory tests may reveal acidosis and an elevated A-a gradient on ABG analysis and evidence of right axis deviation on ECG. An abnormal A-a gradient ($\geq$15 mm Hg) has been reported in only 58% of pregnant women with confirmed PE, however. While an arterial $pO_2 > 85$ mmHg is reassuring, it does not exclude PE. D-dimer cannot currently be used to exclude suspected PE in pregnancy. There are no validated clinical prediction guidelines for determining pretest probability of PE in the pregnant population.

5. Signs and symptoms of DVT are summarized in Chapter 9. If the clinical suspicion for acute VTE is high, consider starting therapeutic anticoagulation immediately to avoid clot propagation and possible repeat PE.

6. In a pregnant woman with suspected PE and signs and symptoms of DVT, bilateral compression ultrasound of the lower extremities can be performed first. Since treatment of DVT and PE is identical, this method allows for possible VTE diagnosis and initiation of treatment without the need for radiation-associated tests.

7. If a DVT is diagnosed, therapeutic anticoagulation should be initiated. Admission is generally warranted for initiation of treatment in pregnancy. Therapeutic subcutaneous low molecular weight heparin (LMWH) is now the treatment of choice for PE in pregnancy. The advantages of LMWH over unfractionated heparin (UFH) include a reduced risk of bleeding, predictable pharmacokinetics allowing weight-based dosing without the need for monitoring, and a reduced risk of heparin-induced thrombocytopenia and heparin-induced osteoporotic fractures. A twice-daily weight-adjusted dosing regimen should be used, such as enoxaparin (Lovenox) 1 mg/kg sc q12h. LMWH does not significantly alter PTT, but serum anti-factor Xa activity can be measured. Therapeutic anticoagulation is achieved with a circulating anti-Xa activity of 0.6–1.0 U/mL; however, routine monitoring of anti-Xa activity may not be justified due to the absence of large studies using clinical end points that demonstrate an optimal therapeutic anti-Xa LMWH range or that dose adjustments increase the safety or efficacy of therapy, the lack of accuracy and reliability of the measurement, the lack of correlation with risk of bleeding and recurrence, and the cost of the assay.

When LMWH cannot be used or when UFH is preferred (e.g., in patients with renal dysfunction and when delivery or surgery may be necessary), UFH can be administered as an initial IV therapy followed by subcutaneous UFH. IV treatment should be initiated with a loading dose of 80 U/kg followed by an initial infusion of 18 U/kg/h. Serum PTT should be checked every 4–6 hours, and the infusion adjusted to maintain PTT at 1.5–2.5 times control. Once a steady state has been achieved, PTT levels should be measured daily. After 5–10 days, IV heparin can be changed to subcuticular (SC) injection (not IM injection because of the risk of hematoma) as follows: begin with 10,000 U SC three times daily and titrate dosage upward depending on the results of PTT; aim for PTT 1.5–2.5 times control. When subcutaneous UFH is used during pregnancy, higher doses and three times daily dosing are usually required to maintain adequate anticoagulation.

Treatment for acute VTE should be continued throughout pregnancy and for at least 6 weeks postpartum (for a minimum total duration of therapy of 3 months).

8. Patients with suspected PE and normal findings on compression ultrasonography require additional diagnostic imaging. A chest radiograph (CXR) can be obtained both to rule out alternative diagnoses (e.g., pulmonary edema) and to selectively triage patients to ventilation-perfusion (V/Q) scanning vs. CT angiography. In women with normal CXR findings, a diagnostic

result is more likely to be obtained with V/Q scan than CT angiography (94% vs 70%, P <0.01), whereas patients with abnormal CXRs have a significantly higher nondiagnostic study rate on V/Q scan than CT angiography (40% vs 16%, P <0.01). Therefore, a normal CXR should prompt further testing with a V/Q scan and an abnormal CXR warrants CT angiography. If the patient is unstable or some studies are not available on a timely basis, empirical initiation of therapy and alternate diagnostic strategies should be considered. For a patient in whom there is a high clinical suspicion of PE and a low risk of bleeding, anticoagulant therapy is recommended while awaiting the outcome of diagnostic tests.

9. To minimize nondiagnostic and repeat studies, CT angiography protocols performed in pregnant women should be specifically adapted and optimized to account for known physiologic changes of pregnancy, such as increases in cardiac output and blood volume that will affect contrast medium dynamics and result in decreased pulmonary arterial opacification. Protocol optimization for the pregnant state include automated bolus triggering, a high iodine flux achieved through high flow rate (4.5–6 mL/s) and/or high iodine concentration (350–400 mg I/mL), and clear breathing instructions to minimize possible Valsalva effects. Although pulmonary angiography was historically considered the reference standard in diagnosis of PE, angiography has now been found to be less sensitive than CT angiography in detection of emboli. At sites with high rates of inadequate CT angiography studies, however, V/Q scan may be a better alternative even in women with abnormal CXRs.

10. Women receiving therapeutic LMWH may be switched to therapeutic UFH in the last month of pregnancy or if delivery appears imminent due to the shorter half-life of UFH, although the benefit of this approach has not been validated by clinical studies. Alternately, therapeutic LMWH can be discontinued 24 hours prior to induction of labor. The purpose of conversion to UFH is primarily to reduce the risk of an epidural or spinal hematoma with regional anesthesia. The pharmacokinetics of subcutaneous UFH and LMWH are quite similar, which may limit the benefit of this approach. The American Society of Regional Anesthesia and Pain Medicine guidelines recommend withholding neuraxial blockade for 24 hours after the last therapeutic dose of LMWH. These guidelines support the use of neuraxial anesthesia in patients receiving dosages of 5,000 units of UFH twice daily, but the safety in patients receiving 10,000 units twice daily or more is unknown. Pregnant women at the highest risk of recurrence (e.g., proximal DVT or PE within 2 weeks) can be switched to therapeutic IV UFH, which is then discontinued 4–6 hours prior to the expected time of delivery or epidural insertion.

According to the American Society of Regional Anesthesia and Pain Medicine, resumption of therapeutic UFH or LMWH should be delayed for 24 hours after delivery, vaginal or cesarean, in women who received neuraxial anesthesia. Otherwise, it can be restarted no sooner than 4–6 hours after a vaginal delivery or 6–12 hours after cesarean delivery. Women who require more than 6 weeks of postpartum therapeutic anticoagulation may be bridged to warfarin. Warfarin, UFH and LMWH are all compatible with breastfeeding.

16 Renal Disease

Confirm the diagnosis of renal disease
- Take a detailed history, perform a physical examination including careful blood pressure assessment, and obtain relevant renal function tests[1]
- Be aware of the normal physiologic changes in the renal system during pregnancy[2,3]
- Consider differential diagnosis[4]

Prognosis and subsequent management depends on the patient's baseline renal status[5]

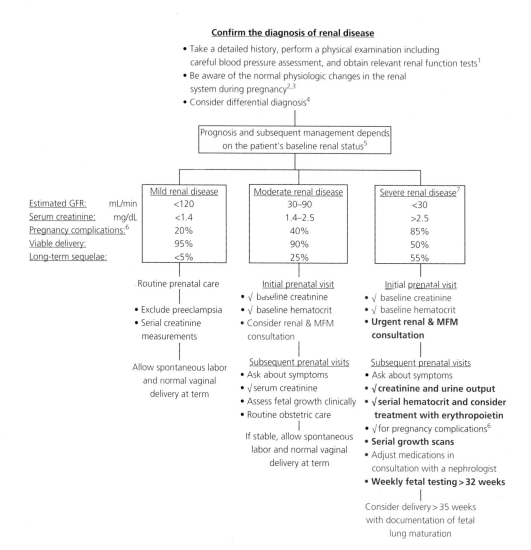

		Mild renal disease	Moderate renal disease	Severe renal disease[7]
Estimated GFR:	mL/min	<120	30–90	<30
Serum creatinine:	mg/dL	<1.4	1.4–2.5	>2.5
Pregnancy complications:[6]		20%	40%	85%
Viable delivery:		95%	90%	50%
Long-term sequelae:		<5%	25%	55%

Mild renal disease

Routine prenatal care

- Exclude preeclampsia
- Serial creatinine measurements

Allow spontaneous labor and normal vaginal delivery at term

Moderate renal disease

Initial prenatal visit
- √ baseline creatinine
- √ baseline hematocrit
- Consider renal & MFM consultation

Subsequent prenatal visits
- Ask about symptoms
- √ serum creatinine
- Assess fetal growth clinically
- Routine obstetric care

If stable, allow spontaneous labor and normal vaginal delivery at term

Severe renal disease

Initial prenatal visit
- √ baseline creatinine
- √ baseline hematocrit
- **Urgent renal & MFM consultation**

Subsequent prenatal visits
- Ask about symptoms
- **√ creatinine and urine output**
- **√ serial hematocrit and consider treatment with erythropoietin**
- √ for pregnancy complications[6]
- **Serial growth scans**
- Adjust medications in consultation with a nephrologist
- **Weekly fetal testing > 32 weeks**

Consider delivery > 35 weeks with documentation of fetal lung maturation

Obstetric Clinical Algorithms, Second Edition. Errol R. Norwitz, George R. Saade, Hugh Miller and Christina M. Davidson.
© 2017 John Wiley & Sons, Ltd. Published 2017 by John Wiley & Sons, Ltd.

1. A number of renal disorders can complicate pregnancy. Asymptomatic bacteriuria (Chapter 21, Asymptomatic Bacteriuria) and urinary tract infection/pyelonephritis (Chapter 22, Urinary Tract Infection/Pyelonephritis) are dealt with elsewhere in this book. Acute and chronic renal disease may be asymptomatic or may present with complaints of oliguria/polyuria, frequency, urgency, and pain or bleeding on urination. Carefully assess blood pressure and consider which medications are appropriate for pregnancy. Renal function tests useful in diagnosing and following renal disease include serum and urine creatinine and urea (blood urea nitrogen (BUN)) measurements, BUN/creatinine ratio, fractional excretion of sodium (FeNa), and 24-hour urinary collections for protein estimation and creatinine clearance. In general, women with mild, well-controlled renal disease tolerate pregnancy well. Women with severe renal disease are at risk of symptomatic deterioration and end-stage renal insufficiency.

2. A number of changes occur in the genitourinary system during pregnancy. The glomerular filtration rate (GFR) increases by 50% early in pregnancy, leading to an increase in creatinine clearance and a 25% decrease in serum creatinine and urea concentrations. The increased GFR results in an increase in filtered sodium, and aldosterone levels increase twofold to threefold to reabsorb this sodium. The increased GFR also results in decreased resorption of glucose; as such, 15% of normal pregnant women exhibit glycosuria. Mild hydronephrosis and hydroureter (Right > Left) are common sonographic findings due both to high levels of progesterone (which is a smooth muscle relaxant) and partial obstruction of the ureters by the gravid uterus at the level of the pelvic brim.

3. As regards the fetal genitourinary system, fetal urination starts early in pregnancy and fetal urine is a major component of amniotic fluid, especially after 16 weeks. Fetal renal function improves slowly as pregnancy progresses. Until delivery, the placenta performs much of the waste disposal responsibilities.

4. The differential diagnosis of intrinsic renal insufficiency includes dehydration, renal artery stenosis, pre-renal disorders (hypovolemic or septic shock, congestive cardiac failure), obstructive uropathy (renal stone, postoperative stricture or obstruction), and endocrine disorders such as Syndrome of Inappropriate ADH secretion (SIADH), diabetes insipidus, hyperaldosteronism, and Cushing syndrome.

5. Pregnancy outcome depends on baseline renal function (above) and on the presence and severity of hypertension. The degree of proteinuria does not correlate with pregnancy outcome. Many of these patients with preexisting renal disease will already be under the care of a nephrologist, but those who are not will significantly benefit from renal consultation. Maternal-fetal medicine (MFM) consultation can also be useful in negotiating the maternal-fetal risks and assisting in the plan of care.

6. Pregnancy-related complications of renal disease include infertility (due usually to chronic anovulation), spontaneous abortion, preeclampsia, intrauterine growth restriction (IUGR), stillbirth/intrauterine fetal demise (IUFD), and spontaneous preterm birth.

7. In women with end-stage renal disease, renal transplantation offers the best chance of a pregnancy success especially if renal function is stable for 1–2 years after transplantation and there is no hypertension. Triple-agent immunosuppression (cyclosporine, azathioprine, and prednisone) should be continued during pregnancy.

17 Seizure Disorder

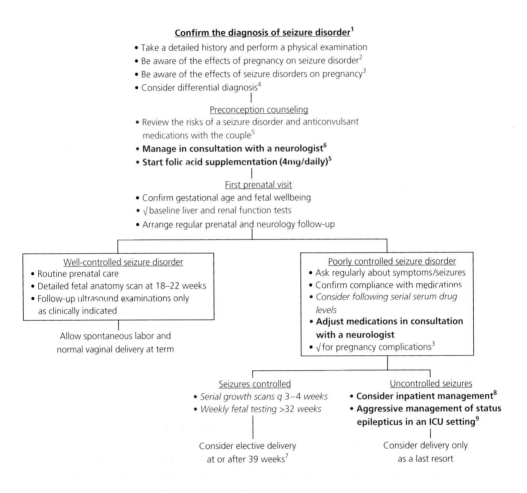

Confirm the diagnosis of seizure disorder[1]
- Take a detailed history and perform a physical examination
- Be aware of the effects of pregnancy on seizure disorder[2]
- Be aware of the effects of seizure disorders on pregnancy[3]
- Consider differential diagnosis[4]

Preconception counseling
- Review the risks of a seizure disorder and anticonvulsant medications with the couple[5]
- **Manage in consultation with a neurologist[6]**
- **Start folic acid supplementation (4mg/daily)[5]**

First prenatal visit
- Confirm gestational age and fetal wellbeing
- √ baseline liver and renal function tests
- Arrange regular prenatal and neurology follow-up

Well-controlled seizure disorder
- Routine prenatal care
- Detailed fetal anatomy scan at 18–22 weeks
- Follow-up ultrasound examinations only as clinically indicated

Allow spontaneous labor and normal vaginal delivery at term

Poorly controlled seizure disorder
- Ask regularly about symptoms/seizures
- Confirm compliance with medications
- *Consider following serial serum drug levels*
- **Adjust medications in consultation with a neurologist**
- √ for pregnancy complications[3]

Seizures controlled
- *Serial growth scans q 3–4 weeks*
- *Weekly fetal testing >32 weeks*

Consider elective delivery at or after 39 weeks[7]

Uncontrolled seizures
- **Consider inpatient management[8]**
- **Aggressive management of status epilepticus in an ICU setting[9]**

Consider delivery only as a last resort

1. Seizure disorders are the most frequently encountered major neurologic condition in pregnancy, affecting 0.3–0.6% of all gestations. Seizures can be classified into primary (idiopathic, epilepsy) or secondary (to trauma, infection, tumors, cerebrovascular disease, drug withdrawal, metabolic disorders, or preeclampsia/eclampsia). Epilepsy is the dominant seizure disorder and the one with which we have the most therapeutic experience.

2. The effect of pregnancy on seizure disorders is variable. High estrogen levels lower the seizure threshold, while progesterone raises it. Seizure frequency is increased in 45% of pregnant women, reduced in 5%, and unchanged

Obstetric Clinical Algorithms, Second Edition. Errol R. Norwitz, George R. Saade, Hugh Miller and Christina M. Davidson.
© 2017 John Wiley & Sons, Ltd. Published 2017 by John Wiley & Sons, Ltd.

in 50%. If seizures are well controlled prior to pregnancy, there is little risk of deterioration. However, if poorly controlled, an increase in seizure frequency can be expected. Moreover, due to a number of factors (including delayed gastric emptying, increase in plasma volume, altered protein binding, and accelerated hepatic metabolism), the pharmacokinetics of antiepileptic drugs (AEDs) change during pregnancy.

3. Obstetric complications are more common in women with epilepsy, including an increased risk of hyperemesis gravidarum, spontaneous abortion, spontaneous preterm delivery, preeclampsia/eclampsia, cesarean delivery, placental abruption, and perinatal mortality. However, the majority (90%) of women with seizure disorders will have an uneventful pregnancy. The most important obstetric complication may be the increased risk of oral contraceptive failure in the setting of many AEDs, which induces the hepatic cytochrome P-450 system.

4. The differential diagnosis of idiopathic seizures (epilepsy) includes drug withdrawal, intracranial lesions (including tumors and intracerebral hemorrhage), trauma, infection, metabolic disorders, and pseudo-seizures. All seizures occurring at >20 weeks in pregnancy should be regarded as preeclampsia/eclampsia until proven otherwise. Seizures associated with hypertensive disease in early pregnancy should exclude gestational trophoblastic disease as an underlying etiology.

5. Women with epilepsy have a twofold to threefold increased incidence of fetal anomalies even off treatment. Moreover, AEDs are teratogenic (see Chapter 55, Screening for Preterm Birth). The incidence of fetal anomalies increases with the number of AEDs: 3–4% with one, 5–6% with two, 10% with three, and 25% with four. Monotherapy is thus recommended. *Valproic acid* is associated with neural tube defect (NTD) in 1% of cases. Risk is greatest from days 17–30 postconception (days 31–44 from LMP). Folic acid (4 mg daily) decreases the incidence of NTD tenfold to a baseline risk of 0.1%. Some 10–30% of women on *phenytoin* will have infants with one or more of the following features: craniofacial abnormalities (cleft lip, epicanthic folds, hypertelorism), cardiac anomalies, limb defects (hypoplasia of distal phalanges, nail hypoplasia), or IUGR. "Fetal hydantoin syndrome" is characterized by all of the above features, and is rare. Exposure to other antiepileptic drugs (trimethadione, phenobarbitol, carbamazepine) can produce similar anomalies.

6. Discontinuation of all medications prior to conception should be considered in women who have been seizure-free for two or more years, although 25–40% of such women will develop a recurrence of their seizures during a subsequent pregnancy.

7. Labor and delivery are an especially susceptible time with respect to generalized tonic-clonic seizures, with occurrence in up to 4% of women with epilepsy. The reasons for this are unclear, but may be related to a reduction in progesterone activity in anticipation of labor, disruption in sleep, and poor compliance with anticonvulsant medications. All medications should be continued during labor and delivery, although benzodiazepines should be used with caution in labor as they can cause maternal and neonatal depression. In most women with epilepsy, labor and delivery are uneventful.

All AEDs cross into breast milk to some degree. The amount of transmission varies with the drug (2% for valproic acid; 30–45% for phenytoin, phenobarbital, and carbamazepine; 90% for ethosuximide). However, the use of such medications is not a contraindication to breastfeeding.

8. Seizures can cause maternal hypoxemia (with or without concurrent aspiration) with resultant fetal injury, and inpatient care may be required to control convulsions. The aim of

therapy is to control convulsions with a single agent using the lowest possible dose, but multiple agents may be required in refractory cases.

9. Status epilepticus refers to repeated convulsions with no intervals of consciousness. It is a medical emergency for both mother and fetus. The management is as for non-pregnant women: maintain maternal vital functions, control convulsions, and prevent subsequent seizures. A transient fetal bradycardia is common in this setting, and every effort should be made to resuscitate the fetus *in utero* before making a decision about delivery. Prolonged seizure activity (>10 minutes) may be associated with placental abruption.

18 Systemic Lupus Erythematosus

Confirm the diagnosis of SLE[1]

- Take a detailed history, perform a physical examination, and obtain relevant immunological tests[2]
- Understand the normal physiologic changes in the immune system during pregnancy[3]
- Be aware of the effects of pregnancy on SLE and SLE on pregnancy[4]
- **Consult an internist, rheumatologist, and/or hematologist**
- Consider the differential diagnosis[5]

Preconception counseling

- Review the risks of SLE and their current medical regimen
- **Patients should have quiescent disease for >6 months and avoid pregnancy with active disease**
- **Manage in consultation with the patient's subspecialist and consider MFM consultation in patients with significant co-morbidities[6]**

First prenatal visit

- √ baseline CBC, creatinine, urinalysis, and 24h urine collection for creatinine clearance and protein estimation
- Adjust medications as needed with appropriate consultation[7]

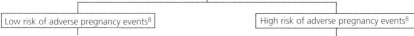

Low risk of adverse pregnancy events[8]	High risk of adverse pregnancy events[8]
- Continue routine prenatal care - Fetal anatomic survey at 18–22 weeks (routine fetal echo is not indicated) - In women with anti-Ro/La antibodies, measure and document fetal heart rate at each prenatal visit - *Consider rheumatology follow-up* - *Serial growth scans* q 3–4 weeks starting at 24 weeks - *Weekly fetal surveillance* from 28–32 weeks	- Continue routine prenatal care - Consider baseline chest x-ray, EKG, and ABG - Fetal anatomic survey at 18–22 weeks (routine fetal echo is not indicated) - Continue baseline therapy[7] - **Regular rheumatology follow-up** - **In women with anti-Ro/La antibodies, measure and document fetal heart rate at each prenatal visit** - *Serial growth scans* q 3–4 weeks starting at 24 weeks - *Weekly fetal surveillance* from 28–32 weeks - √ for pregnancy complications, especially preeclampsia[6]

Recommend routine induction of labor at or after 39 weeks

Consider induction of labor at or after 35 weeks with documentation of fetal lung maturity

Pediatricians at delivery to evaluate for neonatal lupus

1. Systemic lupus erythematosus (SLE) is a chronic inflammatory disease of unknown cause which can affect the skin, joints, kidneys, lungs, nervous system, serous membranes and/or other organs of the body. Immunologic abnormalities, especially the production of a number of antinuclear antibodies, are another prominent feature of the disease. The clinical course of SLE is variable and may be characterized by periods of remissions and chronic or acute relapses.

Obstetric Clinical Algorithms, Second Edition. Errol R. Norwitz, George R. Saade, Hugh Miller and Christina M. Davidson. © 2017 John Wiley & Sons, Ltd. Published 2017 by John Wiley & Sons, Ltd.

2. Patients with SLE are subject to a myriad of symptoms and signs, including a mixture of constitutional complaints (fatigue, malaise, fever, and weight loss, which can be seen in 50–100% of cases) and evidence of skin (photosensitive rash, Raynaud phenomenon, mucocutaneous, alopecia), musculoskeletal (arthralgia or arthritis), gastrointestinal, and serologic involvement (serositis). Some patients have predominately hematologic, renal, or central nervous system (seizures, psychosis) manifestations. Autoantibody testing is indicated, including antinuclear antibodies (ANA), antiphospholipid antibodies (see Chapter 5, APLAS), antibodies to double-stranded DNA, and anti-Smith (Sm) antibodies. Measurement of serum complement levels (total hemolytic complement [CH50], C3, and C4) may also be helpful, since hypocomplementemia is a frequent finding in active SLE. Once the diagnosis is confirmed, check maternal anti-Ro (SS-A) and anti-La (SS-B) antibodies.

3. The maternal immune system remains largely intact throughout pregnancy, and pregnant women should not be considered to be immunosuppressed. The one exception is cellular immunity, which is selectively depressed in pregnancy. As a result, pregnant women may be at increased risk of contracting viral infections and tuberculosis. Fetal humoral immunity consists of immunoglobin G (IgG), which is almost exclusively derived from the mother via receptor-mediated transport beginning at 16 weeks' gestation. The bulk of IgG is acquired in the last 4 weeks of pregnancy. As such, preterm infants have very low circulating IgG levels. IgM is not actively transported across the placenta. As such, IgM levels in the fetus accurately reflect the response of the fetal immune system to infection. B lymphocytes appear in the fetal liver by 9 weeks and in the blood and spleen by 12 weeks. T cells leave the fetal thymus at around 14 weeks. The fetus does not acquire much IgG (passive immunity) from colostrum, although IgA (immunoglobulin A) in breast milk may protect against some enteric infections.

4. Women with SLE are more likely to have pregnancy complications, including spontaneous abortion, gestational hypertension/preeclampsia, preterm birth, cesarean delivery, postpartum hemorrhage, venous thromboembolic disorders (DVT, PE), intrauterine growth restriction (IUGR), and stillbirths and neonatal deaths. Maternal anti-Ro (SS-A) and anti-La (SS-B) antibodies are associated with complete fetal heart block in 5–10% of cases. SLE does not confer risks for other identifiable congenital abnormalities. Understanding the patient's baseline disease, systemic (renal, cardiac and significant autoantibodies) involvement requires close consultation with the patient's subspecialist.

5. The differential diagnosis of SLE is extensive and depends on the dominant clinical manifestations. Other rheumatologic conditions should be considered, including Sjögren's syndrome and rheumatoid arthritis. SLE does not generally worsen in pregnancy. The frequency of exacerbations (or persistently active disease) is dependent in large part on the state of disease activity at the time of conception and on continuation of medications.

6. Patients considering pregnancy should have a careful renal, cardiac and autoantibody evaluation to establish their baseline health. It may also be possible to adjust the patient's medial management in consultation with her subspecialist to an ideal regimen for pregnancy. Patients with active disease should avoid pregnancy and those with recent active disease are well advised to wait until their disease has been quiescent for at least > 6 months.

7. Corticosteroids, antimalarials (chloroquine, hydroxychloroquine), antihypertensives (with the exception of angiotensin converting enzyme [ACE] inhibitors), and select cytotoxic agents (azathioprine) are safe in pregnancy.

Cyclophosphamine, cyclosporine, and penicillamine may have adverse fetal effects, but may be used if indicated. Non-steroidal anti-inflammatory drugs (NSAIDs), mycophenolate, methotrexate, warfarin, anti-TNFα agents, B-cell targeted antibodies (rituximab), and T-cell/B-cell co-stimulation blockers (abatacept) are best avoided in pregnancy, either because they have well-documented adverse effects or because there is little data on their safety in pregnancy.

8. A number of characteristics are associated with high maternal and fetal risk, including: (i) poorly controlled hypertension; (ii) severe pulmonary hypertension (mean pressure >50 mmHg); (iii) restrictive lung disease (forced vital capacity <1 liter); (iv) cardiac failure; (v) chronic renal failure (creatinine >2.8 mg/dL); (vi) history of severe preeclampsia; (vii) stroke within the previous six months; and (viii) severe lupus flare within the previous six months.

19 Thrombocytopenia

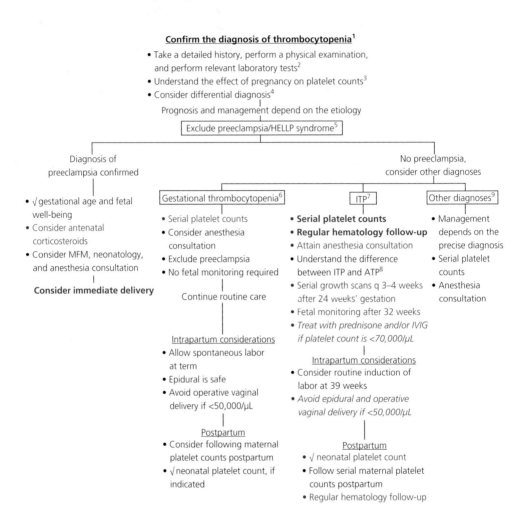

Confirm the diagnosis of thrombocytopenia[1]
- Take a detailed history, perform a physical examination, and perform relevant laboratory tests[2]
- Understand the effect of pregnancy on platelet counts[3]
- Consider differential diagnosis[4]

Prognosis and management depend on the etiology

Exclude preeclampsia/HELLP syndrome[5]

Diagnosis of preeclampsia confirmed
- √ gestational age and fetal well-being
- Consider antenatal corticosteroids
- Consider MFM, neonatology, and anesthesia consultation

Consider immediate delivery

No preeclampsia, consider other diagnoses

Gestational thrombocytopenia[6]
- Serial platelet counts
- Consider anesthesia consultation
- Exclude preeclampsia
- No fetal monitoring required

Continue routine care

Intrapartum considerations
- Allow spontaneous labor at term
- Epidural is safe
- Avoid operative vaginal delivery if <50,000/µL

Postpartum
- Consider following maternal platelet counts postpartum
- √ neonatal platelet count, if indicated

ITP[7]
- **Serial platelet counts**
- **Regular hematology follow-up**
- Attain anesthesia consultation
- Understand the difference between ITP and ATP[8]
- Serial growth scans q 3–4 weeks after 24 weeks' gestation
- Fetal monitoring after 32 weeks
- *Treat with prednisone and/or IVIG if platelet count is <70,000/µL*

Intrapartum considerations
- Consider routine induction of labor at 39 weeks
- *Avoid epidural and operative vaginal delivery if <50,000/µL*

Postpartum
- √ neonatal platelet count
- Follow serial maternal platelet counts postpartum
- Regular hematology follow-up

Other diagnoses[9]
- Management depends on the precise diagnosis
- Serial platelet counts
- Anesthesia consultation

1. Thrombocytopenia (low platelets) complicates 5–15% of all gestations. Unlike nonpregnant women (in whom a cut-off of <150,000 platelets/µL is used), thrombocytopenia in pregnancy is defined as a circulating platelet level of <100,000/µL. Routine CBC measurements at the first prenatal visit and again in the third trimester will identify women with asymptomatic thrombocytopenia.

2. Ask about pre-existing medical and hematologic conditions, medications which can affect platelet counts (such as heparin) or bleeding time, and symptoms of excessive bleeding.

Obstetric Clinical Algorithms, Second Edition. Errol R. Norwitz, George R. Saade, Hugh Miller and Christina M. Davidson.
© 2017 John Wiley & Sons, Ltd. Published 2017 by John Wiley & Sons, Ltd.

Physical examination may reveal a petechial skin rash, subconjunctival hemorrhage, or other evidence of excessive bleeding (bruising, leakage from intravenous sites or bleeding into joints).

3. Although platelet counts are normal in most women during uncomplicated pregnancy, the mean platelet counts of pregnant women are lower than in healthy nonpregnant women, due primarily to hemodilution. Serial platelet counts are more useful than a single measurement.

4. The differential diagnosis of thrombocytopenia in pregnancy includes gestational thrombocytopenia, immune thrombocytopenic purpura (ITP), preeclampsia/HELLP syndrome, coagulopathy (including consumptive coagulopathy), thrombotic thrombocytopenic purpura/hemolytic uremic syndrome (TTP/HUS), and drug-induced thrombocytopenia.

5. See Chapter 12 (Preeclampsia).

6. Gestational thrombocytopenia is defined by five criteria: (i) mild and asymptomatic thrombocytopenia (platelet counts are typically >70,000/μL); (ii) no past history of thrombocytopenia (except during a previous pregnancy); (iii) occurrence during late gestation; (iv) no association with fetal thrombocytopenia (vs 10–15% neonatal thrombocytopenia in patients with ITP); and (v) spontaneous resolution after delivery. It is likely due to hemodilution alone, although an immunologic etiology cannot be definitively excluded. For both mother and infant, routine obstetric management is appropriate. Epidural anesthesia is safe in women with gestational thrombocytopenia who have platelet counts >70,000/μL. Women with documented thrombocytopenia should be followed with platelet counts to determine if spontaneous resolution occurs after delivery. The risk of neonatal bleeding complications (including intracranial hemorrhage) is extremely low. There are no long-term studies to determine whether women with gestational thrombocytopenia have a greater risk of developing ITP.

7. Immune thrombocytopenic purpura (ITP) is a maternal disease characterized by the presence of circulating antiplatelet antibodies. The distinction between gestational thrombocytopenia and ITP is largely empiric, although ITP is the more likely diagnosis if thrombocytopenia occurs early in pregnancy or if the platelet count is very low (<50,000/μL). The prognosis and management depend on the severity of the thrombocytopenia. In addition to maternal bleeding complications, antiplatelet IgG antibodies can cross the placenta and cause fetal thrombocytopenia. At delivery, 10% of infants born to women with ITP will have a platelet count <50,000/μL and 5% will have a count <20,000/μL. The correlation between maternal platelet counts, maternal antiplatelet antibody levels, and fetal platelet counts is poor. Glucocorticoid therapy should be considered if the maternal platelet count is low (<70,000/μL). Intravenous immune globulin (IVIG), plasmapharesis, and splenectomy are rarely necessary in pregnancy. Cesarean delivery has not been shown to improve perinatal outcome and should be reserved for usual obstetric indications. The old practice of percutaneous umbilical blood sampling (PUBS) at 38 weeks to determine the fetal platelet count has a mortality rate of 2%, which is greater than the risk of severe fetal/neonatal intracerebral hemorrhage (<1%), and has therefore been abandoned.

8. Alloimmune thrombocytopenia (ATP, also known as neonatal alloimmune thrombocytopenia (NAIT)) is a condition in which maternal platelet counts are normal, but antiplatelet antibodies (usually anti-PLA1/2) cross the placenta to cause fetal thrombocytopenia and possibly intraventricular hemorrhage. ATP is analogous to Rh disease of platelets. Elective cesarean delivery at 34–36 weeks is recommended.

9. Other causes of thrombocytopenia include drug-induced thrombocytopenia, coagulopathy, and TTP/HUS. TTP/HUS is rare (1 in 25,000) and can occur at any time in pregnancy. There are no pathognomonic findings for TTP/HUS, and the diagnosis is based upon the clinician's judgment after considering the history, physical examination, and laboratory findings. TTP/HUS must be distinguished from preeclampsia. The primary treatment for preeclampsia is delivery; the primary treatment for TTP/HUS is plasma exchange, as it is in nonpregnant patients.

20 Thyroid Dysfunction

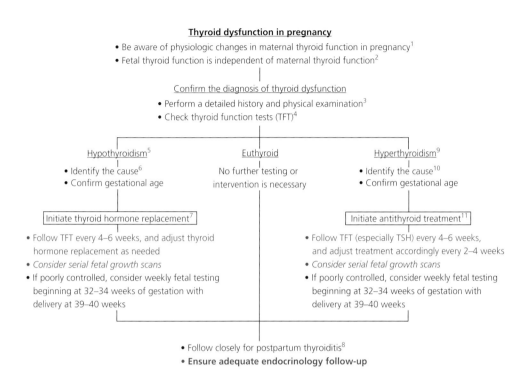

Thyroid dysfunction in pregnancy
- Be aware of physiologic changes in maternal thyroid function in pregnancy[1]
- Fetal thyroid function is independent of maternal thyroid function[2]

Confirm the diagnosis of thyroid dysfunction
- Perform a detailed history and physical examination[3]
- Check thyroid function tests (TFT)[4]

Hypothyroidism[5]
- Identify the cause[6]
- Confirm gestational age

Euthyroid
No further testing or
intervention is necessary

Hyperthyroidism[9]
- Identify the cause[10]
- Confirm gestational age

Initiate thyroid hormone replacement[7]
- Follow TFT every 4–6 weeks, and adjust thyroid hormone replacement as needed
- *Consider serial fetal growth scans*
- If poorly controlled, consider weekly fetal testing beginning at 32–34 weeks of gestation with delivery at 39–40 weeks

Initiate antithyroid treatment[11]
- Follow TFT (especially TSH) every 4–6 weeks, and adjust treatment accordingly every 2–4 weeks
- *Consider serial fetal growth scans*
- If poorly controlled, consider weekly fetal testing beginning at 32–34 weeks of gestation with delivery at 39–40 weeks

- Follow closely for postpartum thyroiditis[8]
- **Ensure adequate endocrinology follow-up**

1. Thyroid functions change in pregnancy. Levothyroxine (T_4) and L-triiodothyronine (T_3) are bound primarily to thyroxine-binding globulin (TBG) with <1% circulating as free (biologically active) hormone. T_4 is a prohormone that is converted to biologically active T_3 in peripheral tissues. High estrogen levels increase TBG production in the liver by 75–100% and stimulate TBG sialylation, which reduces hepatic clearance of T_4 and T_3. The end result is a 10–30% increase in *total* T_4 and T_3 in the maternal circulation during pregnancy, but no change in circulating thyroid stimulating hormone (TSH) or *free* T_4 and T_3. Maternal thyroid volume is 30% greater in the third trimester than in the first trimester. The TSH level decreases in early pregnancy because of weak stimulation of TSH receptors caused by human chorionic gonadotropin (hCG) during the first 12 weeks of gestation. After the first trimester, TSH levels return to baseline values and progressively increase in the third trimester related to placental growth and production of placental deiodinase.

2. <0.1% of thyroid hormone crosses the placenta. As such, fetal thyroid function is entirely independent of maternal thyroid function, although the fetus does require iodine from the maternal diet to make thyroid hormone. Thyroid hormone can be measured in fetal blood

Obstetric Clinical Algorithms, Second Edition. Errol R. Norwitz, George R. Saade, Hugh Miller and Christina M. Davidson.
© 2017 John Wiley & Sons, Ltd. Published 2017 by John Wiley & Sons, Ltd.

as early as 12 weeks' gestation. Before 12 weeks, maternal T4 is especially important for normal fetal brain development.

3. Indicated testing of thyroid function should be performed in women with a personal history of thyroid disease or symptoms of thyroid disease. Initial symptoms of *overt maternal hypothyroidism* include fatigue, constipation, cold intolerance, and muscle cramps. These may progress to insomnia, weight gain, carpal tunnel syndrome, hair loss, voice changes, and intellectual slowness. Such symptoms are commonly attributed to normal pregnancy, however, women who report that such symptoms have worsened over the previous year are more likely to have overt thyroid disease. Common symptoms of *overt maternal hyperthyroidism* include anxiety/nervousness, tremor, tachycardia, insomnia, palpitations, heat intolerance, increased perspiration, weight loss, frequent stools (not diarrhea), and hypertension. Thyroid function studies should also be performed in a pregnant woman with a significant goiter or with distinct nodules. Asymptomatic pregnant women who have a mildly enlarged thyroid, however, do not need thyroid function studies since the thyroid gland enlarges up to 30% during pregnancy. Universal screening for thyroid disease in pregnancy is also not recommended because identification and treatment of maternal subclinical hypothyroidism have not been shown to result in improved neurocognitive function in offspring or an improvement in adverse pregnancy outcomes.

4. Levels of TSH and free T4 should be measured to diagnose thyroid disease in pregnancy, with TSH being the first-line screening test. The American Thyroid Association recommends the following trimester-specific reference ranges for TSH: first trimester: 0.1–2.5 mIU/L; second trimester: 0.2–3.0 mIU/L; third trimester: 0.3–3.0 mIU/L. When the TSH level is abnormally high or low, the free T4 level should be measured next. Overt hyperthyroidism is characterized by a decreased TSH level and an increased free T4 level. In subclinical hyperthyroidism, the TSH level is abnormally low but the free T4 level is within the normal reference range. In rare circumstances, symptomatic hyperthyroidism is caused by abnormally high free T3 levels. Thus, the free T3 should be measured if there is strong clinical suspicion of overt hyperthyroidism and the TSH is low but free T4 is normal. Overt hypothyroidism is characterized by an increased TSH level and a decreased free T4 level; subclinical hypothyroidism is defined as an elevated serum TSH level in the presence of a normal free T4 level.

5. *Maternal overt hypothyroidism* complicates 2–10 per 1,000 pregnancies. Adverse perinatal outcomes such as spontaneous abortion, preeclampsia, preterm birth, abruptio placentae, and fetal death are associated with untreated overt hypothyroidism. Adequate thyroid hormone replacement therapy during pregnancy minimizes the risk of these adverse outcomes.

6. Causes of primary hypothyroidism include: (i) Hashimoto thyroiditis (chronic lymphocytic thyroiditis) which is characterized by hypothyroidism, a firm goiter, and the presence of circulating antithyroglobulin or antimicrosomal antibodies. Measurement of circulating antithyroid antibodies is not helpful in confirming the diagnosis and the results of such testing rarely lead to changes in management; (ii) women previously treated for hyperthyroidism by surgery (thyroidectomy) or ^{131}I ablation may manifest with hypothyroidism and require thyroid hormone replacement; and (iii) endemic iodine deficiency.

7. Start levothyroxine (thyroxine) replacement in dosages of 1–2 micrograms/kg daily or approximately 100 micrograms daily. TSH levels should be measured at 4–6-week intervals, and the levothyroxine dose adjusted by 25–50-microgram increments until the TSH value is normal. Most women will need to increase their dose by 30–50% during pregnancy. Significant hypothyroidism

may develop early in women without thyroid reserve, such as those with a previous thyroidectomy or prior radioiodine ablation; 25% increases in T4 replacement at pregnancy confirmation will reduce this likelihood.

8. *Postpartum thyroiditis* complicates 5–10% of all pregnancies during the first year after childbirth. The etiology is unknown, but it is likely an autoimmune phenomenon. It is characterized by a transient hyperthyroid state occurring 2–3 months postpartum (with dizziness, fatigue, weight loss, palpitations) and/or a transient hypothyroid state 4–8 months postpartum (with fatigue, weight gain, and depression). Treatment may be needed to control symptoms, but can usually be tapered within 1 year.

9. *Maternal overt hyperthyroidism (thyrotoxicosis)* refers to the clinical state resulting from an excess production of and exposure to the thyroid hormone. It complicates 0.2% of all pregnancies. Inadequately treated maternal thyrotoxicosis is associated with a greater risk of severe preeclampsia and maternal heart failure than treated, controlled maternal thyrotoxicosis. Maternal complications of hyperthyroidism include cardiac failure and pulmonary hypertension (8%) as well as thyroid storm (1–2%). Fetal complications include medically indicated preterm birth, low birth weight and fetal loss.

10. Causes of hyperthyroidism include: (i) Graves' disease (>95% of all cases) due to circulating thyroid-stimulating autoantibodies. Ophthalmopathy (lid lag, lid retraction) and dermopathy (localized or pretibial edema) are specific to Graves' disease. In pregnant women with a history of Graves' disease, thyroid-stimulating antibody activity may actually decline, leading to chemical remission during pregnancy. Since IgG antibodies cross the placenta, the fetus is at

risk of thyroid dysfunction. (ii) Toxic multinodular goiter. (iii) Solitary toxic thyroid nodule. (iv) Inflammation (thyroiditis) such as de Quervain thyroiditis is acute in onset with a painful goiter. (v) Hyperemesis gravidarum/gestational trophoblastic neoplasia likely secondary to elevated levels of hCG. Routine measurements of thyroid function are not recommended in patients with hyperemesis gravidarum unless other signs of overt hyperthyroidism are evident. (vi) Metastatic follicular cell carcinoma of the thyroid. (vii) Exogenous T_4 or T_3. (viii) TSH-secreting pituitary adenoma.

11. Either propylthiouracil (PTU) or methimazole, both thioamides, can be used to treat pregnant women with overt hyperthyroidism. PTU blocks the release of hormone from the thyroid gland and (unlike methimazole) also blocks peripheral conversion of T_4 to T_3. Historically, PTU was preferred for this reason and because of the association of methimazole with a rare embryopathy characterized by esophageal or choanal atresia as well as aplasia cutis (a congenital skin defect). More recently, however, PTU has been associated with hepatotoxicity. Thus, in an attempt to balance the rare occurrences of PTU-induced hepatotoxicity and methimazole embryopathy, PTU is now the recommended therapy during the first trimester followed by a switch to methimazole beginning in the second trimester. PTU treatment is initiated at 50–150 mg orally three times daily. Methimazole is initiated at 10–40 mg orally, divided into two or three daily doses. The aim is treatment with the lowest possible thioamide dose to maintain free T4 levels slightly above or in the high-normal range, regardless of TSH levels. Serum free T4 concentrations (not TSH levels) are measured every 2–4 weeks after initiation of therapy, and the thioamide dose should be adjusted accordingly.

SECTION 3
Infectious Complications

21 Asymptomatic Bacteriuria[1]

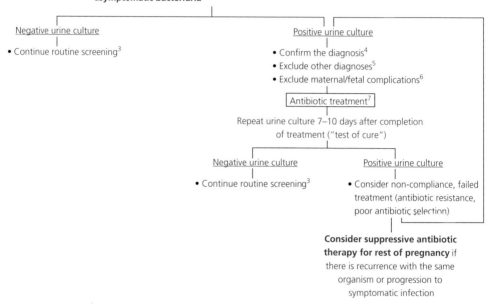

Screening for asymptomatic bacteriuria in pregnancy[2]
- Routine urinalysis and culture in the first trimester for all pregnant women
- Routine urinalysis and urine culture q 3-4 weeks for women at high risk for asymptomatic bacteriuria[3]

Negative urine culture
- Continue routine screening[3]

Positive urine culture
- Confirm the diagnosis[4]
- Exclude other diagnoses[5]
- Exclude maternal/fetal complications[6]

Antibiotic treatment[7]

Repeat urine culture 7–10 days after completion of treatment ("test of cure")

Negative urine culture
- Continue routine screening[3]

Positive urine culture
- Consider non-compliance, failed treatment (antibiotic resistance, poor antibiotic selection)

Consider suppressive antibiotic therapy for rest of pregnancy if there is recurrence with the same organism or progression to symptomatic infection

1. Asymptomatic bacteriuria refers to significant bacterial colonization of the urinary tract in the absence of urinary tract symptoms. The most common pathogen is *E. coli* (65–80%). Asymptomatic bacteriuria complicates 5–10% of all pregnancies. It is not more common in pregnancy than in non-pregnant women, but is more likely to be symptomatic and progress to pyelonephritis during pregnancy.

2. Routine screening and treatment will prevent 80% of pyelonephritis in pregnancy.

3. Women at increased risk for asymptomatic bacteriuria and symptomatic urinary tract infections include women with diabetes mellitus, prior urinary tract infection in the index pregnancy, and sickle cell trait/disease.

4. While the urine dipstix can be positive for nitrates and/or leukocyte esterase, the definitive diagnosis of asymptomatic bacteriuria requires a urinalysis and urine culture demonstrating ≥10,000 CFU/mL of a single pathogenic organism in a midstream clean-catch urine specimen

Obstetric Clinical Algorithms, Second Edition. Errol R. Norwitz, George R. Saade, Hugh Miller and Christina M. Davidson.
© 2017 John Wiley & Sons, Ltd. Published 2017 by John Wiley & Sons, Ltd.

(possibly even lower count in a catheterized sample). Imaging studies are not indicated to confirm the diagnosis.

5. The differential diagnosis of asymptomatic bacteriuria includes contamination with lower genital tract organisms, acute cystitis, and pyelonephritis. Women with asymptomatic bacteriuria are typically asymptomatic with a benign abdominal exam. Women who are symptomatic (with complaints of frequency, urgency, or dysuria) or have clinical evidence of fever or suprapubic/costovertebral angle tenderness should be diagnosed with symptomatic urinary tract infection.

6. Maternal complications include progression to symptomatic urinary infection (cystitis, pyelonephritis), urosepsis, ARDS, preterm labor, transient renal dysfunction, and anemia.

Progression from asymptomatic bacteriuria to pyelonephritis in pregnancy is 13–65% if untreated, but only 2–3% if treated. Fetal complications (sepsis, low birthweight, preterm birth) are rare. Women with asymptomatic bacteriuria are at risk of preterm birth, and treatment with antibiotics decreases this risk.

7. Antibiotic treatment should be continued for 7–10 days because of the high recurrence rate. Adequate treatment options include trimethoprim/sulfamethoxazole 160/180-mg po bid (do not use in first trimester unless it is the only option), nitrofurantoin 100-mg po bid, or cephalexin 500-mg po qid. Aggressive oral hydration should also be recommended. Antibiotic therapy should be adjusted according to culture results, if indicated. Nitrofurantoin 50-100 mg po qhs is the first choice for antibiotic suppression if needed.

22 Urinary Tract Infection/Pyelonephritis

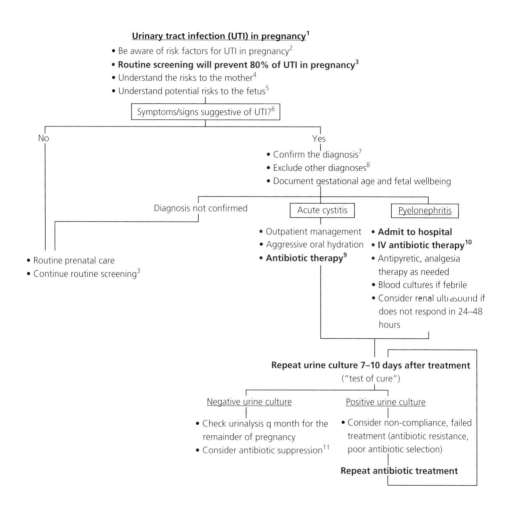

Urinary tract infection (UTI) in pregnancy[1]
- Be aware of risk factors for UTI in pregnancy[2]
- **Routine screening will prevent 80% of UTI in pregnancy[3]**
- Understand the risks to the mother[4]
- Understand potential risks to the fetus[5]

Symptoms/signs suggestive of UTI?[6]

No

Yes
- Confirm the diagnosis[7]
- Exclude other diagnoses[8]
- Document gestational age and fetal wellbeing

Diagnosis not confirmed

- Routine prenatal care
- Continue routine screening[3]

Acute cystitis
- Outpatient management
- Aggressive oral hydration
- **Antibiotic therapy[9]**

Pyelonephritis
- **Admit to hospital**
- **IV antibiotic therapy[10]**
- Antipyretic, analgesia therapy as needed
- Blood cultures if febrile
- Consider renal ultrasound if does not respond in 24–48 hours

Repeat urine culture 7–10 days after treatment
("test of cure")

Negative urine culture
- Check urinalysis q month for the remainder of pregnancy
- Consider antibiotic suppression[11]

Positive urine culture
- Consider non-compliance, failed treatment (antibiotic resistance, poor antibiotic selection)

Repeat antibiotic treatment

1. Urinary tract infections (UTI) include acute cystitis and pyelonephritis, and complicate 3–4% and 1–2% of pregnancies, respectively. The most common pathogens are *Escherichia coli* (80–90%) and *Staphylococcus saprophyticus* (4–7%).

2. Risk factors for UTI in pregnancy include women with diabetes mellitus, prior UTI in the index pregnancy, urinary tract anomalies, and sickle cell trait/disease.

3. See Chapter 21 (Asymptomatic Bacteriuria).

Obstetric Clinical Algorithms, Second Edition. Errol R. Norwitz, George R. Saade, Hugh Miller and Christina M. Davidson.
© 2017 John Wiley & Sons, Ltd. Published 2017 by John Wiley & Sons, Ltd.

4. Risks to the mother of untreated cystitis include progression to pyelonephritis. Complications of pyelonephritis include urosepsis (10–15%) leading to septic shock (1–3%), adult respiratory distress syndrome (ARDS) (2–8%), anemia (25–50%), transient renal dysfunction (25%), and preterm labor.

5. Potential risks to the fetus include preterm birth and low birth weight.

6. Symptoms of acute cystitis include urinary frequency, dysuria, urgency, and suprapubic pain; systemic complaints are usually absent. Physical examination may reveal suprapubic tenderness, but is usually unhelpful. Systemic symptoms of fever, chills, nausea, vomiting, and flank pain suggest a diagnosis of pyelonephritis. In such cases, there may be evidence of flank or costovertebral angle tenderness on physical examination.

7. While the urine dipstix can be positive for nitrates and/or leukocyte esterase, the definitive diagnosis of UTI requires a urinalysis and urine culture with ≥10,000 colony forming units (CFU)/mL of a single pathogenic organism in a midstream clean-catch urine specimen. Imaging studies are not indicated to confirm the diagnosis. If the patient is febrile, obtain blood cultures to exclude urosepsis and antibiotic sensitivities.

8. Differential diagnosis includes contamination with lower genital tract organisms, asymptomatic bacteriuria, and lower genital tract infection (such as bacterial vaginosis or yeast infection). In the setting of pyelonephritis, consider also urosepsis, appendicitis, cholecystitis, and lower lobe pneumonia.

9. Appropriate treatment options for cystitis include trimethoprim/sulfamethoxazole 160/180-mg po bid (do not use in first trimester unless the only option), nitrofurantoin 100-mg po bid, or cephalexin 500-mg po qid. Medications should be adjusted according to culture results. Duration of antibiotic treatment should be 7–10 days. Single-dose therapy is associated with an increased failure rate in pregnancy and is not recommended.

10. Appropriate treatment options for pyelonephritis include: (i) ampicillin 2 g q6h + gentamicin 1.5 mg/kg q8h IV; (ii) cefazolin 1 g q8h IV; (iii) ceftriaxone 12 g q24h IV/IM; (iv) mezlocillin 1–3 g IV q6h; or (v) piperacillin 4 g IV q8h. Antibiotics should be continued until 24–48 hours afebrile. Patient should be switched to oral antibiotic for a total of 10 days.

11. Women who have two or more episodes of acute cystitis or one or more episodes of pyelonephritis should be given suppressive antibiotic therapy (nitrofurantoin 50–100-mg po qhs) for the remainder of the pregnancy and should have urine cultures checked every month until delivery.

23 Lower Genital Tract Infection

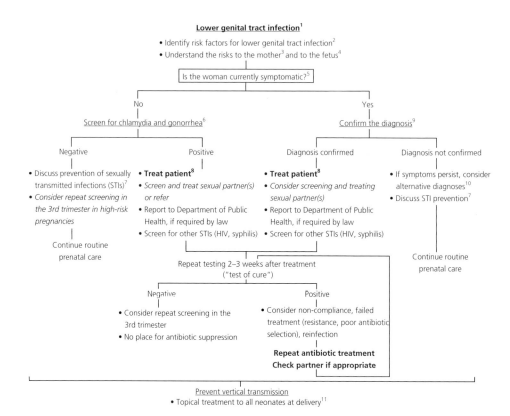

Lower genital tract infection[1]
- Identify risk factors for lower genital tract infection[2]
- Understand the risks to the mother[3] and to the fetus[4]

Is the woman currently symptomatic?[5]

No → Screen for chlamydia and gonorrhea[6]

Yes → Confirm the diagnosis[9]

Negative
- Discuss prevention of sexually transmitted infections (STIs)[7]
- *Consider repeat screening in the 3rd trimester in high-risk pregnancies*

Continue routine prenatal care

Positive
- **Treat patient[8]**
- *Screen and treat sexual partner(s) or refer*
- Report to Department of Public Health, if required by law
- Screen for other STIs (HIV, syphilis)

Diagnosis confirmed
- **Treat patient[8]**
- *Consider screening and treating sexual partner(s)*
- Report to Department of Public Health, if required by law
- Screen for other STIs (HIV, syphilis)

Diagnosis not confirmed
- If symptoms persist, consider alternative diagnoses[10]
- Discuss STI prevention[7]

Continue routine prenatal care

Repeat testing 2–3 weeks after treatment ("test of cure")

Negative
- Consider repeat screening in the 3rd trimester
- No place for antibiotic suppression

Positive
- Consider non-compliance, failed treatment (resistance, poor antibiotic selection), reinfection

Repeat antibiotic treatment
Check partner if appropriate

Prevent vertical transmission
- Topical treatment to all neonates at delivery[11]

1. Lower genital tract infections include: (i) bacterial vaginosis (BV), which refers to an overgrowth of commensal vaginal organisms, including *Bacteroides*, *Peptostreptococcus*, *Gardnerella vaginalis*, *Mycoplasma hominis*, and *Enterobacteriaceae* with a decrease in lactobacillus species. It is not a sexually transmitted infection (STI); (ii) Trichomonas, a predominantly (but not exclusively) STI caused by *Trichomonas vaginalis*; (iii) Gonorrhea, an STI caused by *Neissaria gonorrhea*; and (iv) Chlamydia, the most common STI in the United States, caused by the obligate intracellular parasite, *Chlamydia trachomatis*.

2. Risk factors for lower genital tract infections include multiple sexual partners, unprotected intercourse, other sexually transmitted infections, drug abuse, diabetes, unmarried status, age <20 years, a "high-risk" partner, and late/no prenatal care.

3. Lower genital tract infections are associated with an increased risk of preterm birth, especially

Obstetric Clinical Algorithms, Second Edition. Errol R. Norwitz, George R. Saade, Hugh Miller and Christina M. Davidson.
© 2017 John Wiley & Sons, Ltd. Published 2017 by John Wiley & Sons, Ltd.

if they are symptomatic. However, it is not clear that treatment abrogates this risk. As such, routine screening for lower genital tract infections is not generally recommended in either low- or high-risk pregnancies.

4. Aside from the risk of preterm birth, lower genital tract infections pose little risk to the fetus while *in utero*. They do not generally cause ascending intraamniotic infection. If exposed at delivery, however, such infections (chlamydia, gonorrhea) can cause conjunctivitis and neonatal pneumonia.

5. Most women with lower genital tract infections are asymptomatic (especially chlamydia, gonorrhea, and BV). However, they may present with vulvar itching (pruritis), pain, or burning that may be worse after menses or intercourse (due to a change in vaginal pH). A vaginal discharge and symptoms of dysuria may also be present. Gonorrhea can present with anal or pharyngeal discomfort. Systemic symptoms (low-grade fever, malaise, fatigue, nausea, abdominal pain) are rare, and should prompt a search for alternative causes. The exception is disseminated gonoccocal infection, which can present with fever, chills, small pustular skin lesions, and arthritis of the knees, wrists, and ankles.

6. Because chlamydia and gonorrhea are common, often asymptomatic, and can infect the fetus as it passes through the birth canal, all pregnant women should be screened for these two infections at their first prenatal visit. High-risk women should be screened again in the third trimester. A variety of screening tests are available, including (i) polymerase chain reaction (PCR)-based tests; (ii) antigen detection methods (such as enzyme-linked immunosorbant assay (ELISA) or fluorescein-conjugated antibody test); (iii) cytologic staining; or (v) culture-based protocols using selective culture media. ELISA is most commonly used in low-risk populations. Routine screening for BV and trichomonas is not recommended.

7. Prevention of STIs includes avoidance of unprotected intercourse, routine use of barrier contraception, and stopping drug abuse.

8. Specific treatment depends on the infection: (i) for BV, clindamycin 2% cream vaginally qhs x 7 days in early pregnancy and metronidazole 500 mg po bid or clindamycin 900 mg po bid x 7 days in the latter half of pregnancy (antibiotic therapy is generally deferred if the woman is asymptomatic); (ii) for trichomonas, metronidazole 375–500 mg po bid x 7 days (alternative treatment includes metronidazole 2 g po x 1 dose or vaginal metronidazole/clotrimazole, but failure rate is higher); (iii) for gonorrhea, cefuroxime 400 mg po x 1 or ceftriaxone 125 mg IM x 1 dose (if penicillin-allergic, use spectinomycin 2 g IM x 1 dose; quinolones are contraindicated in pregnancy; consider treating also for presumed chlamydia infection); and (iv) for chlamydia, amoxicillin 500 mg po tid x 7 days, erythromycin 500 mg po qid x 7 days, or azithromycin 1 g po x 1 dose (topical treatment is inadequate).

9. Abdominal exam is typically benign. Speculum exam may reveal cervical erythema (a red, inflamed "strawberry" cervix is suggestive of chlamydia) and/or a cervicovaginal discharge ranging from thin malodorous (BV) to mucopurulent (gonorrhea, chlamydia) to foamy yellow-green with a foul "fishy" odor (trichomonas). Laboratory testing is required to confirm gonorrhea or chlamydia infection. Confirmation of trichomonas infection requires a wet smear of cervicovaginal discharge showing motile, flagellated, pear-shaped organisms. BV is a clinical diagnosis requiring at least two of the following criteria: wet mount positive for clue cells, decrease in lactobacilli, a positive "whiff test" (fishy odor) on mixture with potassium hydroxide, and vaginal pH >4.5.

10. Alternative diagnoses include urinary tract infection, ruptured membranes, foreign body, non-specific cervicitis, herpes, and candidal (yeast) infection.

11. All infants should receive erythromycin ointment applied to their eyes within 1 hour of birth to prevent conjunctivitis from chlamydia or gonorrhea.

24 Group B β-Hemolytic Streptococcus[1]

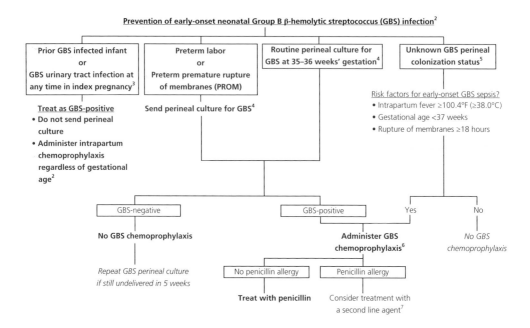

Prevention of early-onset neonatal Group B β-hemolytic streptococcus (GBS) infection[2]

Prior GBS infected infant
or
GBS urinary tract infection at any time in index pregnancy[3]

Treat as GBS-positive
• Do not send perineal culture
• Administer intrapartum chemoprophylaxis regardless of gestational age[2]

Preterm labor
or
Preterm premature rupture of membranes (PROM)

Send perineal culture for GBS[4]

Routine perineal culture for GBS at 35–36 weeks' gestation[4]

Unknown GBS perineal colonization status[5]

Risk factors for early-onset GBS sepsis?
• Intrapartum fever ≥100.4°F (≥38.0°C)
• Gestational age <37 weeks
• Rupture of membranes ≥18 hours

GBS-negative

No GBS chemoprophylaxis

Repeat GBS perineal culture if still undelivered in 5 weeks

GBS-positive

Administer GBS chemoprophylaxis[6]

No penicillin allergy

Treat with penicillin

Penicillin allergy

Consider treatment with a second line agent[7]

Yes

No

No GBS chemoprophylaxis

1. Group B β-hemolytic streptococcus (GBS), also known as *Streptococcus agalactiae*, is an encapsulated gram-positive coccus that colonizes the gastro-intestinal and lower genital tracts of 20% (range, 15–40%) of pregnant women. It is not a sexually transmitted infection. Although women whose genital tracts are colonized with GBS are typically asymptomatic, 50% of fetuses passing through a colonized birth canal will themselves be colonized with GBS and some will develop infection (also known as invasive GBS disease).

2. GBS is the most common cause of bacterial infection in the first 90 days of life. Two clinically distinct neonatal GBS infections have been identified: (i) Early-onset neonatal GBS infection (80% of all GBS infection) results from GBS transmission during labor or delivery. It is characterized by signs of serious infection (respiratory distress, apnea, pneumonia, or septic shock) within one week of delivery, although it presents most often within 6–12 hours of birth. The mortality rate is 5–25% and surviving infants frequently exhibit neurological sequelae. The overall rate of early-onset neonatal GBS infection is 1–3 per 1,000 live births, but is increased to 10 per 1,000 deliveries in women colonized with GBS and may be as high as 40–50 per 1,000 preterm births. This infection can be effectively prevented by intrapartum antibiotic chemoprophylaxis. (ii) Late-onset neonatal GBS infection (20%) is a hospital-acquired (nosocomial) or community-acquired infection. It

Obstetric Clinical Algorithms, Second Edition. Errol R. Norwitz, George R. Saade, Hugh Miller and Christina M. Davidson.
© 2017 John Wiley & Sons, Ltd. Published 2017 by John Wiley & Sons, Ltd.

presents more than a week after birth, usually as meningitis. The mortality rate is lower than for early onset disease, but neurological sequelae are equally common. This infection cannot be effectively prevented by intrapartum antibiotic chemotherapy.

3. Women who have had a prior infant affected with early-onset GBS infection (not simply GBS colonization in a prior pregnancy) or had a GBS urinary tract infection in the index pregnancy have a high perineal colonization rate at delivery. As such, they should be regarded as GBS-positive and should all receive intrapartum chemoprophylaxis. It is not necessary to check a routine GBS perineal culture in such women.

4. The Centers for Disease Control and Prevention (CDC) in the United States recommend that all pregnant women have a perineal culture at 35–36 weeks' gestation. Although GBS colonizes the lower genital tract of 20% of pregnant women at any one time, it is not the same 20% of women throughout pregnancy with an 8–10% crossover of GBS carrier status each trimester. This is why determination of GBS carrier status cannot be done at the first prenatal visit. GBS colonization increases as one moves from the cervix to the introitus. As such, the GBS culture should be taken by swabbing the lower vagina, perineum and perianal area (not the cervix) and the swab should be placed briefly into the anal canal. A speculum should not be used. This perineal culture should be inoculated into selective broth media (either Todd-Hewitt broth or selective blood agar), stored at room temperature, and transported to the laboratory ideally within 8 hours of collection. Results should be available within 48 hours. Cultures sent at 35–36 weeks are reliable for 5 weeks and have been shown to accurately reflect GBS carrier status at delivery. Rapid screening tests for GBS carrier status in labor have been developed, but are more difficult to perform, not available in all hospitals at all times, and have a poor sensitivity in identifying women with light (low-level) GBS colonization.

5. This group includes women presenting with preterm labor or preterm PROM prior to routine GBS perineal culture as well as women at term who did not have a routine GBS culture sent. The management of such women depends on the presence or absence of a series of risks factors (listed above). Reliance on a risk factor-based protocol (as in the United Kingdom) results in treatment of 20–25% of women in labor with prevention of 65–70% of early-onset GBS disease. The culture-based protocol (as recommended by CDC in the United States) results in treatment of 15–20% of women in labor with prevention of 70–80% of early-onset GBS disease.

6. A number of strategies have been developed to prevent early-onset neonatal GBS infection. Intrapartum—but not antepartum—antibiotic chemoprophylaxis can prevent early-onset GBS infection in GBS-positive women. Penicillin G (5 million units IV followed by 2.5 million units every 4 hours) is the treatment of choice. Ampicillin (2 g IV load followed by 1 g every 4 hours) is an alternative prophylactic regimen, but is not recommended because it has a wider spectrum of action and is therefore more likely to cause antibiotic resistance. To date, there have been no cases of GBS resistance to penicillin or ampicillin. A minimum of 4 hours of antibiotic chemoprophylaxis is recommended. Delivery prior to one completed hour of chemoprophylaxis may be associated with a higher incidence of early-onset neonatal GBS infection. Antibiotics should be continued until delivery is complete. Only women with chorioamnionitis require antibiotic treatment beyond delivery.

7. A number of second-line antibiotics have been recommended for GBS chemoprophylaxis in women who are allergic to penicillin, including clindamycin (900 mg IV every 8 hours),

erythromycin (500 mg IV every 6 hours), a second-generation cephalosporin (such as cefazolin 2 g IV followed by 1 g every 8 hours), and vancomycin (1 g every 12 hours). Approximately 20–30% of GBS isolates are resistant to erythromycin and 10–20% are resistant to clindamycin, and these rates appear to be increasing. In GBS-positive women who have a history of severe penicillin allergy (e.g., bronchospasm, urticaria, angioedema, hypotension, or shock within 30 minutes of drug administration), antimicrobial susceptibility of the GBS isolates should be done. If resistance to erythromycin or clindamycin is documented, vancomycin should be administered. An alternative approach is to perform penicillin skin testing in such woman, but this is rarely done. In women who have an allergy to penicillin that is not severe, treatment with cefazolin 2 g IV followed by 1 g every 8 hours is recommended.

25 Hepatitis B

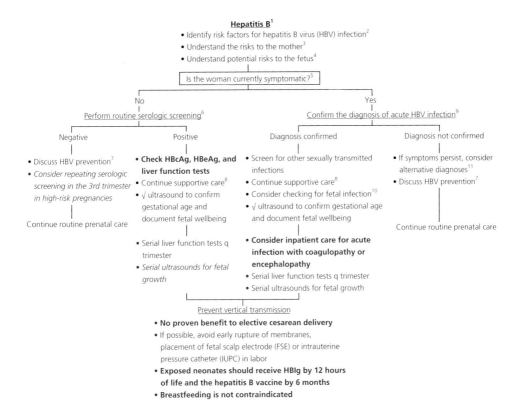

Hepatitis B[1]
- Identify risk factors for hepatitis B virus (HBV) infection[2]
- Understand the risks to the mother[3]
- Understand potential risks to the fetus[4]

Is the woman currently symptomatic?[5]

No

Perform routine serologic screening[6]

Negative
- Discuss HBV prevention[7]
- *Consider repeating serologic screening in the 3rd trimester in high-risk pregnancies*

Continue routine prenatal care

Positive
- **Check HBcAg, HBeAg, and liver function tests**
- Continue supportive care[8]
- √ ultrasound to confirm gestational age and document fetal wellbeing
- Serial liver function tests q trimester
- *Serial ultrasounds for fetal growth*

Yes

Confirm the diagnosis of acute HBV infection[9]

Diagnosis confirmed
- Screen for other sexually transmitted infections
- Continue supportive care[8]
- Consider checking for fetal infection[10]
- √ ultrasound to confirm gestational age and document fetal wellbeing
- **Consider inpatient care for acute infection with coagulopathy or encephalopathy**
- Serial liver function tests q trimester
- Serial ultrasounds for fetal growth

Diagnosis not confirmed
- If symptoms persist, consider alternative diagnoses[11]
- Discuss HBV prevention[7]

Continue routine prenatal care

Prevent vertical transmission
- **No proven benefit to elective cesarean delivery**
- If possible, avoid early rupture of membranes, placement of fetal scalp electrode (FSE) or intrauterine pressure catheter (IUPC) in labor
- **Exposed neonates should receive HBIg by 12 hours of life and the hepatitis B vaccine by 6 months**
- **Breastfeeding is not contraindicated**

1. Viral hepatitis is caused by members of the hepatitis family of small DNA viruses. Approximately 80–85% of individuals infected with hepatitis B virus (HBV) clear the infection and develop lifelong protective immunity as evidenced by the presence of anti-hepatitis B surface antibodies (HBsAb); 10–15% remain chronically infected with detectable hepatitis B surface antigen (HBsAg) but have normal hepatic function; and 5–10% are chronically infected with persistent viral replication, elevated liver function tests, and measurable HBeAg expression (a marker of high infectivity). Acute hepatitis B occurs in 1 in 1,000 pregnancies, and chronic hepatitis B is seen in 10 in 1,000 pregnancies.

2. Risk factors for acute HBV infection include intravenous drug abuse, multiple sexual partners, household or occupational exposure (especially working in a hemodialysis unit), intravenous drug abuse, prior blood transfusion, and chronic

Obstetric Clinical Algorithms, Second Edition. Errol R. Norwitz, George R. Saade, Hugh Miller and Christina M. Davidson.
© 2017 John Wiley & Sons, Ltd. Published 2017 by John Wiley & Sons, Ltd.

hospitalization. Risk factors for chronic HBV carrier status include infant or early childhood exposure, immunosuppression, and endemic home origin such as Asia or Latin America.

3. Acute viral hepatitis is the most common cause of jaundice in pregnancy. Other manifestations include: right upper quadrant pain, elevated liver function tests, and (rarely) coagulopathy and encephalopathy. Serious long-term complications include cirrhosis and hepatocellular carcinoma.

4. The risk to the fetus of acquiring HBV infection is related primarily to two factors: (i) gestational age (10% risk if infected in the first trimester versus 90% if infected in the third trimester); and (ii) maternal infectivity status (10–20% if HBsAg-positive only versus 90% if HBsAg-positive and HBeAg-positive). Every effort should be made to avoid amniocentesis.

5. Women with acute HBV infection are often asymptomatic. Symptoms may include low-grade fever, malaise, fatigue, nausea, abdominal pain, and jaundice.

6. Serologic screening is recommended for all pregnant women at their first prenatal visit regardless of their risk status. The clinically relevant antigens include: (i) surface antigen (HBsAg), which is found on the viral surface and free in maternal serum; (ii) core antigen (HBcAg), which is found in hepatocytes; and (iii) envelope antigen (HBeAg), which is only expressed in the setting of a high viral load and is a marker of high infectivity. Routine serologic screening includes HBsAg only. If the HBsAg screen is positive, then HBcAg and HBeAg serology should be sent along with liver function tests (transaminase levels, bilirubin) and coagulation profile. There is no place for imaging studies to confirm the diagnosis of viral hepatitis, although a right upper quadrant ultrasound may be useful in excluding other diagnoses (such as gallbladder disease).

7. Prevention of maternal HBV infection includes avoidance of unprotected intercourse, routine use of barrier contraception, and stopping IV drug abuse. If an exposure is documented, hepatitis B immunoglobulin (HBIg) 0.06 mL/kg IM should be administered with 12 hours, and the hepatitis B vaccine should be offered (two injections 6 months apart). Reducing perinatal transmission is critical to reducing newborn HBV infection and is achieved by administering HBIg and the first dose of a three-dose series of HBV vaccine prophylactically within 12 hours of birth. Prevention also extends to all obstetrical providers who in addition to adhering to standard blood-borne pathogen precautions should receive the hepatitis B virus vaccine series.

8. The management of maternal HBV infection is primarily supportive. Antiviral treatment with interferon-alpha may be recommended in non-pregnant women with chronic hepatitis, but is contraindicated in pregnancy. Lamivudine (100–150 mg daily) can decrease viral load and reduce vertical transmission. It should be started in the 3rd trimester if the viral load is >10^6 copies/mL.

9. Physical examination is often unhelpful, but may show evidence of jaundice or abdominal tenderness. Maternal hepatitis B infection is typically confirmed by serologic testing.

10. Fetal infection can be confirmed by detection of viral particles or DNA in fetal serum, amniotic fluid, or placental tissues; however, invasive prenatal testing is not routinely recommended.

11. Differential diagnosis includes other viral hepatitis infections (such as hepatitis A, C, and D), cytomegalovirus hepatitis, pancreatitis, gallbladder disease, cholestasis of pregnancy, severe preeclampsia/HELLP (hemolysis, elevated liver enzymes, low platelets) syndrome, and acute fatty liver of pregnancy.

26 Herpes Simplex Virus

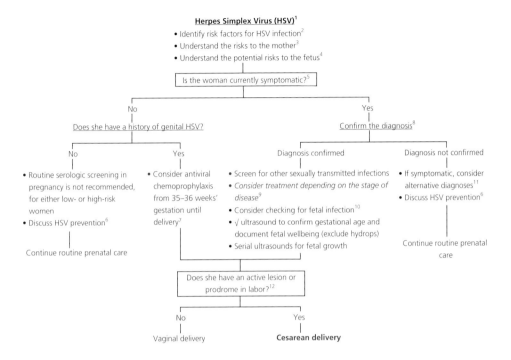

Herpes Simplex Virus (HSV)[1]
- Identify risk factors for HSV infection[2]
- Understand the risks to the mother[3]
- Understand the potential risks to the fetus[4]

Is the woman currently symptomatic?[5]

No

Does she have a history of genital HSV?

No
- Routine serologic screening in pregnancy is not recommended, for either low- or high-risk women
- Discuss HSV prevention[6]

Continue routine prenatal care

Yes
- Consider antiviral chemoprophylaxis from 35–36 weeks' gestation until delivery[7]

Yes

Confirm the diagnosis[8]

Diagnosis confirmed
- Screen for other sexually transmitted infections
- *Consider treatment depending on the stage of disease[9]*
- Consider checking for fetal infection[10]
- √ ultrasound to confirm gestational age and document fetal wellbeing (exclude hydrops)
- Serial ultrasounds for fetal growth

Diagnosis not confirmed
- If symptomatic, consider alternative diagnoses[11]
- Discuss HSV prevention[6]

Continue routine prenatal care

Does she have an active lesion or prodrome in labor?[12]

No
Vaginal delivery

Yes
Cesarean delivery

---

1. HSV is caused by members of the herpesviridae family of DNA viruses. There are two major serotypes: (i) HSV-1 which causes conjunctivitis, stomatitis, and gingivitis as well as 20% of genital infections; and (ii) HSV-2 which accounts for 80% of genital infections. It is the most common viral pathogen in the United States with over 45 million people infected and more than 500,000 new cases annually.

2. Risk factors include multiple sexual partners, unprotected intercourse, multiparity, other sexually transmitted infection, a history of recent exposure to HSV or intercourse with an HSV-positive partner, and history of prior HSV infection.

3. Maternal complications include localized erythema, swelling, and pain. Serious complications such as hepatitis, encephalitis, and death are rare.

4. There are 1,500–2,000 cases of neonatal HSV infection in the United States annually, and most are due to HSV-2. First episode primary infection leads to a viremia and an increased risk of vertical transmission; however, *in utero* HSV infection is rare. Most neonatal infections result from contact

---

Obstetric Clinical Algorithms, Second Edition. Errol R. Norwitz, George R. Saade, Hugh Miller and Christina M. Davidson.
© 2017 John Wiley & Sons, Ltd. Published 2017 by John Wiley & Sons, Ltd.

with infected secretions at the time of vaginal delivery. Indeed, neonatal disease occurs in 30–60% of infants exposed to HSV at vaginal delivery. Recurrent HSV is not associated with viremia; as such, the fetus is not at risk if the fetal membranes remain intact and there is no labor. If the fetus is infected *in utero*, complications may include preterm birth, intrauterine fetal demise or neonatal mortality (15–60%), localized infection (skin, eye, mouth, CNS), or disseminated HSV.

5. Symptoms depend on the stage of the disease: (i) First episode primary infection refers to the first clinical presentation in the absence of circulating anti-HSV IgG. Typical symptoms include painful vesicles on the vulva, vagina, and/or cervix that develop 2–14 days after exposure along with tender adenopathy and systemic symptoms (low-grade fever, malaise) in two-thirds of cases. The lesions resolve spontaneously in 3–4 weeks without treatment. Primary infections that occur in proximity to delivery represent the greatest risk for subsequent neonatal infection due to asymptomatic viral shedding and the absence of anti-HSV antibodies. (ii) First episode non-primary infection refers to the first clinical presentation, but in the presence of anti-HSV IgG suggesting evidence of prior infection. (iii) Recurrent infection refers to reactivation of dormant virus, and symptoms are generally less severe with no systemic features.

6. Prevention of HSV includes avoiding contact with infected persons and the routine use of barrier contraception. There is no vaccine or immune globulin available. Of note, anti-HSV-1 IgG does not prevent primary infection with HSV-2, and vice versa.

7. Antiviral chemoprophylaxis starting at 35–36 weeks' gestation until delivery is recommended for women at risk of viral shedding at delivery to decrease the likelihood of a lesion in labor requiring cesarean delivery. Whether this decreases the rate of neonatal infection is not known.

8. Maternal HSV infection can be confirmed by viral isolation from vesicular fluid or infected tissues, but problems with specimen sampling and transportation limit the sensitivity to 60–70%. Serologic testing is often performed, but is of limited utility. Such testing does not easily distinguish between anti-HSV-1 and anti-HSV-2 antibodies, and in excess of 30% of all pregnant women have anti-HSV-2 IgG.

9. The management of maternal HSV infection is primarily supportive. Antiviral treatment of first episode primary HSV can decrease the severity and duration of symptoms in the mother, but does not prevent fetal infection. Acyclovir is the treatment of choice; alternatives include valacyclovir and famciclovir. Topical is less effective than oral treatment and is therefore not recommended. Disseminated disease should be treated with intravenous (IV) acyclovir in an intensive care unit (ICU) setting. It is unclear whether antiviral treatment decreases the severity or duration of symptoms in recurrent HSV infections, although it may abort an outbreak if given during the clinical prodrome or within one day of the onset of lesions.

10. Fetal infection can be confirmed by detection of viral particles or DNA in fetal serum, amniotic fluid, or placental tissues; however, invasive prenatal testing is not routinely recommended.

11. Differential diagnosis includes other herpes virus infections, such as varicella zoster.

12. To prevent vertical transmission, cesarean delivery should be recommended for all women with an active genital lesion or clinical prodrome in labor. Due to the low yield of viral cultures and poor correlation between culture and asymptomatic viral shedding in labor, screening for viral shedding in labor is not recommended.

27 Human Immunodeficiency Virus

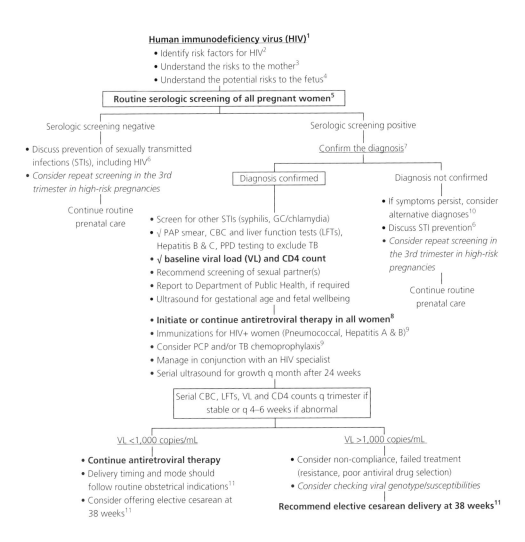

Human immunodeficiency virus (HIV)[1]
- Identify risk factors for HIV[2]
- Understand the risks to the mother[3]
- Understand the potential risks to the fetus[4]

Routine serologic screening of all pregnant women[5]

Serologic screening negative

- Discuss prevention of sexually transmitted infections (STIs), including HIV[6]
- *Consider repeat screening in the 3rd trimester in high-risk pregnancies*

Continue routine prenatal care

Serologic screening positive

Confirm the diagnosis[7]

Diagnosis confirmed

- Screen for other STIs (syphilis, GC/chlamydia)
- √ PAP smear, CBC and liver function tests (LFTs), Hepatitis B & C, PPD testing to exclude TB
- **√ baseline viral load (VL) and CD4 count**
- Recommend screening of sexual partner(s)
- Report to Department of Public Health, if required
- Ultrasound for gestational age and fetal wellbeing
- **Initiate or continue antiretroviral therapy in all women[8]**
- Immunizations for HIV+ women (Pneumococcal, Hepatitis A & B)[9]
- Consider PCP and/or TB chemoprophylaxis[9]
- Manage in conjunction with an HIV specialist
- Serial ultrasound for growth q month after 24 weeks

Diagnosis not confirmed

- If symptoms persist, consider alternative diagnoses[10]
- Discuss STI prevention[6]
- *Consider repeat screening in the 3rd trimester in high-risk pregnancies*

Continue routine prenatal care

Serial CBC, LFTs, VL and CD4 counts q trimester if stable or q 4–6 weeks if abnormal

VL <1,000 copies/mL

- **Continue antiretroviral therapy**
- Delivery timing and mode should follow routine obstetrical indications[11]
- Consider offering elective cesarean at 38 weeks[11]

VL >1,000 copies/mL

- Consider non-compliance, failed treatment (resistance, poor antiviral drug selection)
- *Consider checking viral genotype/susceptibilities*

Recommend elective cesarean delivery at 38 weeks[11]

1. HIV is a single-stranded DNA virus that causes acquired immune deficiency system (AIDS). In women, it is primarily (although not exclusively) a sexually transmitted infection (STI) acquired through heterosexual intercourse. It can also be acquired through blood transfusion, intravenous drug abuse, or transplacental infection (perinatal or vertical transmission). Once acquired, it cannot be eradicated.

2. Risk factors for HIV include prostitution/multiple sexual partners, unprotected intercourse,

Obstetric Clinical Algorithms, Second Edition. Errol R. Norwitz, George R. Saade, Hugh Miller and Christina M. Davidson.
© 2017 John Wiley & Sons, Ltd. Published 2017 by John Wiley & Sons, Ltd.

other sexually transmitted infections, drug abuse, HIV-positive/bisexual partner, late/no prenatal care, new immigrant from a high prevalence area (such as Africa), and a prior blood transfusion (especially before 1985).

3. HIV causes AIDS. Pregnancy does not increase progression to AIDS. Pregnant women with HIV should receive pneumococcal and hepatitis A & B inactivated vaccines to reduce the risk of acquiring these infections during pregnancy. HIV in pregnancy is associated with an increased risk of preterm birth, preterm premature rupture of membranes (PROM) and possibly poor fetal growth in women receiving combination antiretroviral (ARV) therapy. Routine fundal height measurements or interval ultrasound assessment should be used to monitor fetal growth.

4. The major risk to the fetus is vertical transmission. HIV-positive infants may develop AIDS with a high mortality rate. Baseline rates of vertical transmission without treatment range from 20–30%. The risk is highest during labor and delivery. Monotherapy with zidovudine (ZDV), formerly (azidothymidine (AZT)) administration to the mother throughout pregnancy, during labor, and in the first 6 weeks of newborn life can reduce vertical transmission to around 8%, but is no longer the mainstay of treatment. Three-drug combination antiretroviral therapy (ART) is now the gold-standard and can reduce the perinatal transmission rate to 1%. Perinatal transmission is related to the circulating viral load (VL). If the circulating VL is undetectable (<50 copies/mL), the risk of perinatal transmission decreases to <1%.

5. HIV-positive women who are on ART and found to be pregnant may need their regimen adjusted. For the majority of women, pregnancy is an opportunity for universal screening, regardless of risk. Pregnant women with HIV are generally asymptomatic and may or may not have risk factors. Physical examination is usually unhelpful, but may identify non-specific features (weight loss, skin lesions) or evidence of thrush, vaginitis, cervical lesion, or generalized lymphadenopathy. Now that combination ART can effectively prevent vertical transmission, all pregnant women should be screened for HIV at their first prenatal visit with an opt-out approach. It may be valuable to rescreen high-risk patients again in later pregnancy. This would include patients with a history of STIs, opportunistic infections (such as *pneumocystis carinii* pneumonia (PCP)), or cervical dysplasia/cancer that may suggest the diagnosis of HIV. The traditional ELISA for HIV has been supplanted by newer combination antigen-antibody testing (see below).

6. Prevention of HIV includes avoidance of unprotected intercourse, routine use of barrier contraception, and stopping drug abuse/needle sharing. Needle exchange programs have been shown to be effective in preventing HIV infection.

7. To confirm the diagnosis, the US Centers for Disease Control and Prevention (CDC) recommend the fourth-generation assay that detects HIV p24 antigen and HIV1/2 antibodies, which can be processed more quickly and is more likely to detect early infection. HIV-1/HIV-2 differentiation immunoassay in combination with the viral load (HIV RNA level) is used to confirm the screening results and determine which HIV serotype is involved. Women who were not antenatally tested or whose HIV status is unknown when presenting with labor should be offered rapid screening (results in < 1 hr) and receive immediate antiretroviral prophylaxis prior to laboratory confirmation.

8. HIV-positive women who become pregnant should generally continue their ART in consultation with their HIV specialist. For women with a new diagnosis of HIV, multi-drug ART is recommended to arrest maternal HIV disease and reduce perinatal transmission by achieving an undetectable VL. HIV-positive women should be treated in pregnancy with three-drug combination

ART that addresses drug safety, known toxicity, efficacy, and pragmatic considerations such as convenience, adherence potential, tolerability, potential for drug interactions with other medications, and the resistance characteristics of the specific HIV serotype in an effort to maximally reduce VL. Because these ART regimens are complicated, rapidly changing over time, and require long-term compliance, it is advisable to involve an HIV specialist. Multi-drug ART includes nucleoside inhibitors (AZT, DDI, 3TC, D4T), protease inhibitors (indinavir, nelfinavir, ritonivir, sequanavir), and/or other drugs (nivaripine, delacirone, etacirenz). Some drugs (such as efavirenz) are best avoided pre-conceptually and in the first trimester, because of the risk of neural tube defect (NTD). Similarly, other ART (darunavir, dolutegravir, and elvitegravir) are best avoided because of the lack of experience in pregnancy. Treatment should include AZT since it is best proven to prevent vertical transmission. Women should be followed closely for drug side-effects (such as rash, bone marrow depression, and liver dysfunction).

9. If CD4 count is <200 cells/mm³, PCP chemoprophylaxis (bactrim, inhaled pentamidine) is indicated. If CD4<50 cells/mm³, administer TB prophylaxis.

10. Alternative diagnoses include, among others, viral hepatitis, pneumonia, and anorexia.

11. Women on combination ART with a low VL (<1,000 copies/mL) should be allowed to deliver vaginally, regardless of duration of labor or rupture of membranes since there is no evidence that perinatal transmission is reduced when delivered by cesarean. There also appears to be no benefit in adding intrapartum ZDV in these women provided they are consistently taking their ART and VL is low. The plan of care should be discussed with the patient with input from her HIV specialist. In contrast, in women with an elevated VL (>1,000 copies/mL), elective cesarean delivery at 38 0/7 weeks will decrease vertical transmission to <1% (range, 0–2%). Amniocentesis for fetal lung maturity testing is not required. However, once there is rupture of membranes or labor, the protective effect appears to disappear. If a vaginal delivery is planned, every effort should be made to avoid early amniotomy, prolonged rupture of membranes, and fetal scalp electrode placement. All infants born to HIV-infected mothers should receive ART prophylaxis, typically in the form of ZDV for 6 weeks after birth to decrease the risk of acquiring HIV.

28 Parvovirus B19

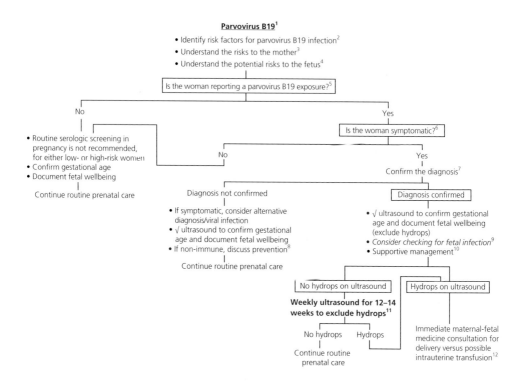

Parvovirus B19[1]
- Identify risk factors for parvovirus B19 infection[2]
- Understand the risks to the mother[3]
- Understand the potential risks to the fetus[4]

Is the woman reporting a parvovirus B19 exposure?[5]

No
- Routine serologic screening in pregnancy is not recommended, for either low- or high-risk women
- Confirm gestational age
- Document fetal wellbeing

Continue routine prenatal care

Yes

Is the woman symptomatic?[6]

No

Yes
Confirm the diagnosis[7]

Diagnosis not confirmed
- If symptomatic, consider alternative diagnosis/viral infection
- √ ultrasound to confirm gestational age and document fetal wellbeing
- If non-immune, discuss prevention[8]

Continue routine prenatal care

Diagnosis confirmed
- √ ultrasound to confirm gestational age and document fetal wellbeing (exclude hydrops)
- Consider checking for fetal infection[9]
- Supportive management[10]

No hydrops on ultrasound

Weekly ultrasound for 12–14 weeks to exclude hydrops[11]

No hydrops — Continue routine prenatal care

Hydrops

Hydrops on ultrasound

Immediate maternal-fetal medicine consultation for delivery versus possible intrauterine transfusion[12]

1. Parvovirus B19 is a single-stranded DNA virus that causes fifth disease (erythema infectiosum). It is transmitted by hand-to-mouth contact and respiratory secretions. The incubation period is 5–10 days in length, although the infectious period is usually past once clinical manifestations are present.

2. Risk factors include frequent contact with children aged 5–18 years old in the home or in the workplace. Professions at risk are those who have regular contact with young children (such as teachers, daycare providers), are of Caucasian ethnicity, and age <30 years. Non-immune fetal hydrops due to acute parvovirus B19 infection does not recur in subsequent pregnancies; as such, a history of such an event should be regarded as protective.

3. Fifth disease is a common, self-limiting illness of childhood presenting with a reticular facial and truncal rash, mild upper respiratory tract symptoms, and a low-grade fever. Adults with fifth disease may present with a self-limiting arthropathy and, rarely, can develop a transient aplastic crisis and cardiac failure.

Obstetric Clinical Algorithms, Second Edition. Errol R. Norwitz, George R. Saade, Hugh Miller and Christina M. Davidson.
© 2017 John Wiley & Sons, Ltd. Published 2017 by John Wiley & Sons, Ltd.

4. Transplacental passage of parvovirus B19 is high (33%), but the risk of fetal morbidity and mortality is low, estimated at 3% for household contact and <1% for school contact. Serious fetal sequelae usually occur with infection prior to 20 weeks' gestation, and may include anemia (due to parvovirus-induced bone marrow suppression), non-immune hydrops (associated with a fetal hematocrit <15% [normal is approximately 50%]), stillbirth, and spontaneous abortion. If the fetus survives, its long-term development appears to be normal. Of note, parvovirus B19 is not a teratogen, and exposure in early pregnancy has not been associated with any structural defects.

5. Approximately 40–50% of reproductive-age women have not previously been exposed to parvovirus B19. In susceptible women, exposure results in seroconversion in 50–70% of cases if the contact is household member and in 20% of cases if the exposure occurs at school.

6. Symptoms/signs may include a low-grade fever, joint pains, and a characteristic "slapped-cheek" facial rash.

7. Maternal parvovirus B19 infection is usually confirmed by serologic testing in 80–90% of suspected cases, but can be confirmed by polymerase chain reaction (PCR) or direct visualization of viral particles in infected tissues. Positive IgM can be detected within two weeks of exposure and often before symptoms appear. A fourfold increase in IgG titers over a period of 4–6 weeks is diagnostic of acute parvovirus B19 infection. Anti-parvovirus B19 IgM persists only for a few months, whereas IgG persists for life

8. If a woman is known to be non-immune, she should be counseled to avoid exposure if possible. There is no vaccine or immune globulin available.

9. Fetal infection can be confirmed by detection of viral particles or PCR for small amounts of DNA in fetal serum, amniotic fluid, or placental tissues; however, invasive prenatal testing is not routinely recommended.

10. The management of maternal parvovirus B19 infection is primarily supportive. There is no effective treatment and no vaccine.

11. In pregnancies with confirmed maternal parvovirus B19 infection, weekly ultrasound surveillance for 12–14 weeks is indicated to watch for the development of non-immune hydrops. The fetal hydrops results from severe anemia (hematocrit <15%) due to parvovirus-induced bone marrow suppression. After 14 weeks, the likelihood of this event is minimal and surveillance can be discontinued. Ultrasound examination should include middle cerebral artery (MCA) peak velocity measurement to identify fetuses with anemia.

12. Should hydrops develop, management options are limited to either immediate delivery if the gestational age is favorable (>34–36 weeks) or percutaneous umbilical blood sampling (PUBS) to confirm the diagnosis, to exclude other causes of non-immune hydrops, and possibly to perform an intrauterine transfusion (IUT) to correct the anemia and reverse the hydropic changes. Serial (weekly) IUTs may be required until the parvovirus infection resolves.

29 Syphilis

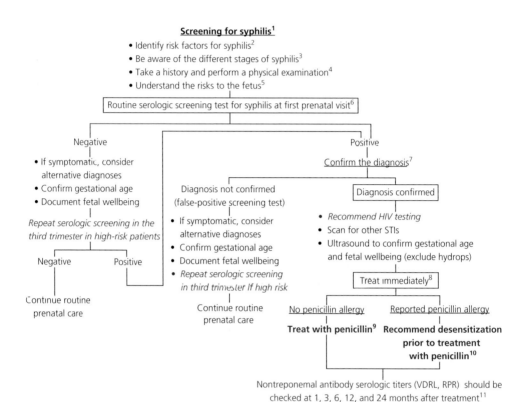

Screening for syphilis[1]
- Identify risk factors for syphilis[2]
- Be aware of the different stages of syphilis[3]
- Take a history and perform a physical examination[4]
- Understand the risks to the fetus[5]

Routine serologic screening test for syphilis at first prenatal visit[6]

Negative
- If symptomatic, consider alternative diagnoses
- Confirm gestational age
- Document fetal wellbeing

Repeat serologic screening in the third trimester in high-risk patients

Negative | Positive

Continue routine prenatal care

Positive

Confirm the diagnosis[7]

Diagnosis not confirmed (false-positive screening test)
- If symptomatic, consider alternative diagnoses
- Confirm gestational age
- Document fetal wellbeing
- *Repeat serologic screening in third trimester If high risk*

Continue routine prenatal care

Diagnosis confirmed
- *Recommend HIV testing*
- Scan for other STIs
- Ultrasound to confirm gestational age and fetal wellbeing (exclude hydrops)

Treat immediately[8]

No penicillin allergy
Treat with penicillin[9]

Reported penicillin allergy
Recommend desensitization prior to treatment with penicillin[10]

Nontreponemal antibody serologic titers (VDRL, RPR) should be checked at 1, 3, 6, 12, and 24 months after treatment[11]

1. Syphilis is a chronic infection caused by the spirochete *Treponema pallidum*. It is sexually acquired (except for cases of vertical transmission) with an incubation period of 10–90 days (average 21 days). If untreated in pregnancy, there is a high risk of fetal infection.

2. Risk factors include sexual promiscuity, illicit drug use, HIV, no prenatal care, poor socio-economic status, black or Hispanic ethnicity, and age <25 years.

3. Early syphilis (<1 year) includes primary, secondary, and early latent. Latent syphilis refers to asymptomatic infection with positive serology and no physical findings. It is divided into early (<1 year) and late latent (>1 year). Tertiary syphilis occurs after early or latent syphilis, and typically involves the central nervous system (CNS), the cardiovascular system, or skin and subcutaneous tissues. It can arise as soon as 1 year after initial infection or up to 25–30 years later.

Obstetric Clinical Algorithms, Second Edition. Errol R. Norwitz, George R. Saade, Hugh Miller and Christina M. Davidson.
© 2017 John Wiley & Sons, Ltd. Published 2017 by John Wiley & Sons, Ltd.

4. History should include questions about risk factors (above). Clinical manifestations depend on the stage of the disease, and are not altered by pregnancy:

- *Primary syphilis* is characterized by a papule at the site of inoculation, which ulcerates to produce the classic painless chancer with a raised, indurated margin and regional lymphadenopathy. Chancer heals spontaneously in 3–6 weeks even in the absence of treatment.
- *Secondary syphilis* is a disseminated systemic process that begins 6 weeks to 6 months after the chancer in 25% of untreated patients. Findings may include a generalized maculopapular skin rash (involving the palms, soles, and mucous membranes), generalized lymphadenopathy, fever, pharyngitis, weight loss, and genital lesions (condylomata lata). The rash resolves spontaneously in 2–6 weeks. Neurologic manifestations are rare.
- *Latent syphilis* is usually subclinical, although clinical relapses may occur.
- *Tertiary syphilis* is characterized by slowly progressive signs and symptoms, including gumma formation, cardiovascular disease, and/or CNS changes (neurosyphilis). Such manifestations usually develop 5–20 years after the disease has become latent.

5. *Treponema pallidum* crosses the placenta. Vertical transmission can occur at any time in pregnancy and any stage of the disease, but is most common with primary, secondary or early latent disease (40–50%) compared with late latent or tertiary disease (10%). Fetal infection causes intrauterine growth restriction (IUGR), preterm birth, stillbirth, hydrops fetalis, low birthweight, neonatal death, and congenital anomalies. Only 20% of children born to mothers with untreated syphilis will be normal.

6. All pregnant women should have blood taken for serologic screening for syphilis at their first prenatal. Nontreponemal antibody tests should be used for screening, either the Venereal Disease Research Laboratory (VDRL) or rapid plasma reagin (RPR) test. These tests are inexpensive and easy to perform. A positive test should include report of an antibody titer.

7. *Treponema pallidum* cannot be cultured in the laboratory. Confirmation of the diagnosis relies on direct visualization of the organism (by dark-field microscopy or direct fluorescent antibody staining of scrapings or body secretions) or, more commonly, by serologic testing using specific treponemal antibody tests (e.g. fluorescent treponemal antibody absorption (FTA-ABS), microhemagglutination assay for antibodies to *T. pallidum* (MHA-TP) or *T. pallidum* particle agglutination assay (TPPA)). Rarely, examination of the cerebrospinal fluid may be needed. CSF abnormalities suggestive of infection include an elevated white cell count (>5 cells/μL), elevated total protein (>45 mg/dL), normal glucose concentrations, and a positive CSF VDRL.

8. Treatment of maternal syphilis is critical to prevent congenital infection: 70–100% of infants born to untreated mothers will be infected vs 1–2% of those born to women adequately treated in pregnancy. Note that treatment may precipitate the Jarisch–Herxheimer reaction due to the release of large amounts of treponemal antigen, which, in the latter half of pregnancy, can lead to uterine contractions, preterm labor, and/or nonreassuring fetal testing.

9. *Penicillin is the treatment of choice for syphilis in pregnancy* to treat maternal disease, prevent vertical transmission, and treat established fetal disease. No penicillin-resistant strains of *T. pallidum* have yet been identified. Second-line agents are not recommended in pregnancy because they are ineffective (erythromycin, clindamycin), contraindicated (tetracycline), or lack sufficient data regarding efficacy (ceftriaxone,

azithromycin). The penicillin regimen depends on the stage of disease: (i) benzathine penicillin 2.4 mU intramuscular injection (IMI) x 1 for early disease; (ii) benzathine penicillin 2.4 mU IMI weekly x 3 for latent disease.

10. Approximately 5–10% of pregnant women report an allergy to penicillin. Skin testing to document a true penicillin allergy should be performed in all such women, except those who have had a documented anaphylactic reaction to penicillin. The only satisfactory treatment for penicillin-allergic pregnant patients with syphi-lis is inpatient desensitization (either oral or subcutaneous) followed by penicillin therapy.

11. Nontreponemal antibody serologic titers (VDRL, RPR) should decrease fourfold by 6 months and become nonreactive by 12–24 months after treatment. Titers that show a fourfold rise or do not decrease appropriately suggest either treat-ment failure or reinfection. Such women should be treated again, their partners should be treated, and consideration should be given to performing a lumbar puncture to evaluate for CNS involvement.

30 Tuberculosis[1]

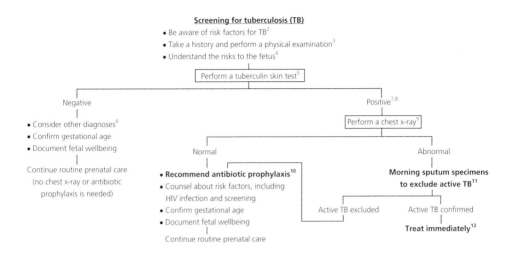

Screening for tuberculosis (TB)
- Be aware of risk factors for TB[2]
- Take a history and perform a physical examination[3]
- Understand the risks to the fetus[4]

Perform a tuberculin skin test[5]

Negative
- Consider other diagnoses[6]
- Confirm gestational age
- Document fetal wellbeing

Continue routine prenatal care
(no chest x-ray or antibiotic
prophylaxis is needed)

Positive[7,8]

Perform a chest x-ray[9]

Normal
- **Recommend antibiotic prophylaxis**[10]
- Counsel about risk factors, including HIV infection and screening
- Confirm gestational age
- Document fetal wellbeing

Continue routine prenatal care

Abnormal

Morning sputum specimens to exclude active TB[11]

Active TB excluded

Active TB confirmed

Treat immediately[12]

1. Tuberculosis (TB) refers to infection with the organism, *Myobacterium tuberculosis*. Most cases of TB in immunocompetent adults involve the lungs, but it can affect any organ system. Although it is now rare in developed countries, TB remains one of the leading causes of morbidity and mortality worldwide.

2. Risk factors for TB include: (i) a prior history of TB; (ii) a history of a positive tuberculin skin test; (iii) new immigrants (<5 years) from countries with a high prevalence of TB; (iv) travel to a high-prevalence area; (v) HIV infection; and (vi) a history of homelessness or incarceration. Pregnancy itself does not predispose to infection with TB, although it may be associated with a higher rate of reactivation in women previously infected with TB.

3. A history should include questions about risk factors for TB (above). Symptoms may be non-specific, including fever, weight loss, malaise, and sweats (especially drenching "night sweats"). In pulmonary TB, additional symptoms may include cough, hemoptysis (coughing blood), and shortness of breath. In extra-pulmonary TB, symptoms may include local swelling or pain, a chronically-draining lesion, headache, or confusion. However, most infected women are symptomatic. Physical findings may include focal rales on pulmonary examination, evidence of pleural effusion, or a focal mass or lymphadenopathy.

4. Congenital disease resulting from transplacental transmission of TB is rare and occurs almost exclusively when the placenta is actively infected, which is seen more commonly with maternal extra-pulmonary disease. As such, pulmonary TB alone poses little risk to the fetus. The greatest risk in women with pulmonary TB is transmission to the infant shortly after birth. Thus, the potential infectiousness of the mother should be resolved prior to delivery.

Obstetric Clinical Algorithms, Second Edition. Errol R. Norwitz, George R. Saade, Hugh Miller and Christina M. Davidson.
© 2017 John Wiley & Sons, Ltd. Published 2017 by John Wiley & Sons, Ltd.

5. All pregnant women at risk should be screened for exposure to TB. Exceptions include: (i) low-risk women who have already had such testing within the preceding year; and (ii) asymptomatic women who have previously had a positive tuberculin test and who have completed a full course of antibiotic prophylaxis. Pregnancy itself does not alter the response to the tuberculin skin test. Such testing involves intradermal (not subcutaneous) injection of purified protein derivative (PPD), also called the tuberculin skin testing (TST), which measures the extent of induration (skin thickening, not redness) at the injection site 72 hours later.

6. If the patient has pulmonary symptoms, consider other diagnoses such as pneumonia (coccidioidomycosis), asthma, and pulmonary embolism.

7. Interpretation of the PPD test depends on the risk status of the patient: (i) in very high-risk women (HIV positive, abnormal chest x-ray, recent contact with an active case of TB), use ≥5 mm induration as positive; (ii) in high-risk women (foreign-born, IV drug use, medical conditions or immunosuppressant medications increasing the risk of TB), use ≥10 mm induration as positive; (iii) in low-risk women (no risk factors), use ≥15 mm induration as positive. A positive PPD test implies that a woman has been <u>exposed</u> to *M. tuberculosis*, it does not mean that she has TB <u>infection</u>. The QuantiFERON®-TB Gold In-Tube test (QFT-GIT) and the T-SPOT®.TB test (T-Spot) are the two FDA-approved interferon gamma release assays (IGRAs) that have emerged as an alternate testing strategy for patients who have previously received a BCG vaccination, or are unlikely to return for their follow-up reading of their TST. It is not generally recommended or necessary to get a TST and IGRA.

8. The Bacillus Calmette-Guérin (BCG) vaccination is commonly used in developing countries. It does not prevent pulmonary TB, but does prevent complications such as TB meningitis. To maintain its efficacy, BCG should be boosted every 5 years. If >5 years has passed, a positive PPD cannot be attributed to BCG.

9. Chest x-ray is not a good screening tool for TB infection in low-risk populations, but is useful in PPD-positive and symptomatic patients. A normal chest x-ray is reassuring. However, an abnormal x-ray cannot accurately distinguish between old and active disease. Women may be reluctant to have a chest x-ray in pregnancy. While it does expose the fetus to ionizing radiation, the amount is so small (<1 mRad) as to be non-significant. ACOG has stated that up to 5 Rad (5,000 mRad) is completely safe in pregnancy. Waiting until after 12 weeks and appropriate shielding of the abdomen are reasonable recommendations. If a woman declines a chest x-ray in pregnancy, she should be separated from her baby immediately after birth until active TB infection can be excluded.

10. Women who are PPD-positive with a normal chest x-ray require antibiotic prophylaxis. The recommended regimen is isoniazid (INH) 300 mg/day with pyridoxine (to decrease the incidence of INH neurotoxicity) for 9 months. Prophylaxis can be deferred in women over the age of 35. Although INH crosses the placenta, there is no increased toxicity to the fetus. As such, INH can be started in pregnancy. Indeed, if the patient is very high-risk (see above), INH should be started immediately. Alternatively, it can be deferred until 6 weeks' postpartum; it is not recommended to start INH prophylaxis in the immediate postpartum period because of the increased risk of hepatic toxicity. Breastfeeding is not contraindicated.

11. An abnormal x-ray cannot accurately distinguish between old infection (scarring) and active disease. As such, active pulmonary TB disease must be excluded in all asymptomatic patients who are PPD-positive with an abnormal chest x-ray. This is done by sputum examination for *M. tuberculosis*. Three negative early morning sputum specimens effectively

exclude the diagnosis of active disease. While the sputum is being evaluated, patients should be started on treatment with INH and ethambutol, and, if in hospital, should be maintained on contact precautions and in a laminar flow room.

12. If sputum examination confirms active TB, the benefits of treatment in pregnancy dramatically outweigh any potential drug toxicity. Pregnancy does not affect the response to medications, but standard regimens should be modified (e.g., streptomycin is not used because of possible ototoxicity in the fetus). Pregnant women should be treated with a combination of INH, rifampin, and ethambutol for 9 months. Pyrazinamide should be added if drug-resistant TB is suspected.

31 Chorioamnionitis (Intraamniotic Infection)[1]

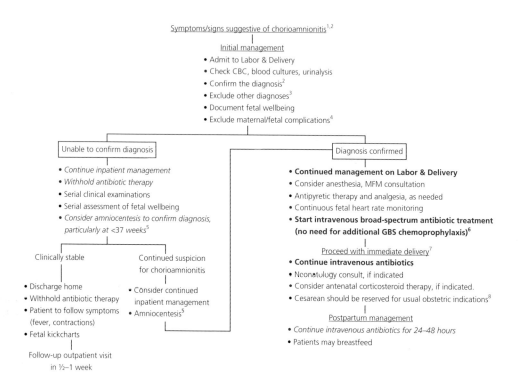

Symptoms/signs suggestive of chorioamnionitis[1,2]

Initial management
- Admit to Labor & Delivery
- Check CBC, blood cultures, urinalysis
- Confirm the diagnosis[2]
- Exclude other diagnoses[3]
- Document fetal wellbeing
- Exclude maternal/fetal complications[4]

Unable to confirm diagnosis
- *Continue inpatient management*
- *Withhold antibiotic therapy*
- Serial clinical examinations
- Serial assessment of fetal wellbeing
- *Consider amniocentesis to confirm diagnosis, particularly at <37 weeks[5]*

Clinically stable
- Discharge home
- Withhold antibiotic therapy
- Patient to follow symptoms (fever, contractions)
- Fetal kickcharts

Follow-up outpatient visit in ½–1 week

Continued suspicion for chorioamnionitis
- Consider continued inpatient management
- Amniocentesis[5]

Diagnosis confirmed
- **Continued management on Labor & Delivery**
- Consider anesthesia, MFM consultation
- Antipyretic therapy and analgesia, as needed
- Continuous fetal heart rate monitoring
- **Start intravenous broad-spectrum antibiotic treatment (no need for additional GBS chemoprophylaxis)[6]**

Proceed with immediate delivery[7]
- **Continue intravenous antibiotics**
- Neonatology consult, if indicated
- Consider antenatal corticosteroid therapy, if indicated.
- Cesarean should be reserved for usual obstetric indications[8]

Postpartum management
- *Continue intravenous antibiotics for 24–48 hours*
- Patients may breastfeed

1. Chorioamnionitis or intraamniotic infection (IAI) is usually an ascending infection by organisms of the lower genital tract. As such, most intraamniotic infections are polymicrobial, including such organisms as *E. coli*, Klebsiella, Bacteroides, GBS, Fusobacterium, Clostridium, and Peptostreptococcus. Mild subclinical infections may be associated with Mycoplasma, Ureaplasma, and Fusobacterium. Risk factors for chorioamnionitis at term include prolonged rupture of the fetal membranes (>24 hours), multiple digital vaginal examinations, and active vaginal infection (such as bacterial vaginosis). Over 50% of pPROM are associated with occult IAI and 20–30% of preterm labor has been attributed to IAI, often in the absence of symptoms other than preterm labor. In rare instances (such as listeriosis), maternal bacteremia can seed the amniotic space. Chorioamnionitis complicates 14% of all pregnancies.

2. Chorioamnionitis is a <u>clinical</u> diagnosis characterized by maternal fever ≥38°C (>100.4°F orally) and one or more of the following features: fetal tachycardia (>160 bpm), maternal

---

Obstetric Clinical Algorithms, Second Edition. Errol R. Norwitz, George R. Saade, Hugh Miller and Christina M. Davidson.
© 2017 John Wiley & Sons, Ltd. Published 2017 by John Wiley & Sons, Ltd.

tachycardia (>100 bpm), uterine tenderness (typically fundal tenderness between contractions), or foul odor of the amniotic fluid. Constitutional symptoms (chills, malaise), uterine contractions, and an elevated white cell count are common findings, but are not required for the diagnosis. There is no place for radiologic imaging studies to confirm the diagnosis. Intraamniotic infection with *Listeria monocytogenes* is unusual in that the mother is often asymptomatic. Amniocentesis remains the gold standard for diagnosing IAI when the clinical findings suggest significant risk.

3. The differential diagnosis of chorioamnionitis includes labor and other infectious/inflammatory conditions such as appendicitis, urinary tract infection (cystitis, pyelonephritis), and inflammatory bowel disease.

4. Maternal complications include preterm labor and delivery, increased cesarean delivery rate, postpartum endometritis, pulmonary edema, sepsis, acute respiratory distress syndrome (ARDS), and death. Fetal complications include prematurity, fetal/neonatal sepsis, and increased risk of cerebral palsy.

5. Definitive diagnosis requires a positive amniotic fluid culture obtained by transabdominal amniocentesis. Other features of the amniotic fluid that may suggest infection include glucose ≤20-mg/dL, leukocytes, and bacteria on Gram stain. Gram stain alone has a sensitivity of only 30–50%. In the setting of equivocal symptoms, a definitive diagnosis by amniocentesis can be valuable in guiding the plan of care.

6. Although chorioamnionitis cannot be managed expectantly with antibiotics, prompt administration of antibiotics will reduce neonatal sepsis, maternal febrile morbidity, and duration of hospitalization. Intravenous ampicillin 2 g q4–6 h plus gentamycin 1.5 mg/kg q8h (after confirmation of normal renal function) are the antibiotics of choice prior to delivery. In penicillin-allergic patients, vancomycin 1 g intravenously q12h should be used instead of ampicillin. Clindamycin or metronidazole should be added immediately after clamping of the cord to further cover anaerobic organisms. Although antibiotics have traditionally been continued until the patient was afebrile and asymptomatic for 24–48 h postpartum, newer evidence suggests that a single dose of antibiotics beyond delivery may be sufficient, particularly for vaginal deliveries. Longer antibiotic therapy may be required if blood cultures are positive.

7. Once the diagnosis of chorioamnionitis has been established, delivery should be affected regardless of gestational age. Ideally, delivery should be achieved within 12–18 hours, but labor can be continued beyond that time so long as the fetal status is reassuring. Maternal prognosis is good with prompt diagnosis and treatment. Neonatal mortality and morbidity are related primarily to gestational age.

8. Chorioamnionitis is an indication for delivery, but is not in of itself an indication for cesarean delivery. However, pregnancies complicated by chorioamnionitis are more likely to be delivered abdominally, usually due to non-reassuring fetal testing.

SECTION 4
Antenatal Complications

32 Advanced Maternal Age

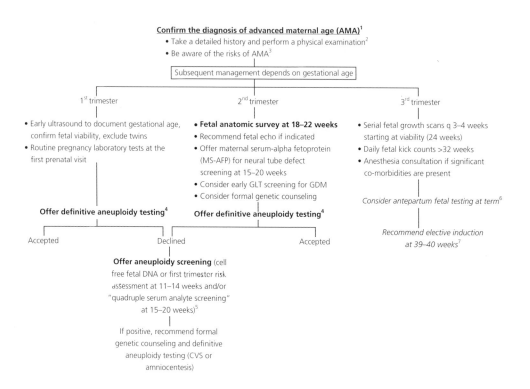

Confirm the diagnosis of advanced maternal age (AMA)[1]
- Take a detailed history and perform a physical examination[2]
- Be aware of the risks of AMA[3]

Subsequent management depends on gestational age

1st trimester
- Early ultrasound to document gestational age, confirm fetal viability, exclude twins
- Routine pregnancy laboratory tests at the first prenatal visit

Offer definitive aneuploidy testing[4]

Accepted | Declined

Offer aneuploidy screening (cell free fetal DNA or first trimester risk assessment at 11–14 weeks and/or "quadruple serum analyte screening" at 15–20 weeks)[5]

If positive, recommend formal genetic counseling and definitive aneuploidy testing (CVS or amniocentesis)

2nd trimester
- **Fetal anatomic survey at 18–22 weeks**
- Recommend fetal echo if indicated
- Offer maternal serum-alpha fetoprotein (MS-AFP) for neural tube defect screening at 15–20 weeks
- Consider early GLT screening for GDM
- Consider formal genetic counseling

Offer definitive aneuploidy testing[4]

Accepted

3rd trimester
- Serial fetal growth scans q 3–4 weeks starting at viability (24 weeks)
- Daily fetal kick counts >32 weeks
- Anesthesia consultation if significant co-morbidities are present

Consider antepartum fetal testing at term[6]

Recommend elective induction at 39–40 weeks[7]

1. Advanced maternal age (AMA) refers to a woman who is age 35 or older on her estimated date of delivery. Over the last 30 years, there has been a 30% increase in first births among women aged 35–39 years in the USA and an even higher increase (70%) among women aged 40–45 years. This change in maternal demographics poses new challenges for prenatal care. It is not clear whether the entity of "advanced paternal age" exists, although there is evidence to suggest that pregnancies fathered by men over 65 years of age are at increased risk of autosomal dominant genetic disorders (such as achondroplasia) and autism.

2. Confirm maternal age. Obtain further details about the timing and mode of conception. For example, if the pregnancy is the result of *in vitro* fertilization with donor oocytes, then the risks of fetal aneuploidy are related to the "age" of the oocytes (i.e., the age of the donor) and not the age of the woman carrying the pregnancy. Physical examination should be focused on identifying underlying co-morbid medical conditions.

Obstetric Clinical Algorithms, Second Edition. Errol R. Norwitz, George R. Saade, Hugh Miller and Christina M. Davidson.
© 2017 John Wiley & Sons, Ltd. Published 2017 by John Wiley & Sons, Ltd.

3. AMA has long been known to be a risk factor for fetal aneuploidy, including trisomy 21 (Down syndrome), trisomy 13, and trisomy 18. In this regard, there is nothing magical about age 35 at delivery. The risk of fetal aneuploidy does not jump up after that date, but increases exponentially with advancing maternal age. The reason that age 35 at delivery was chosen to define AMA, is that the risk of identifying a fetal aneuploidy by the 2nd trimester genetic amniocentesis at that maternal age is approximately equal to the procedure-related pregnancy loss rate of amniocentesis (originally estimated at 1 in 270).

In addition to the risk of fetal aneuploidy, AMA is also an independent risk factor for other adverse pregnancy events, including higher rates of spontaneous abortion, spontaneous preterm birth, gestational diabetes mellitus (GDM), gestational hypertension/preeclampsia, placenta previa, intrauterine growth restriction (IUGR), and stillbirth/intrauterine fetal death (IUFD). Other maternal complications include an increased risk of cesarean delivery and postpartum hemorrhage. The reason for these increased risks is not clear, although some of these complications can be attributed to the higher incidence of maternal medical disorders with advancing age. The risks of AMA should be reviewed with the couple at their first prenatal visit.

4. In the 1st trimester, chorionic villous sampling (CVS) can be offered for karyotype analysis at 11–14 weeks' gestation. Early amniocentesis (<15 weeks) is associated with increased pregnancy loss and is therefore not recommended. After 15 weeks, ultrasound-guided amniocentesis can be performed and amniocytes isolated for karyotype analysis (see Chapter 53, Prenatal Diagnosis). The procedure-related pregnancy loss rate for both of these procedures is estimated at 1 in 400.

5. See Chapter 53, Prenatal Diagnosis.

6. The role of routine antenatal fetal testing in pregnancies complicated by AMA in the absence of another obstetric indication (such as hypertension or IUGR) is not clear. Although there are no clear guidelines, some authorities would recommend weekly non-stress testing (NST) with an assessment of amniotic fluid volume (BPP or AFI) starting at 37–38 weeks.

7. Elective induction of labor should be offered to all AMA women at or after 39 weeks' gestation with or without cervical ripening. If the patient declines, continued expectant management with fetal testing is appropriate with induction at 40 weeks, but no later than 41 weeks.

33 Antepartum Fetal Testing[1]

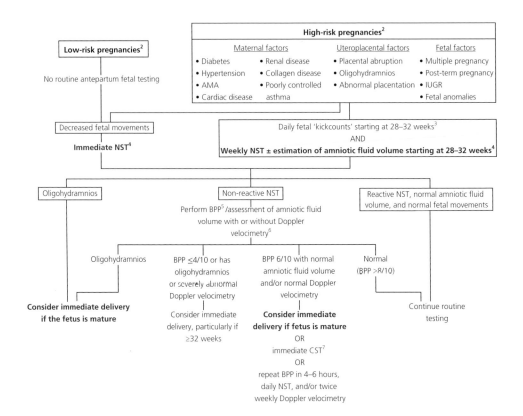

1. Obstetric care providers have two patients: the mother and fetus. Assessment of maternal well-being is relatively easy, but fetal well-being is far more difficult to assess. A number of tests have been developed to confirm fetal well-being prior to the onset of labor. There are many causes of irreversible neonatal cerebral injury, including congenital abnormalities, intracerebral hemorrhage, hypoxic ischemic injury, infection, drugs, trauma, hypotension, and metabolic derangements (such as hypoglycemia and thyroid dysfunction). Antenatal fetal testing cannot predict or reliably detect all of these causes. Moreover, the predictive value of these tests depends on gestational age, the presence or absence of congenital anomalies, and underlying clinical risk factors.

The goal of antepartum fetal surveillance is early identification of a fetus at risk for preventable morbidity or mortality due specifically to uteroplacental insufficiency. All antenatal fetal tests make the following assumptions: (i) that pregnancies may be complicated by progressive fetal asphyxia which can lead to fetal death or

Obstetric Clinical Algorithms, Second Edition. Errol R. Norwitz, George R. Saade, Hugh Miller and Christina M. Davidson.
© 2017 John Wiley & Sons, Ltd. Published 2017 by John Wiley & Sons, Ltd.

permanent handicap; (ii) that current antenatal tests can adequately discriminate between asphyxiated and non-asphyxiated fetuses; and (iii) that detection of asphyxia at an early stage can lead to an intervention which is capable of reducing the likelihood of an adverse perinatal outcome. Unfortunately, it is not clear whether any of these assumptions are true.

2. The designation "low-risk" and "high-risk" pregnancies refer to whether or not pregnancies are at risk of uteroplacental insufficiency. This list is not exhaustive.

3. Fetal movement charts ("kickcounts") involve counting the time it takes the fetus to kick 10 times ("count-to-ten") or counting all fetal movements in 1 hour. Measurements should be repeated twice daily. Use of "kickcounts" in high-risk pregnancies after 28–32 weeks can decrease perinatal mortality fourfold. Although decreased fetal movements may be a sign of fetal compromise, other factors associated with decreased fetal movements include advancing gestational age, oligohydramnios, smoking, and antenatal corticosteroid therapy.

4. Non-stress test (NST), also known as cardiotocography (CTG), refers to changes in the fetal heart rate pattern with time. It reflects maturity of the fetal autonomic nervous system. NST is non-invasive, simple to perform, readily available, and inexpensive. Interpretation is largely subjective. A "reactive" NST (R-NST)—defined as an NST with a normal baseline heart rate (110–160 bpm), moderate variability, and at least two accelerations in 20 min each lasting ≥15 sec and peaking at ≥15 bpm above baseline (or ≥10 bpm for ≥10 sec if <32 weeks)—is reassuring and is associated with normal neurologic outcome. If less than 2 accelerations occur in the first 20 minutes, the monitoring should be extended another 20 minutes before it is called non-reactive. The same criteria should be used for the second 20 minutes. In high-risk pregnancies, weekly NST after 32 weeks has been shown to decrease perinatal mortality. A non-reactive NST (NR-NST) should be interpreted in light of gestational age. Once a R-NST has been documented, it should remain so throughout gestation. A NR-NST at term is associated with poor perinatal outcome in only 20% of cases. Vibroacoustic stimulation (VAS) refers to the response of the fetal heart rate to a vibroacoustic stimulus. An acceleration on NST (≥15 bpm for ≥15 sec) is a positive result. It is a useful adjunct to decrease the time to achieve a R-NST and to decrease the proportion of NR-NST at term, thereby precluding the need for further testing. Variables decelerations may be noted on the NST. Non-repetitive variables decelerations (less than 3 in 20 minutes) lasting less than 30 seconds are not associated with fetal compromise. Repetitive variables or those lasting more than 1 minute should lead to further evaluation.

5. Biophysical profile (BPP) refers to a sonographic scoring system designed to assess fetal well-being. The five variables described in the original BPP include: NST, fetal movement, fetal tone, amniotic fluid volume, and fetal breathing; 2 points are awarded if the variable is present or normal; 0 points if absent or abnormal. Amniotic fluid volume is the most important variable. More recently, BPP is interpreted without the NST.

6. Umbilical artery Doppler velocimetry measurements reflect resistance to blood flow from the fetus to the placenta. Absent or reversed end-diastolic flow (so-called severely abnormal Doppler velocimetry) is associated with poor perinatal outcome in the setting of IUGR. It is unclear how to interpret these data in the setting of a normally grown fetus. Abnormal flow in the fetal middle cerebral artery (MCA) and/or ductus venosus may help in the timing of delivery of IUGR fetuses.

7. Contraction stress test (CST), also known as the oxytocin stimulation test (OST), refers to

the response of the fetal heart rate to artificially induced uterine contractions. A minimum of three uterine contractions in 10 min are required to interpret the test. A negative CST (i.e., no decelerations with contractions) is reassuring. A positive CST (i.e., repetitive late or severe variable decelerations with ≥50% of contractions) is associated with adverse perinatal outcome in 35–40% of cases. Although the false-positive rate exceeds 50%, a positive CST should result in immediate and urgent delivery. An equivocal CST should be repeated in 24–72 hours. Because this test is time-consuming, requires skilled nursing care, and may precipitate "fetal distress" requiring emergent cesarean delivery, it is rarely used in clinical practice.

34 Breast Lesions

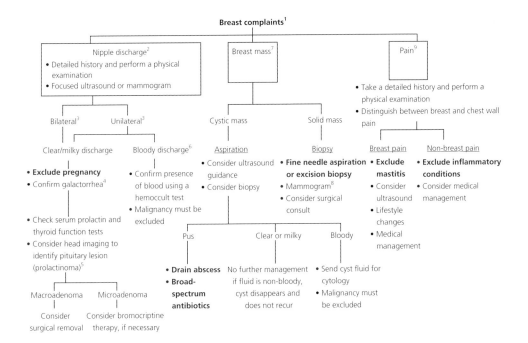

1. A wide range of disorders can present with symptoms relating to the breast, including developmental disorders and diseases of infectious, endocrine, and neoplastic etiology. The presenting symptoms fall into four main categories: pruritus, pain (mastalgia), nipple discharge, and breast masses. Careful attention to history and physical exam as well as selective use of laboratory and imaging studies will allow definitive diagnosis. While the majority of breast conditions are benign, an underlying malignancy should always be excluded. Breast discomfort (mastalgia) may be cyclic or non-cyclic. Cyclic mastalgia (breast pain that varies with the menstrual cycle) is not related to cancer, but may be severe enough to require symptomatic

treatment. Non-cyclic mastalgia should be evaluated further to exclude mastitis, abscess, fat necrosis, or trauma. Persistent severe localized breast pain warrants serial clinical breast exams and interval mammograms with or without guided biopsy to exclude malignancy.

2. A detailed history should be taken regarding the character, timing, color, and consistency of the discharge. Spontaneous discharge more likely represents an intraductal growth, whereas discharge only upon stimulation or squeezing of the nipple is less concerning. A thorough clinical breast exam should be performed. Breast imaging is recommended either in the form of a focused ultrasound (which is useful for ductal

Obstetric Clinical Algorithms, Second Edition. Errol R. Norwitz, George R. Saade, Hugh Miller and Christina M. Davidson.
© 2017 John Wiley & Sons, Ltd. Published 2017 by John Wiley & Sons, Ltd.

disease) or mammography (which is preferred in women ≥30 years old). Ductography is technically challenging, but may be useful in some situations. MRI and MRI ductography are gaining popularity as the technology improves.

3. Bilateral nipple discharge almost always represents benign disease. Non-milky, non-bloody bilateral nipple discharge is symptomatic of duct ectasia (plasma cell mastitis) in most cases. Unilateral nipple discharge raises concern about malignancy, but may represent a benign condition (such as intraductal papilloma). Pathologic examination of biopsy material is required to distinguish between these possibilities.

4. Galactorrhea refers to an inappropriate production of milk by the breast. It typically presents as a painless, milky discharge from the breasts bilaterally. Microscopic examination of the discharge will stain positive for fat droplets. It may occur during pregnancy or may represent an underlying endocrine disorder. Women with galactorrhea typically have elevated serum prolactin levels. Causes of elevated prolactin levels include prolactinoma, underlying medical conditions (hypothyroidism, renal failure, encephalitis, meningitis, craniopharyngioma, hypothalamic tumors, hydrocephalus), medications (oral contraceptives, anabolic steroids, medroxyprogesterone acetate, reserpine, omeprazole, calcium channel blockers, opiates, antiemetics, phenothiazines, tricyclic antidepressants, butyrophenones), and other substances (marijuana, alcohol). If pituitary macroadenoma is excluded, the patient has normal menstrual cycles, and the galactorrhea is not socially embarrassing, no treatment is necessary. If one of these medications is implicated, it may be possible to change or discontinue the medication in consultation with the prescribing provider. Dopamine agonists are considered first-line therapy when medical management is warranted. Cabergoline (0.25 mg twice weekly) has replaced bromocriptine as the drug of choice due to better efficacy and fewer side effects. Symptoms typically resolve within 2–3 weeks and, in the case of a macroadenoma, regression can occur within 6 weeks, but may take as long as 6 months. Fewer than 10% of patients will require long-term dopamine agonist therapy.

5. Prolactinoma is a prolactin-secreting adenoma of the pituitary gland. Dopamine agonists are usually adequate to control symptoms and cause tumor regression (see above). Transsphenoidal resection of the adenoma should be reserved for patients who have macroadenomas (>1.0 cm), have failed medical treatment, or have symptoms of headache or evidence of visual field defects (bitemporal hemianopia).

6. A bloody nipple discharge is concerning for cancer. While only 4% of spontaneous, unilateral, bloody discharge represent cancer, a history of a bloody nipple discharge (whether unilateral or bilateral) should be thoroughly evaluated to exclude malignancy. Any elicited discharge should be examined for the presence of blood (by guiac testing) and managed in concert with the physical findings and breast imaging. A unilateral papilloma arising from the duct is the most likely cause and should be thoroughly evaluated by core needle biopsy to exclude atypia, ductal carcinoma in situ (DCIS), and frank ductal carcinoma. Ductography may be useful in some cases. Cytology alone is no longer considered sufficiently sensitive, specific, or cost-effective.

7. While not all breast masses are cancer, it should be remembered that a palpable mass is the most common presenting symptom of breast cancer. Therefore, reports of a suspected breast mass should always be taken seriously. A detailed history should be taken regarding the timing, character, and consistency of the mass. Associated clinical features may include nipple discharge and pain. The patient's age, parity, menopausal status, personal or family history of cancer, and medication history should also be recorded. The presence of constitutional symptoms (weight loss, anorexia) should be

evaluated, since these may point to an underlying malignancy. A detailed clinical breast exam may confirm the presence of the mass as well as its location, size, mobility, consistency, and nodularity. The overlying skin and axillary and supraclavicular lymph nodes should also be examined. Aspiration, imaging (mammography, ultrasound), and biopsy may be necessary to determine what the mass represents.

8. Mammography and directed breast biopsies have led to the increased detection of subclinical abnormalities (such as clustered microcalicifications or asymmetric densities) that may reflect precancerous disease or early breast cancer. Approximately 30% of all biopsies of mammographically abnormal lesions are found to be malignant. Indeed, 35–50% of early breast cancers are detectable only by mammography. Biopsy of the abnormality may be indicated if the diagnostic mammogram remains suspicious. A negative mammogram does not exclude cancer, since upwards of 40% of breast cancers are detectable only by palpation. A screening mammogram is not routinely indicated in young women (<28 years) or in pregnancy, because of the density of the breast tissue.

9. A detailed history and a careful physical examination will determine if the pain is cyclical (usually worse during the luteal phase of the menstrual cycle), bilateral, its severity, and the presence or absence of associated symptoms. Breast pain can have a significant impact on both physical and sexual quality of life. Non-cyclical pain can be a consequence of breast size or inflammatory conditions such as mastitis, ductal ectasia, and hidradenitis suppurativa. It can also be associated with the chest wall, either musculoskeletal or costochondritis (Tietze's syndrome). In rare cases, cholecystitis or ischemic heart disease can masquerade as chest-wall pain. Ultrasound is frequently more helpful in women <30 years old with denser breasts, whereas abnormalities on mammography may be diagnostic at any age, depending on the findings. In the absence of a treatable lesion, dietary changes, increased breast support, or nonsteroidal anti-inflammatory drugs (NSAIDs) can be considered as first-line medical management. In more severe cases of mastalgia, danazol (the only FDA-approved treatment) or tamoxifen should be considered, while recognizing their significant side effects and reproductive implications.

35 Cervical Insufficiency

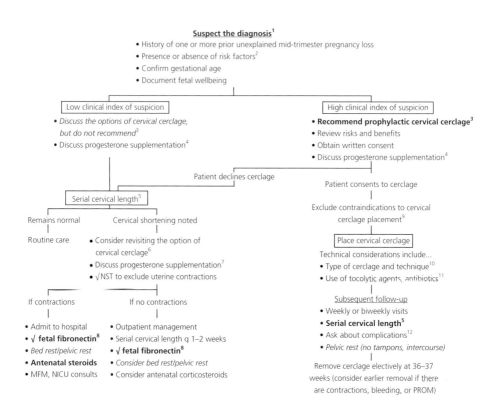

Suspect the diagnosis[1]
- History of one or more prior unexplained mid-trimester pregnancy loss
- Presence or absence of risk factors[2]
- Confirm gestational age
- Document fetal wellbeing

Low clinical index of suspicion
- *Discuss the options of cervical cerclage, but do not recommend[3]*
- Discuss progesterone supplementation[4]

High clinical index of suspicion
- **Recommend prophylactic cervical cerclage[3]**
- Review risks and benefits
- Obtain written consent
- Discuss progesterone supplementation[4]

Patient declines cerclage

Patient consents to cerclage

Serial cervical length[5]

Exclude contraindications to cervical cerclage placement[9]

Remains normal — Cervical shortening noted

Routine care

- Consider revisiting the option of cervical cerclage[6]
- Discuss progesterone supplementation[7]
- √NST to exclude uterine contractions

Place cervical cerclage

Technical considerations include...
- Type of cerclage and technique[10]
- Use of tocolytic agents, antibiotics[11]

If contractions

If no contractions

- Admit to hospital
- **√ fetal fibronectin[8]**
- *Bed rest/pelvic rest*
- **Antenatal steroids**
- MFM, NICU consults

- Outpatient management
- Serial cervical length q 1–2 weeks
- **√ fetal fibronectin[8]**
- *Consider bed rest/pelvic rest*
- Consider antenatal corticosteroids

Subsequent follow-up
- Weekly or biweekly visits
- **Serial cervical length[5]**
- Ask about complications[12]
- *Pelvic rest (no tampons, intercourse)*

Remove cerclage electively at 36–37 weeks (consider earlier removal if there are contractions, bleeding, or PROM)

1. Cervical insufficiency (also known as cervical incompetence (CI)) refers to a <u>functional</u> weakness of the cervix resulting in a failure to carry a pregnancy till term. CI is a <u>clinical</u> diagnosis characterized by acute, painless dilatation of the cervix usually in the mid-trimester (16–24 weeks) culminating in membrane prolapse and/or pPROM with resultant preterm and often previable delivery. Symptoms may include watery discharge, pelvic pressure, vaginal bleeding, or pPROM, but most women are asymptomatic. Uterine contractions are typically absent or minimal. The cause is not known. There is no test in the non-pregnant state that can confirm the diagnosis. CI complicates 0.1–2% of all pregnancies, and is responsible for 15% of births between 16–28 weeks' gestation.

2. Risk factors for CI include a prior history of CI, *in utero* diethylstilbestrol (DES) exposure,

Obstetric Clinical Algorithms, Second Edition. Errol R. Norwitz, George R. Saade, Hugh Miller and Christina M. Davidson.
© 2017 John Wiley & Sons, Ltd. Published 2017 by John Wiley & Sons, Ltd.

connective tissue disorders (Ehlers-Danlos syndrome), cervical hypoplasia, (possibly) prior cervical surgery (cone biopsy, LEEP), and (possibly) ≥2 late D&E procedures. Most patients with CI have no identifiable risk factors.

3. Prophylactic (elective) cerclage placement at 13–16 weeks is the appropriate treatment for CI, because of the 15–30% risk of recurrence. If the prior preterm birth was due to preterm labor and not CI, then elective cerclage is not indicated. In women with prior spontaneous preterm birth, serial cervical length measurements with cerclage placement, if shortened, are recommended. Elective cerclage has only been proven effective in women with ≥2 mid-trimester pregnancy losses due to CI. Prophylactic cerclage is not indicated for multiple pregnancies or a history of *in utero* DES exposure in the absence of a prior pregnancy loss.

4. Progesterone supplementation (17α-hydroxyprogesterone caproate 250 mg IM weekly starting between 16 and 20 weeks through 36 weeks) can prevent preterm birth in women with prior spontaneous preterm birth of a liveborn singleton between 20 weeks and 36 weeks 6 days. This option should be discussed and the discussion documented.

5. Cervical length (CL) should be measured serially in women at high risk for preterm birth, including a baseline measurement at 16–18 weeks and q 1–2 weeks thereafter depending on the clinical setting. Measurements can be discontinued at 24 weeks. Mean CL at 22–24 weeks is 3.5 cm (10th–90th percentile is 2.5–4.5 cm). A CL of <2.5 cm is abnormal. A CL of <1.5 cm occurs in <2% of women, but is associated with a 60% and 90% risk of preterm birth <28 weeks and <32 weeks, respectively.

6. Cervical cerclage placement for either asymptomatic cervical shortening (salvage/rescue cerclage) or premature effacement and/or dilatation of the cervix (emergent cerclage) is

controversial. The weight of evidence in the literature suggests that there is no benefit from such procedures.

7. It remains controversial as to whether progesterone supplementation administered vaginally can prevent preterm birth in some women at high risk by virtue of a short cervix (<1.5 cm) measured on transvaginal ultrasound in the mid-trimester.

8. See Chapter 55 (Screening for Preterm Birth).

9. Absolute contraindications to cerclage include uterine contractions/preterm labor, intraamniotic/vaginal infection, ruptured membranes, IUFD, major fetal structural/chromosomal anomaly incompatible with life, absence of patient consent, and ≥28 weeks' gestation. Relative contraindications include unexplained vaginal bleeding, IUGR, advanced cervical dilatation with prolapsing membranes (because of 50% risk of rupture of membranes), and ≥24 weeks' gestation.

10. Written consent is required. An ultrasound should be performed prior to placement to confirm fetal viability and exclude major structural anomalies. Regional anesthesia is preferred. A postoperative ultrasound is recommended to confirm fetal well-being. The decision of which non-absorbable suture and transvaginal cerclage technique to use (Shirodkar, McDonald) is best left to the discretion of the care provider. Shirodkar cerclage is a single suture placed around the cervix at the level of the internal os after surgically reflecting the bladder anteriorly and rectum posteriorly. McDonald cerclage is one or more purse-string sutures around the cervix placed without dissection of the bladder or rectum. These two types of cerclages are likely equally effective. Transabdominal cerclage is a more invasive procedure requiring a laparotomy for placement and subsequent cesarean delivery, and should therefore be reserved for women in whom a transvaginal cerclage is technically

impossible to place or who have failed previous transvaginal cerclage placements.

11. There are insufficient data to recommend routine use of prophylactic antibiotics or tocolytic medications for elective cerclage placement, although there may be some benefit for emergency cerclage.

12. Short-term complications (<24 hours) include excessive blood loss, PROM, and pregnancy loss (3–20%). Long-term complications include cervical lacerations (3–4%), chorioamnionitis (4%), cervical stenosis (1%), and bladder pain and migration of the suture (rare). Puerperal infection is two-fold more common in women with a cerclage (6%).

36 First-trimester Vaginal Bleeding

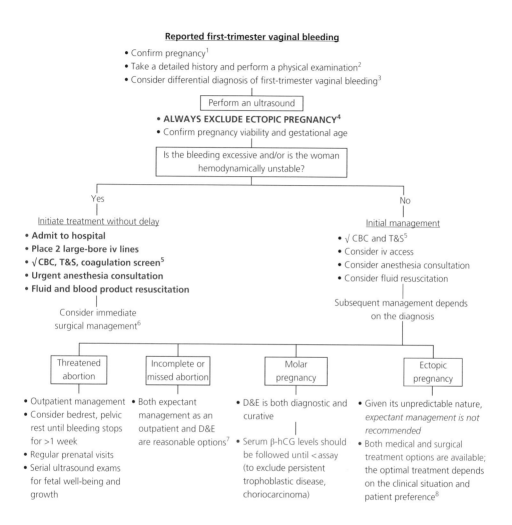

<u>Reported first-trimester vaginal bleeding</u>
- Confirm pregnancy[1]
- Take a detailed history and perform a physical examination[2]
- Consider differential diagnosis of first-trimester vaginal bleeding[3]

Perform an ultrasound
- **ALWAYS EXCLUDE ECTOPIC PREGNANCY[4]**
- Confirm pregnancy viability and gestational age

Is the bleeding excessive and/or is the woman hemodynamically unstable?

Yes

<u>Initiate treatment without delay</u>
- **Admit to hospital**
- **Place 2 large-bore iv lines**
- **√ CBC, T&S, coagulation screen[5]**
- **Urgent anesthesia consultation**
- **Fluid and blood product resuscitation**

Consider immediate surgical management[6]

No

<u>Initial management</u>
- √ CBC and T&S[5]
- Consider iv access
- Consider anesthesia consultation
- Consider fluid resuscitation

Subsequent management depends on the diagnosis

Threatened abortion	Incomplete or missed abortion	Molar pregnancy	Ectopic pregnancy
• Outpatient management • Consider bedrest, pelvic rest until bleeding stops for >1 week • Regular prenatal visits • Serial ultrasound exams for fetal well-being and growth	• Both expectant management as an outpatient and D&E are reasonable options[7]	• D&E is both diagnostic and curative • Serum β-hCG levels should be followed until < assay (to exclude persistent trophoblastic disease, choriocarcinoma)	• Given its unpredictable nature, *expectant management is not recommended* • Both medical and surgical treatment options are available; the optimal treatment depends on the clinical situation and patient preference[8]

1. A positive serum β-hCG (>5 mIU/mL) confirms the presence of trophoblast tissue (although, in the case of complete abortion, the tissue may already have been passed). Very high levels of β-hCG suggest a molar pregnancy. Very rarely, β-hCG may be a marker of an ovarian tumor.

2. Bleeding in the first trimester is common; 15–20% of clinically diagnosed pregnancies end in miscarriage. The timing, extent, and severity of the bleeding should be documented. Maternal vital signs should be taken to rule out hemodynamic instability. Speculum examination allows

Obstetric Clinical Algorithms, Second Edition. Errol R. Norwitz, George R. Saade, Hugh Miller and Christina M. Davidson.
© 2017 John Wiley & Sons, Ltd. Published 2017 by John Wiley & Sons, Ltd.

visualization of the cervix and potentially the location of products of conception. Bimanual exam may help estimate gestational age and identify an adnexal mass or tenderness.

3. The differential diagnosis of first-trimester vaginal bleeding includes: (i) a threatened abortion (defined as a viable intrauterine pregnancy <20 weeks with a closed cervix), incomplete abortion (viable intrauterine pregnancy with an open cervix), missed abortion (nonviable intrauterine pregnancy) or complete abortion (complete passage of an intrauterine pregnancy and closure of the cervix); (ii) ectopic pregnancy (implantation of the pregnancy outside the uterine cavity, including fallopian tubes, cornua, cervix or ovary); (iii) gestational trophoblastic disease (including molar pregnancy); and (iv) less commonly, an "implantation bleed," a cervical or vaginal lesion (such as a cervical erosion or postcoital bleeding), and rectal bleeding (hemorrhoids).

4. All first-trimester vaginal bleeding should be regarded as an *ectopic pregnancy* until proven otherwise. Failure to promptly diagnose and manage an ectopic pregnancy can be catastrophic. Ectopic pregnancy accounts for 10% of all pregnancy-related maternal deaths, and is the most common cause of maternal death in the first half of pregnancy. Abdominal pain, absence of menses, and irregular vaginal bleeding (usually spotting) are the main symptoms. The most common presenting sign in a woman with symptomatic ectopic pregnancy is abdominal tenderness, and 50% will have a palpable adnexal mass. Ruptured ectopic pregnancies cause shoulder pain in 10–20% of cases as a result of diaphragmatic irritation from the hemoperitoneum. Profound intraperitoneal hemorrhage can lead to tachycardia and hypotension. The amount of vaginal bleeding is not a reliable indicator of the severity of the hemorrhage since bleeding is often concealed. The primary goal of ultrasound is to confirm the presence of an intrauterine pregnancy, which should be evident by transabdominal

ultrasound at a serum β-hCG level of ≥6000 mIU/mL and by transvaginal ultrasound at a serum β-hCG level of ≥1200 mIU/mL (approximately 5 weeks from LMP). The absence of an intrauterine pregnancy on ultrasound with a positive serum β-hCG level should raise the suspicion of an ectopic pregnancy. Only rarely will the ectopic pregnancy itself be visible on ultrasound. The presence of free fluid (blood) in the abdomen suggests a ruptured ectopic or ruptured ovarian cyst.

5. If the patient is Rh negative, she should receive anti-Rh[D]-immunoglobulin (RhoGAM) 300 μg IM to prevent Rh isoimmunization.

6. The nature of the surgical procedure will depend on the diagnosis: (i) D&E if an incomplete abortion is suspected; and (ii) laparoscopy and/or explorative laparotomy if a ruptured ectopic pregnancy or ovarian cyst is diagnosed.

7. If the patient is hemodynamically stable with minimal bleeding, expectant management on an outpatient basis is reasonable and will likely avoid a surgical procedure. Only 10% of such women will subsequently require a D&E for excessive vaginal bleeding.

8. Goals of management for an ectopic pregnancy are to prevent maternal mortality, reduce morbidity, and preserve fertility. Once the diagnosis is confirmed, expectant management is rarely justified. Most (95%) ectopic pregnancies occur in the fallopian tubes. Treatment options for such pregnancies include:

• *Methotrexate (MTX)* (50 mg/m^2 im) is an effective treatment for patients who are hemodynamically stable without evidence of rupture, who are compliant, and who meet the selection criteria (below). The dose is administered on day 1, but serum β-hCG levels typically continue to rise for several days thereafter. An acceptable response to MTX therapy is defined as a ≥15% decrease in serum β-hCG levels from day 4 to day 7. β-hCG levels should thereafter be followed weekly. Most cases will be successfully treated with one dose of MTX, but up to 25% will require two or more doses if the serial β-hCG levels plateau or rise. Patients with a gestational sac >3.5 cm, starting β-hCG > 6000 mIU/mL or fetal cardiac motion evident on ultrasound are at higher risk for MTX failure and should be considered for surgical management. Side-effects of MTX are generally mild and include nausea, vomiting, bloating, and transient transaminitis. Increased abdominal pain will occur in up to 75% of patients due to tubal abortion and serosal irritation or distension of the fallopian tube. All MTX patients should be closely monitored due to the risk of rupture and hemorrhage.

- *Surgical therapy.* Definitive surgery (salpingectomy) is the treatment of choice for women who are not hemodynamically stable or where the fallopian tube is significantly damaged. Conservative surgery may be appropriate for the hemodynamically stable patient. Laparoscopic salpingostomy and removal of the products of conception are the most common conservative surgical procedure. The injection of vasopressin prior to the linear incision can be used to decrease bleeding. Serum β-hCG levels must be followed until undetectable in conservatively managed patients, because 5–10% will develop a persistent ectopic pregnancy which may require further treatment with MTX. Failure to achieve hemostasis is the only indication for oophorectomy.

37 Higher-Order Multifetal Pregnancy

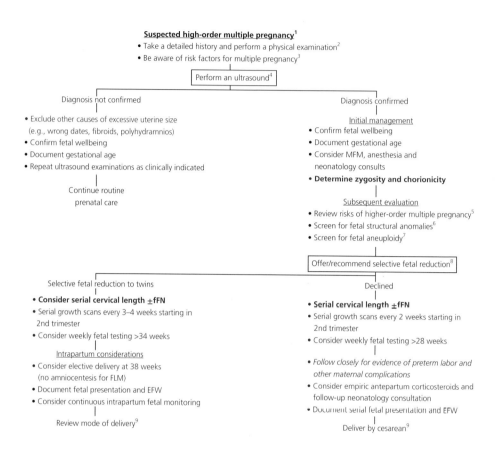

Suspected high-order multiple pregnancy[1]
- Take a detailed history and perform a physical examination[2]
- Be aware of risk factors for multiple pregnancy[3]

Perform an ultrasound[4]

Diagnosis not confirmed
- Exclude other causes of excessive uterine size
  (e.g., wrong dates, fibroids, polyhydramnios)
- Confirm fetal wellbeing
- Document gestational age
- Repeat ultrasound examinations as clinically indicated

Continue routine
prenatal care

Diagnosis confirmed

Initial management
- Confirm fetal wellbeing
- Document gestational age
- Consider MFM, anesthesia and
  neonatology consults
- **Determine zygosity and chorionicity**

Subsequent evaluation
- Review risks of higher-order multiple pregnancy[5]
- Screen for fetal structural anomalies[6]
- Screen for fetal aneuploidy[7]

Offer/recommend selective fetal reduction[8]

Selective fetal reduction to twins
- **Consider serial cervical length ±fFN**
- Serial growth scans every 3–4 weeks starting in
  2nd trimester
- Consider weekly fetal testing >34 weeks

Intrapartum considerations
- Consider elective delivery at 38 weeks
  (no amniocentesis for FLM)
- Document fetal presentation and EFW
- Consider continuous intrapartum fetal monitoring

Review mode of delivery[9]

Declined
- **Serial cervical length ±fFN**
- Serial growth scans every 2 weeks starting in
  2nd trimester
- Consider weekly fetal testing >28 weeks

- *Follow closely for evidence of preterm labor and
  other maternal complications*
- Consider empiric antepartum corticosteroids and
  follow-up neonatology consultation
- Document serial fetal presentation and EFW

Deliver by cesarean[9]

1. Multifetal pregnancies complicate 3% of all deliveries. The numbers had been steadily increasing until recent changes in assisted reproductive technology (ART) that have led to a reduction in the number of embryos transfer during IVF. Higher-order multifetal pregnancies (triplets and up) constitute 0.1–0.3% of all births.

2. Multifetal pregnancy should be excluded in all patients who have undergone ART and suspected in women with excessive symptoms of pregnancy (e.g., nausea and vomiting) or uterine size larger than expected for gestational age.

3. The major risk factor for high-order multifetal pregnancy is ART. In this regard, ovulation induction/intrauterine insemination poses a higher risk than *in vitro* fertilization. Minor risk factors include a family or personal history of multifetal pregnancy (except monozygous twins), advanced maternal age, and African-American ethnicity.

Obstetric Clinical Algorithms, Second Edition. Errol R. Norwitz, George R. Saade, Hugh Miller and Christina M. Davidson.
© 2017 John Wiley & Sons, Ltd. Published 2017 by John Wiley & Sons, Ltd.

4. Ultrasound will confirm the diagnosis, gestational age, fetal well-being, and chorionicity (arrangement of placenta/fetal membranes). Since high-order multifetal pregnancy can contain monozygous pairs, it is imperative that chorionicity be carefully established as soon as possible by someone who is specially trained and credentialed in advanced ultrasound, such as a MFM subspecialist.

5. Antepartum complications develop in 80% of multifetal pregnancies versus 20–30% of singleton gestations. Preterm delivery is the most common complication and the risk of preterm delivery increases as fetal number increases: the average length of gestation is 40 weeks in singletons, 37 weeks in twins, 33 weeks in triplets, and 29 weeks in quadruplets. Fetal growth discordance (defined as ≥25% difference in EFW) is associated with a significant increase in perinatal mortality. Maternal complications include an increased risk of gestational diabetes, preeclampsia, preterm premature rupture of membranes, anemia, cholestasis of pregnancy, cesarean delivery (due primarily to malpresentation), and postpartum hemorrhage. Other fetal complications include an increased risk of fetal structural anomalies, intrauterine fetal demise (IUFD) of one or both twins (see Chapter 39, Intrauterine Fetal Demise), twin-to-twin transfusion syndrome (TTTS), twins reverse arterial perfusion (TRAP) sequence, and cord entanglement in the case of monochorionic-monoamniotic pair (see Chapter 57).

6. Multifetal pregnancies are at increased risk of fetal structural anomalies compared with singletons. A detailed fetal anatomic survey of each fetus is indicated at 18–20 weeks. Fetal echocardiography is not routinely recommended in multiple pregnancies, but is indicated if the conception was by ART.

7. Maternal serum alpha-fetoprotein (MS-AFP), "quadruple panel" serum analyte screening (MS-AFP, estriol, hCG, and inhibin A), and first trimester risk assessment (nuchal translucency (NT) + serum PAPP-A and β-hCG) have not been adequately validated in higher-order multiple pregnancies. As such, NT alone has become the preferred aneuploidy screening test for higher-order multiple pregnancies. Chorionic villous sampling (CVS) and amniocentesis can be offered for definitive karyotype analysis, but are associated with procedure-related pregnancy loss rate (estimated at 1 in 400).

8. Spontaneous reduction in the first trimester occurs in 10–15% of higher-order multifetal pregnancies. If not, the option of multifetal pregnancy reduction (MFPR) to twins at 10–13 weeks should be offered. The benefits of MFPR include increased length of gestation, increased birth weight, and reduced prematurity and perinatal mortality and mortality. For quadruplet pregnancies and upward, the benefits of MFPR clearly outweigh the risks. In the absence of fetal anomaly, no clear benefit has been demonstrated for reduction of twins to a singleton. A recent Cochrane Review concluded that triplet pregnancies benefit from selective reduction to twins, with a reduction in pregnancy loss, antenatal complications, preterm birth, and neonatal death. The procedure-related pregnancy loss rate prior to 20 weeks may be as high as 15% (range: 5–35%), which is comparable to the background spontaneous loss rate for higher-order multiple pregnancies. However, the fetal loss rate increases with advancing gestation at the time of the reduction. MFPR should be distinguished from selective fetal reduction in which one fetus is selectively terminated because of a known structural or chromosomal abnormality.

9. Route of delivery depends on fetal number, gestational age, EFW, presentation, and maternal and fetal wellbeing (see Chapter 63, Cesarean Delivery). Cesarean delivery has traditionally been recommended for all higher-order multifetal pregnancies, although vaginal delivery may be appropriate in selected patients.

38 Hyperemesis Gravidarum

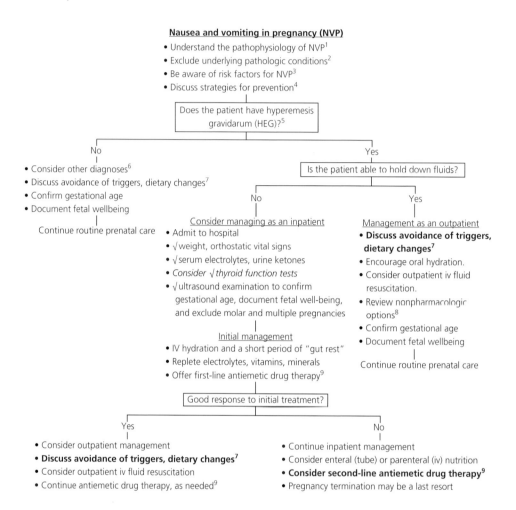

Nausea and vomiting in pregnancy (NVP)
- Understand the pathophysiology of NVP[1]
- Exclude underlying pathologic conditions[2]
- Be aware of risk factors for NVP[3]
- Discuss strategies for prevention[4]

Does the patient have hyperemesis gravidarum (HEG)?[5]

No
- Consider other diagnoses[6]
- Discuss avoidance of triggers, dietary changes[7]
- Confirm gestational age
- Document fetal wellbeing

Continue routine prenatal care

Yes

Is the patient able to hold down fluids?

No

Consider managing as an inpatient
- Admit to hospital
- √ weight, orthostatic vital signs
- √ serum electrolytes, urine ketones
- *Consider √ thyroid function tests*
- √ ultrasound examination to confirm gestational age, document fetal well-being, and exclude molar and multiple pregnancies

Initial management
- IV hydration and a short period of "gut rest"
- Replete electrolytes, vitamins, minerals
- Offer first-line antiemetic drug therapy[9]

Yes

Management as an outpatient
- **Discuss avoidance of triggers, dietary changes[7]**
- Encourage oral hydration.
- Consider outpatient iv fluid resuscitation.
- Review nonpharmacologic options[8]
- Confirm gestational age
- Document fetal wellbeing

Continue routine prenatal care

Good response to initial treatment?

Yes
- Consider outpatient management
- **Discuss avoidance of triggers, dietary changes[7]**
- Consider outpatient iv fluid resuscitation
- Continue antiemetic drug therapy, as needed[9]

No
- Continue inpatient management
- Consider enteral (tube) or parenteral (iv) nutrition
- **Consider second-line antiemetic drug therapy[9]**
- Pregnancy termination may be a last resort

1. Some degree of nausea and vomiting in pregnancy (NVP) or "morning sickness" occurs in >80% of all pregnancies. The mean onset of symptoms is 5–6 weeks, peaking at 9 weeks, and usually abating by 16–18 weeks; however, symptoms continue into the third trimester in 15–20% of women and 5% have symptoms that persist to term. The cause of NVP is not known, although it is thought to be related to hCG production. NVP is not a sign of an unhealthy pregnancy; in fact, pregnancies complicated by NVP have a better outcome than

Obstetric Clinical Algorithms, Second Edition. Errol R. Norwitz, George R. Saade, Hugh Miller and Christina M. Davidson.
© 2017 John Wiley & Sons, Ltd. Published 2017 by John Wiley & Sons, Ltd.

those that are not, with lower rates of miscarriage and stillbirth.

2. Conditions that may present with severe NVP include molar pregnancy, higher-order multiple pregnancy, and women with theca lutein cysts. An ultrasound can exclude these underlying conditions.

3. Risk factors for NVP include: (i) severe NVP in a prior pregnancy (recurrence rate is 15–20%); (ii) nausea and vomiting after estrogen exposure (such as combined oral contraceptive pill), with motion sickness, with migraine, or with exposure to certain tastes; (iii) a pre-existing psychiatric disorder; and (iv) diabetes. A number of protective factors have also been identified, including anosmia (inability to smell), advanced maternal age, and smoking.

4. Several strategies have been tried to prevent NVP, but most have been shown to be no better than placebo. The only intervention that may be somewhat effective in preventing NVP is multivitamin supplementation from the time of conception.

5. Hyperemesis gravidarum (HEG) refers to the severe end of the spectrum of NVP, and complicates 0.3–2% of all pregnancies. It is a <u>clinical diagnosis</u> made in the first trimester and characterized by three criteria: (i) persistent vomiting; (ii) weight loss >5% of pre-pregnancy body weight; and (iii) ketonuria. A number of other laboratory abnormalities have been described in the setting of HEG, including electrolyte derangements (hypokalemia, metabolic alkalosis), hemoconcentration (increase in hematocrit), abnormal liver enzyme (elevated ALT and mild hyperbilirubinemia), and hyperthyroidism (mildly elevated free T_4 and depressed TSH, although patients are clinically euthyroid and do not need treatment). However, none of these abnormalities is diagnostic of HEG.

6. The differential diagnosis of HEG is extensive, and includes medication-induced nausea and vomiting, infections (gastroenteritis), small bowel obstruction, peptic ulcer disease, inflammatory bowel disease, and (rarely) central nervous system disorders, malignancies, and endocrine/metabolic derangements. After 20 weeks, preeclampsia must always be excluded. NVP predating pregnancy or with abdominal pain, fever or neurologic signs suggests an alternative cause.

7. Patients should be counselled about avoidance of environmental triggers for NVP, including odors (coffee, perfume, food, smoke), noise, and visual or physical motion (flickering lights). Dietary changes may relieve NVP in some women, such as frequent, small, high-carbohydrate/low-fat meals; elimination of spicy foods; eating salty or high-protein meals and cold, carbonated, or sour fluids (ginger ale, lemonade). Powdered ginger (1 g daily) and foods containing ginger (ginger lollipops) have been shown to be effective in mild NVP.

8. Nonpharmacologic interventions (such as acupuncture, acupressure wristbands, hypnosis, and psychotherapy) have been proposed to treat mild NVP, but with variable results. Meta-analyses of randomized trials show no significant benefit over sham therapy.

9. Several drugs have been shown to be more effective than placebo in treating NVP with few side-effects and no increased risk of congenital anomalies. A stepwise approach to antiemetic therapy is recommended. *First-line agents* include: (i) pyridoxine (vitamin B6) (10–25 mg q 8 h po) with or without the antihistamine doxylamine succinate (20 mg); (ii) antihistamines (H_1-receptor antagonists) such as promethazine (12.5–25 mg q 4 h po/im/pr). *Second-line agents* include: (i) the selective 5-HT3 serotonin receptor antagonist ondansetron (8 mg q 12 h po/im); (ii) dopamine antagonists

such as metoclopramide (5–10 mg q 8 h po/iv), prochlorperazine (5–10 mg q 3–4 h po/im or 25 mg q 12 h pr), phenothiazines or droperidol; and (iii) a short course of corticosteroids (methylprednisolone 16 mg q 8 h po/iv 3 3–14 days).

The efficacy of corticosteroids is unproven and it has been associated with preterm premature rupture of membranes (PPROM) and oral clefts when administered <10 weeks of gestation; as such, they should be used only as a last resort.

39 Intrauterine Fetal Demise

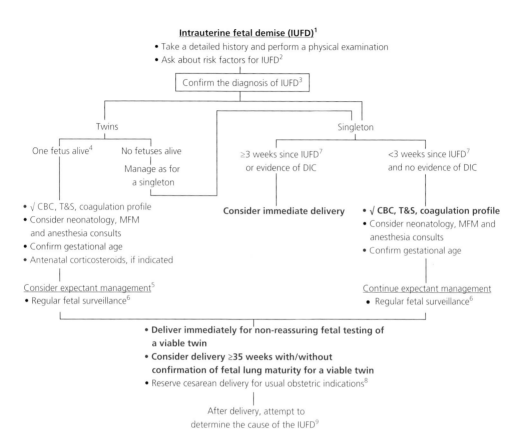

Intrauterine fetal demise (IUFD)[1]
- Take a detailed history and perform a physical examination
- Ask about risk factors for IUFD[2]

Confirm the diagnosis of IUFD[3]

Twins

One fetus alive[4]   No fetuses alive
                      |
                  Manage as for
                   a singleton

- √ CBC, T&S, coagulation profile
- Consider neonatology, MFM and anesthesia consults
- Confirm gestational age
- Antenatal corticosteroids, if indicated

Consider expectant management[5]
- Regular fetal surveillance[6]

Singleton

≥3 weeks since IUFD[7]   <3 weeks since IUFD[7]
or evidence of DIC   and no evidence of DIC

Consider immediate delivery

- √ CBC, T&S, coagulation profile
- Consider neonatology, MFM and anesthesia consults
- Confirm gestational age

Continue expectant management
- Regular fetal surveillance[6]

- **Deliver immediately for non-reassuring fetal testing of a viable twin**
- **Consider delivery ≥35 weeks with/without confirmation of fetal lung maturity for a viable twin**
- Reserve cesarean delivery for usual obstetric indications[8]

After delivery, attempt to
determine the cause of the IUFD[9]

1. Intrauterine fetal demise (IUFD) or stillbirth is defined in the United States as fetal demise after 20 weeks' gestation and prior to delivery.

2. Risk factors for IUFD include extremes of maternal age, multiple pregnancy, post-term pregnancy, male fetus, fetal macrosomia, and maternal disease such as pregestational diabetes, systemic lupus erythematosus (SLE), and preeclampsia.

3. The inability to identify fetal heart tones or the absence of uterine growth may suggest the diagnosis. Ultrasound is the gold standard to confirm an IUFD by documenting the absence of fetal cardiac activity. Other sonographic findings in later pregnancy may include scalp edema, overlapping skull sutures, and fetal maceration.

4. The death of one twin confers an increased risk of major morbidity onto the surviving twin,

Obstetric Clinical Algorithms, Second Edition. Errol R. Norwitz, George R. Saade, Hugh Miller and Christina M. Davidson.
© 2017 John Wiley & Sons, Ltd. Published 2017 by John Wiley & Sons, Ltd.

including IUFD, neurologic injury, multiorgan system failure, thrombosis, distal limb necrosis, placental abruption, and premature labor.

5. Prognosis for the surviving twin depends on the cause of death, gestational age, chorionicity, and time interval between death of the first twin and delivery of the second. Dizygous twin pregnancies do not share a circulation, and death of one twin may have little impact on the surviving twin. The dead twin may be resorbed completely or become compressed and incorporated into the fetal membranes (*fetus papyraceus*). Disseminated intravascular coagulopathy (DIC) in the surviving fetus and/or mother is rare. On the other hand, some degree of shared circulation can be demonstrated in many monozygous twin pregnancies, and the death of one fetus in this setting carries an increased risk of death of its co-twin due to profound hypotension and/or transfer of thromboplastic proteins from the dead fetus to the live fetus. If it survives, the co-twin has a 40% risk of developing neurologic injury (multicystic encephalomalacia), which may not be prevented by immediate delivery. Therefore, management of a surviving co-twin depends primarily on chorionicity and gestational age.

6. Fetal surveillance should be instituted, including daily kickcharts and weekly or twice weekly non-stress testing/biophysical profile.

7. Approximately 20–25% of women who retain a dead singleton fetus for longer than 3 weeks will develop DIC due to excessive consumption of clotting factors. Therefore, delivery should be affected within this time period.

8. Every effort should be made to avoid cesarean delivery in the setting of IUFD. As such, expectant management is often recommended. Latency (the period from fetal demise to delivery) varies, depending on the underlying cause and gestational age. In general, the earlier the gestational age, the longer the latency period. Overall, >90% of women will go into spontaneous labor within 2 weeks of a singleton fetal death. However, many women find the prospect of carrying a dead fetus distressing and want the pregnancy terminated as soon as possible. Management options include surgical dilatation and evacuation or induction of labor with cervical ripening, if indicated.

9. Causes of IUFD can be identified in only around 50% of cases. Pathologic examination of the fetus (autopsy) and placenta/fetal membranes is the single most useful test to identify a cause for the IUFD. Fetal karyotyping (with or without chromosomal microarray) should be considered in all cases of fetal death to identify chromosomal abnormalities, particularly in cases with documented fetal structural abnormalities. Approximately 5–10% of stillborn fetuses have an abnormal karyotype. Amniocentesis may be recommended to salvage viable amniocytes for cytogenetic analysis prior to delivery. Trafficking of fetal cells into the maternal circulation occurs in all pregnancies, but is usually minimal (<0.1 mL total volume). In rare instances, fetal-maternal hemorrhage may be massive, leading to fetal demise. The Kleihauer-Betke (acid elution) test or flow cytometric analysis of maternal blood may allow for an estimation of the volume of fetal blood in the maternal circulation, but should ideally be drawn within hours of the suspected bleeding episode due to the rapid clearance of fetal cells from maternal circulation. Intraamniotic infection resulting in fetal death is usually evident on clinical exam. Placental membrane culture and autopsy examination of the fetus, the placenta/fetal membranes, and the umbilical cord may be useful. Fetal X-rays or MRI may sometimes be valuable if autopsy is declined. Other conditions that should be considered in the setting of IUFD include preeclampsia (especially in the setting of intrauterine growth restriction) and maternal diabetes.

40 Fetal Growth Restriction[1]

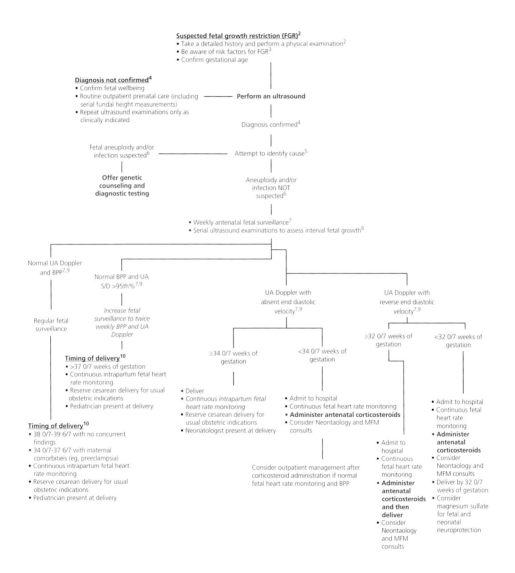

Suspected fetal growth restriction (FGR)[2]
- Take a detailed history and perform a physical examination[2]
- Be aware of risk factors for FGR[3]
- Confirm gestational age

Diagnosis not confirmed[4]
- Confirm fetal wellbeing
- Routine outpatient prenatal care (including serial fundal height measurements)
- Repeat ultrasound examinations only as clinically indicated

— **Perform an ultrasound**

Diagnosis confirmed[4]

Fetal aneuploidy and/or infection suspected[6] ——— Attempt to identify cause[5]

Offer genetic counseling and diagnostic testing

Aneuploidy and/or infection NOT suspected[6]

- Weekly antenatal fetal surveillance[7]
- Serial ultrasound examinations to assess interval fetal growth[8]

Normal UA Doppler and BPP[7,9]

Normal BPP and UA S/D >95th%[7,9]

UA Doppler with absent end diastolic velocity[7,9]

UA Doppler with reverse end diastolic velocity[7,9]

Regular fetal surveillance

Increase fetal surveillance to twice weekly BPP and UA Doppler

≥34 0/7 weeks of gestation

<34 0/7 weeks of gestation

≥32 0/7 weeks of gestation

<32 0/7 weeks of gestation

Timing of delivery[10]
- >37 0/7 weeks of gestation
- Continuous intrapartum fetal heart rate monitoring
- Reserve cesarean delivery for usual obstetric indications
- Pediatrician present at delivery

- Deliver
- *Continuous intrapartum fetal heart rate monitoring*
- *Reserve cesarean delivery for usual obstetric indications*
- *Neonatologist present at delivery*

- Admit to hospital
- Continuous fetal heart rate monitoring
- **Administer antenatal corticosteroids**
- Consider Neontaology and MFM consults

- Admit to hospital
- Continuous fetal heart rate monitoring
- **Administer antenatal corticosteroids**

Timing of delivery[10]
- 38 0/7-39 6/7 with no concurrent findings
- 34 0/7-37 6/7 with maternal comorbitieis (eg, preeclampsia)
- Continuous intrapartum fetal heart rate monitoring
- Reserve cesarean delivery for usual obstetric indications
- Pediatrician present at delivery

- Admit to hospital
- Continuous fetal heart rate monitoring
- **Administer antenatal corticosteroids and then deliver**
- Consider Neontaology and MFM consults

- Admit to hospital
- Continuous fetal heart rate monitoring
- **Administer antenatal corticosteroids**
- Consider Neontaology and MFM consults
- Deliver by 32 0/7 weeks of gestation
- Consider magnesium sulfate for fetal and neonatal neuroprotection

Consider outpatient management after corticosteroid administration if normal fetal heart rate monitoring and BPP

Obstetric Clinical Algorithms, Second Edition. Errol R. Norwitz, George R. Saade, Hugh Miller and Christina M. Davidson.
© 2017 John Wiley & Sons, Ltd. Published 2017 by John Wiley & Sons, Ltd.

1. ACOG defines fetal growth restriction (FGR) as fetuses with an estimated fetal weight (EFW) <10th percentile for gestational age; the term small for gestational age (SGA) is reserved for *newborns* with birth weight <10th percentile for gestational age. Several studies have shown that customized birth weight percentiles more accurately reflect the potential for adverse outcome. Findings from a recent study suggest that the only ultrasound EFW consistently and significantly associated with adverse compared to normal outcome was that of the <3rd percentile.

FGR can be subdivided into asymmetric and symmetric growth restriction. With symmetric growth restriction, the weight and skeletal dimensions are both below normal, whereas asymmetrically small FGR infants have normal skeletal measurements and head size, but the weight is below normal due to decreased abdominal circumference. The symmetrically small fetus (20–30%) is usually the result of some factor that influences growth in early pregnancy, most commonly fetal aneuploidy, malformations, or infection. The FGR fetus with an asymmetric growth pattern is most commonly the result of placental disease.

In the United States, approximately 4–8% of fetuses are diagnosed with FGR. FGR fetuses have higher rates of perinatal morbidity and mortality as compared with appropriate for gestational age (AGA) fetuses for any given gestational age. Neonatal morbidity associated with FGR includes meconium aspiration syndrome, hypoglycemia, polycythemia, and neonatal asphyxia. Premature FGR infants are also at increased risk of mortality, necrotizing enterocolitis, and need for neonatal respiratory support. Long-term studies show a twofold increased incidence of cerebral dysfunction (ranging from minor learning disability to cerebral palsy) in FGR infants delivered at term, and an even higher incidence if the infant was born preterm. Epidemiologic studies also suggest that these infants may be at higher risk for developing chronic disease in adulthood such as type 2 diabetes mellitus, obesity, stroke, and coronary heart disease.

2. The clinical diagnosis of FGR is difficult, and physical examination alone will fail to identify up to 50% of FGR fetuses. Fundal height measured in centimeters between 24–38 weeks approximates the gestational age and is used to screen for FGR, using a discrepancy of greater than 3. A single fundal height measurement at 32–34 weeks of gestation has been reported to be 65–85% sensitive and 96% specific for detecting FGR. Fundal height measurements are limited by maternal obesity and uterine leiomyomas.

3. FGR can be the result of maternal, fetal, and/or placental factors. Maternal etiologies include pre-existing medical conditions such as pregestational diabetes mellitus, renal insufficiency, autoimmune disease (e.g., SLE), cyanotic cardiac disease, antiphospholipid antibody syndrome and chronic hypertension; hypertensive disorders of pregnancy (e.g., gestational hypertension or preeclampsia) are additional causes. Maternal substance use and abuse (e.g., tobacco, alcohol, cocaine, or narcotics), teratogen exposure (antithrombotic drugs), and infectious diseases (e.g., malaria, cytomegalovirus, rubella, toxoplasmosis, or syphilis) can also result in FGR.

4. FGR is a radiologic diagnosis. The diagnosis is made when sonographic EFW is <10th percentile for gestational age, using the biparietal diameter (BPD), head circumference (HC), abdominal circumference (AC), and femur diaphysis length (FDL). As such, accurate gestational age dating is a prerequisite for the diagnosis. FGR likely represents the clinical end-point of many different fetal, uteroplacental, and maternal conditions.

5. Every effort should be made to determine the cause prior to delivery. Since FGR fetuses have a high incidence of structural and genetic abnormalities, investigations should include a detailed fetal anatomic survey. The placenta and umbilical cord should also be closely inspected

since certain placental disorders (e.g., abruption, infarction, circumvallate shape, hemangioma, and chorioangioma) and umbilical cord disorders (e.g., single umbilical artery, velamentous or marginal cord insertion) are associated with FGR. In addition, preeclampsia and antiphospholipid antibody syndrome should be excluded.

6. The risk of aneuploidy is increased if fetal structural abnormalities are present and/or if fetal growth restriction is detected earlier in gestation (onset in the midtrimester); in these settings, genetic counselling and prenatal diagnostic testing (amniocentesis for karyotype and PCR for cytomegalovirus and toxoplasmosis; or noninvasive prenatal diagnosis with maternal cell-free fetal DNA testing) should be offered. Management should then be directed at the underlying etiology, if identified.

7. Fetal surveillance should be instituted once FGR has been diagnosed and the gestational age is such that delivery would be considered for perinatal benefit. Antenatal surveillance should include daily fetal kickcounts and either (i) weekly or twice-weekly non-stress test (NST) with amniotic fluid assessment (modified biophysical profile); or (ii) weekly or twice-weekly biophysical profile (BPP) with NST. Doppler evaluation of the umbilical artery should also be performed at least once weekly, with the systolic to diastolic (S/D) ratio being the most common quantitative measurement. Doppler velocimetry of the umbilical artery assesses the resistance to blood perfusion of the fetoplacental unit. Maternal or placental conditions that obliterate placental vessels result in a progressive decrease in end-diastolic flow in the umbilical artery Doppler waveform until absent, and then reversed, flow during diastole is evident. Reversed end-diastolic flow in the umbilical arterial circulation represents an advanced stage of placental compromise and has been associated with obliteration of >70% of arteries in placental tertiary villi. Absent or reversed end-diastolic flow in the umbilical artery is commonly associated with severe (birth weight <3rd percentile) FGR and oligohydramnios. Umbilical artery Doppler evaluation of the fetus with suspected FGR can help differentiate the hypoxic growth-restricted fetus from the nonhypoxic small fetus, and thereby reduce perinatal mortality and unnecessary interventions. Clinical management based on Doppler evaluation of the umbilical artery in fetuses with FGR is associated with fewer perinatal deaths and fewer inductions of labor and cesarean deliveries.

8. Serial growth scans should be performed every 3 to 4 weeks. Ultrasound assessment of growth performed more frequently than every 2 weeks may be associated with inherent error in ultasonographic measurements and is not recommended.

9. Umbilical artery Doppler blood flow studies can be used clinically to guide interventions such as the frequency and type of other fetal testing, hospitalization, antenatal corticosteroid administration, and delivery. Experts have recommended Doppler surveillance up to 2–3 times per week when FGR is complicated by oligohydramnios or absent or reversed umbilical artery end-diastolic flow. Doppler changes precede deteriorating BPP scores in fetuses with severe FGR, primarily during the week before delivery. The umbilical artery Doppler changes occur approximately 4 days before BPP deterioration. Fetal breathing movement begins to diminish 2–3 days before delivery; amniotic fluid volume begins to decrease within 24 hours; composite BPP score decreases abruptly on the day of delivery, with loss of fetal movement and tone. FGR fetuses with normal BPP and Doppler velocimetry can be monitored as outpatients. Once absent or reverse end-diastolic blood flow is noted in the umbilical artery, the patients are admitted to the hospital for prolonged fetal monitoring, administration of antenatal corticosteroids, and possible delivery. Although there are no randomized studies to

guide the decision to hospitalize, admission may also be offered once fetal testing more often than 3 times per week is deemed necessary.

10. According to ACOG, FGR fetuses should be delivered when the risk of fetal death exceeds that of neonatal death. The risk of fetal death among FGR fetuses at <3rd percentile is three-fold higher than that of fetuses between the 3rd and 5th centile and 4- to 7-fold higher than fetuses between the 5th and 10th centile. The decision to deliver is frequently based on "non-reassuring fetal assessment" or lack of fetal growth over a 3–4-week interval. For a single-ton gestation with FGR, delivery is recommended between 38 0/7–39 6/7 weeks with no concurrent findings and between 34 0/7–37 6/7 weeks with concurrent findings including oligohydramnios, abnormal Doppler findings, or maternal comorbidities (e.g., preeclampsia).

41 Isoimmunization

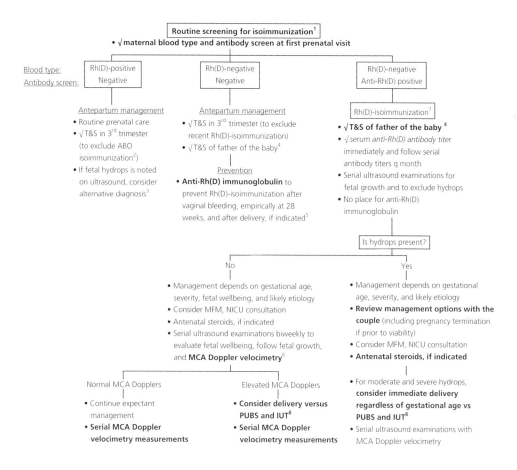

Routine screening for isoimmunization[1]
• √ maternal blood type and antibody screen at first prenatal visit

Blood type:
Antibody screen:

Rh(D)-positive
Negative

Antepartum management
• Routine prenatal care
• √ T&S in 3rd trimester (to exclude ABO isoimmunization[2])
• If fetal hydrops is noted on ultrasound, consider alternative diagnosis[3]

Rh(D)-negative
Negative

Antepartum management
• √ T&S in 3rd trimester (to exclude recent Rh(D)-isoimmunization)
• √ T&S of father of the baby[4]

Prevention
• **Anti-Rh(D) immunoglobulin** to prevent Rh(D)-isoimmunization after vaginal bleeding, empirically at 28 weeks, and after delivery, if indicated[5]

Rh(D)-negative
Anti-Rh(D) positive

Rh(D)-isoimmunization[7]
• **√ T&S of father of the baby [4]**
• √ *serum anti-Rh(D) antibody titer* immediately and follow serial antibody titers q month
• Serial ultrasound examinations for fetal growth and to exclude hydrops
• No place for anti-Rh(D) immunoglobulin

Is hydrops present?

No
• Management depends on gestational age, severity, fetal wellbeing, and likely etiology
• Consider MFM, NICU consultation
• Antenatal steroids, if indicated
• Serial ultrasound examinations biweekly to evaluate fetal wellbeing, follow fetal growth, and **MCA Doppler velocimetry**[6]

Normal MCA Dopplers
• Continue expectant management
• **Serial MCA Doppler velocimetry measurements**

Elevated MCA Dopplers
• **Consider delivery versus PUBS and IUT**[8]
• **Serial MCA Doppler velocimetry measurements**

Yes
• Management depends on gestational age, severity, and likely etiology
• **Review management options with the couple** (including pregnancy termination if prior to viability)
• Consider MFM, NICU consultation
• **Antenatal steroids, if indicated**

• For moderate and severe hydrops, **consider immediate delivery regardless of gestational age vs PUBS and IUT**[8]
• Serial ultrasound examinations with MCA Doppler velocimetry

1. Isoimmunization occurs when fetal erythrocytes express a protein that is not present on maternal erythrocytes. Since there is constant trafficking of fetal cells across the placenta into the maternal circulation, the maternal immune system can become sensitized and produce antibodies against these 'foreign' proteins. Maternal IgG antibodies can cross the placenta and destroy fetal erythrocytes leading to fetal anemia and high-output cardiac failure, known as immune hydrops fetalis. Immune hydrops is associated with a fetal hematocrit <15% (normal, 50%). The most antigenic protein on the surface of erythrocytes is D, also known as rhesus D or (Rh)D. Other antigens that can cause severe immune hydrops include Kell ("Kell kills"), Rh-E, Rh-c, and Duffy ("Duffy dies"). Antigens causing less severe hydrops include ABO, Rh-e,

Obstetric Clinical Algorithms, Second Edition. Errol R. Norwitz, George R. Saade, Hugh Miller and Christina M. Davidson.
© 2017 John Wiley & Sons, Ltd. Published 2017 by John Wiley & Sons, Ltd.

Rh-C, Fy^a, Ce, k, and s. Lewis^{a,b} incompatibility can cause mild anemia but not hydrops ("Lewis lives") because they are primarily IgM antibodies, which do not cross the placenta.

2. Since the introduction of anti-(Rh)D immunoglobulin, 60% of immune hydrops is due to ABO incompatibility, which cannot be effectively prevented.

3. Hydrops fetalis (Latin for "edema of the fetus") is a radiologic diagnosis requiring the presence of an abnormal accumulation of fluid in more than one fetal extravascular compartment, including ascites, pericardial effusion, pleural effusion, and/or subcutaneous edema. Polyhydramnios is seen in 50–75% of cases. Hydrops is a rare but very serious complication of pregnancy with a high perinatal mortality (>50%). Of all cases of fetal hydrops, 90% are due to a non-immune cause and 10% have an immune etiology. Non-immune hydrops may be due to fetal cardiac abnormalities (20–35%), chromosomal anomalies such as Turner syndrome (15%), hematological aberrations such as α-thalassemia (10%), and other causes (infections such as CMV or parvovirus B19, twin-to-twin transfusion, vascular malformations, placental anomalies, congenital metabolic disorders); 50–60% have no clear explanation.

4. If the father of the baby is Rh(D)-negative, then the fetus must be Rh(D)-negative and Rh(D) sensitization will not occur. However, because of the well-documented 10% likelihood of non-paternity in a clinic population, anti-(Rh)D immunoglobulin is often still recommended. Fetal Rh(D) status can be confirmed by amniocentesis or, more recently, through the evaluation cell-free fetal DNA in the maternal circulation.

5. Exposure of Rh(D)-negative women to as little as 0.25 mL of Rh(D)-positive blood may induce an antibody response. Since the initial immune response is IgM (which does not cross the placenta), the index pregnancy is rarely affected. However, immunization in subsequent pregnancies will trigger an IgG response that will cross the placenta and cause hemolysis. Risk factors for Rh(D) sensitization include mismatched blood transfusion (95% sensitization rate), pregnancy (16–18% sensitization rate following normal pregnancy without anti-Rh(D) IgG, 1.3% with anti-Rh(D) IgG at delivery, 0.13% with anti-Rh(D) IgG at delivery and empirically at 28 weeks), abortion (3–6%), CVS/amniocentesis (1–3%), and ectopic pregnancy (<1%). Passive immunization with anti-Rh(D) IgG can destroy fetal erythrocytes before they evoke a maternal immune response. Anti-Rh(D) IgG should be given within 72 hours of potential exposure. 300 μg (U.S.) or 500 IU (U.K.) given intramuscularly will cover up to 30 mL of fetal whole blood or 15 mL of fetal red blood cells.

6. Immune-mediated fetal hemolysis results in release of bile pigment into amniotic fluid that can be measured as the change in optical density at wavelength 450 nm (ΔOD_{450}). Traditionally, the degree of hemolysis was measured by serial amniocentesis every 1–2 weeks starting in the mid 2nd trimester. Amniotic fluid ΔOD_{450} measurements were then plotted against gestational age (Liley curve) in an attempt to predict fetal outcome. If the ΔOD_{450} rose into the upper 80% of zone 2 or into zone 3 of the Liley curve, prompt intervention was indicated. However, this test has been replaced almost entirely with non-invasive measurements of peak systolic velocity (PSV) in the middle cerebral artery (MCA) of the fetus using Doppler velocimetry. An elevated MCA PSV for gestational age has been shown to accurately identify fetuses with severe anemia requiring intervention.

7. Unlike ABO, the (Rh)D antigen is expressed only on primate erythrocytes. It is evident by 38 days of intrauterine life. Mutation in the D gene

on chromosome 1 results in lack of expression of D antigen on circulating erythrocytes. Such individuals are regarded as Rh(D)-negative. This mutation arose first in the Basque region of Spain, and the difference in prevalence of Rh(D)-negative individuals between the races may reflect the amount of Spanish blood in their ancestry: Caucasians, 15%; African-Americans, 8%; African, 4%; Native American, 1%; and Asian, <<1%.

8. Percutaneous umbilical blood sampling (PUBS) involves ultrasound-guided aspiration of fetal blood from the umbilical cord. Advantages include the ability to get a rapid fetal karyotype and to measure several hematological, immunological, and acid/base parameters in the fetus. Intrauterine fetal blood transfusions (IUT) can also be performed, but has a procedure-related fetal loss rate of 1–5% and is therefore rarely performed after 32 weeks.

42 Macrosomia

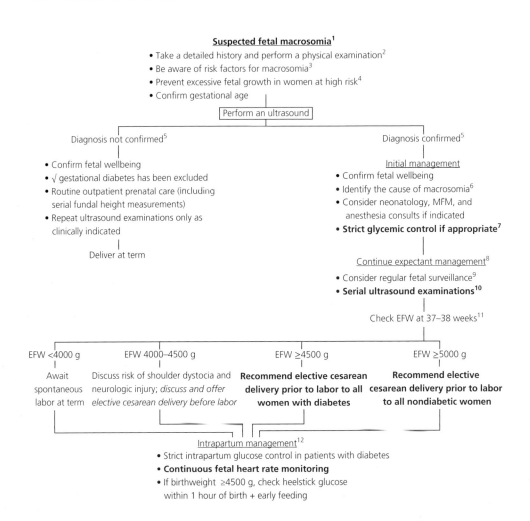

Suspected fetal macrosomia[1]
- Take a detailed history and perform a physical examination[2]
- Be aware of risk factors for macrosomia[3]
- Prevent excessive fetal growth in women at high risk[4]
- Confirm gestational age

Perform an ultrasound

Diagnosis not confirmed[5]
- Confirm fetal wellbeing
- √ gestational diabetes has been excluded
- Routine outpatient prenatal care (including serial fundal height measurements)
- Repeat ultrasound examinations only as clinically indicated

Deliver at term

Diagnosis confirmed[5]

Initial management
- Confirm fetal wellbeing
- Identify the cause of macrosomia[6]
- Consider neonatology, MFM, and anesthesia consults if indicated
- **Strict glycemic control if appropriate[7]**

Continue expectant management[8]
- Consider regular fetal surveillance[9]
- **Serial ultrasound examinations[10]**

Check EFW at 37–38 weeks[11]

EFW <4000 g	EFW 4000–4500 g	EFW ≥4500 g	EFW ≥5000 g
Await spontaneous labor at term	Discuss risk of shoulder dystocia and neurologic injury; *discuss and offer elective cesarean delivery before labor*	**Recommend elective cesarean delivery prior to labor to all women with diabetes**	**Recommend elective cesarean delivery prior to labor to all nondiabetic women**

Intrapartum management[12]
- Strict intrapartum glucose control in patients with diabetes
- **Continuous fetal heart rate monitoring**
- If birthweight ≥4500 g, check heelstick glucose within 1 hour of birth + early feeding

1. Fetal macrosomia is defined most commonly as an estimated fetal weight (EFW) – not birth weight – of ≥4500 g (10 lb 8 oz). It is a single cut-off independent of gestational age or diabetic status. It should be distinguished from "large for gestational age" (LGA), which refers to a fetus with an EFW of >90th percentile for gestational age. Macrosomic fetuses have an increased risk of intrauterine and neonatal death as well as birth trauma, especially shoulder dystocia and resultant neurologic (brachial plexus) injury. Other neonatal complications include hypoglycemia,

Obstetric Clinical Algorithms, Second Edition. Errol R. Norwitz, George R. Saade, Hugh Miller and Christina M. Davidson.
© 2017 John Wiley & Sons, Ltd. Published 2017 by John Wiley & Sons, Ltd.

polycythemia, hypocalcemia, and jaundice. In developing countries, 5% of infants weigh >4000 g at delivery and 0.5% weigh >4500 g.

2. The clinical diagnosis of fetal macrosomia is difficult, and physical examination alone will fail to identify over 50% of such fetuses. If the fundal height measurement is significantly greater than expected (>3–4 cm for gestational age), an ultrasound examination should be considered.

3. Although a number of factors have been associated with fetal macrosomia, most women with risk factors have normal-weight babies. Risk factors include: (i) maternal diabetes (seen in 35–40% of macrosomic infants); (ii) post-term pregnancy (10–20%) – of all pregnancies continuing beyond 42 weeks' gestation, 2.5% are complicated by macrosomia; (iii) maternal obesity defined as a pre-pregnancy BMI >30 kg/m^2 (10–20%) – moreover, clinical and ultrasound estimation of fetal weight is far more difficult and less accurate in obese women; and (iv) other risk factors (such as multiparity, a prior macrosomic infant, a male infant, increased maternal height, advanced maternal age, and Beckwith–Wiedemann syndrome (pancreatic islet cell hyperplasia)).

4. Meticulous glycemic control throughout pregnancy in women with pregestational or gestational diabetes mellitus (GDM) can effectively reduce the incidence of fetal macrosomia.

5. Clinical estimation of fetal weight based on fundal height measurements and abdominal palpation (Leopold's maneuvers) is largely subjective, poorly reproducible, and depends on the experience of the obstetric care provider. It is especially unreliable in women with uterine fibroids and obesity, and in multiple pregnancies. For all these reasons, ultrasound is often used to estimate fetal weight. It should be noted, however, that ultrasound is accurate only to within 15–20% of actual fetal weight. Indeed, studies have shown that ultrasound is no more accurate in predicting actual fetal weight than a clinical examination by an experienced obstetrician or than the estimate of the mother, providing she has had a previous child.

6. Most cases of macrosomia have no known cause. A detailed perinatal ultrasound should be performed to confirm gestational age, exclude other causes of a large fundal height (twins, fibroids, polyhydramnios), and to identify any fetal structural anomalies. In all cases, GDM should be excluded.

7. In women with GDM, the goal of antepartum management is to maintain strict glycemic control throughout gestation, defined as fasting blood glucose <95 mg/dL and 1 hour postprandial <140 mg/dL. This is typically achieved through a diabetic diet, moderate exercise, four times daily glucose monitoring, and additional treatment (oral hypoglycemic agents, insulin) as needed.

8. Because of the association between fetal macrosomia and birth trauma as well as peripartum maternal complications (including cesarean delivery, postpartum hemorrhage, severe perineal trauma, and puerperal infection), early induction of labor is often recommended with a view to maximizing the probability of a vaginal delivery. However, induction of labor for so-called "impending macrosomia" does not decrease the cesarean delivery rate. As such, this approach should not be encouraged.

9. Although the benefit is unclear in the absence of diabetes, most authorities recommend regular fetal surveillance in pregnancies complicated by fetal macrosomia, including daily kickcounts and weekly or twice-weekly nonstress testing and/or biophysical profile.

10. Serial growth scans of the fetus should be performed every 2–3 weeks. More regular ultrasound examinations may be indicated to document amniotic fluid volume.

11. To prevent birth trauma, elective (prophylactic) cesarean delivery should be offered before the onset of labor at or after 39 weeks to diabetic women with an EFW ≥ 4500 g and nondiabetic women with an EFW ≥ 5000 g. An elective delivery prior to 39 weeks requires confirmation of fetal lung maturity.

12. Because of the risk of shoulder dystocia, attempted vaginal delivery of a macrosomic infant should take place in a controlled fashion, with immediate access to anesthesia staff and a neonatal resuscitation team. It may be prudent to avoid assisted vaginal delivery in this setting.

43 Medically-Indicated Late Preterm and Early Term Delivery

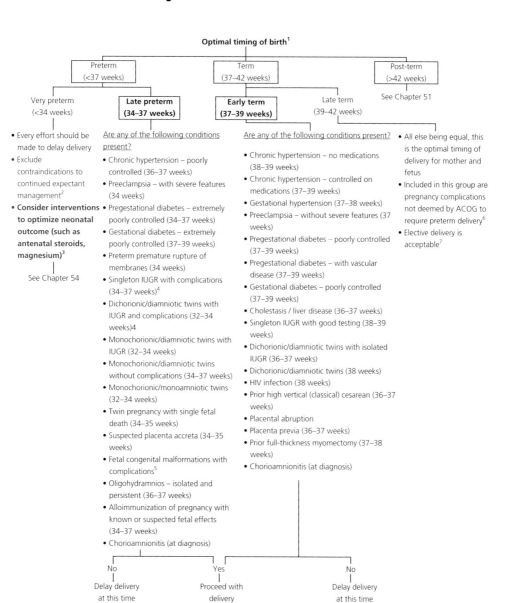

Optimal timing of birth[1]

Preterm (<37 weeks) → Very preterm (<34 weeks) / **Late preterm (34–37 weeks)**

Term (37–42 weeks) → **Early term (37–39 weeks)** / Late term (39–42 weeks)

Post-term (>42 weeks) → See Chapter 51

Very preterm (<34 weeks)
- Every effort should be made to delay delivery
- Exclude contraindications to continued expectant management[2]
- **Consider interventions to optimize neonatal outcome (such as antenatal steroids, magnesium)[3]**

See Chapter 54

Late preterm (34–37 weeks)
Are any of the following conditions present?
- Chronic hypertension – poorly controlled (36–37 weeks)
- Preeclampsia – with severe features (34 weeks)
- Pregestational diabetes – extremely poorly controlled (34–37 weeks)
- Gestational diabetes – extremely poorly controlled (37–39 weeks)
- Preterm premature rupture of membranes (34 weeks)
- Singleton IUGR with complications (34–37 weeks)[4]
- Dichorionic/diamniotic twins with IUGR and complications (32–34 weeks)4
- Monochorionic/diamniotic twins with IUGR (32–34 weeks)
- Monochorionic/diamniotic twins without complications (34–37 weeks)
- Monochorionic/monoamniotic twins (32–34 weeks)
- Twin pregnancy with single fetal death (34–35 weeks)
- Suspected placenta accreta (34–35 weeks)
- Fetal congenital malformations with complications[5]
- Oligohydramnios – isolated and persistent (36–37 weeks)
- Alloimmunization of pregnancy with known or suspected fetal effects (34–37 weeks)
- Chorioamnionitis (at diagnosis)

Early term (37–39 weeks)
Are any of the following conditions present?
- Chronic hypertension – no medications (38–39 weeks)
- Chronic hypertension – controlled on medications (37–39 weeks)
- Gestational hypertension (37–38 weeks)
- Preeclampsia – without severe features (37 weeks)
- Pregestational diabetes – poorly controlled (37–39 weeks)
- Pregestational diabetes – with vascular disease (37–39 weeks)
- Gestational diabetes – poorly controlled (37–39 weeks)
- Cholestasis / liver disease (36–37 weeks)
- Singleton IUGR with good testing (38–39 weeks)
- Dichorionic/diamniotic twins with isolated IUGR (36–37 weeks)
- Dichorionic/diamniotic twins (38 weeks)
- HIV infection (38 weeks)
- Prior high vertical (classical) cesarean (36–37 weeks)
- Placental abruption
- Placenta previa (36–37 weeks)
- Prior full-thickness myomectomy (37–38 weeks)
- Chorioamnionitis (at diagnosis)

Late term (39–42 weeks)
- All else being equal, this is the optimal timing of delivery for mother and fetus
- Included in this group are pregnancy complications not deemed by ACOG to require preterm delivery[6]
- Elective delivery is acceptable[7]

No → Delay delivery at this time

Yes → Proceed with delivery

No → Delay delivery at this time

Obstetric Clinical Algorithms, Second Edition. Errol R. Norwitz, George R. Saade, Hugh Miller and Christina M. Davidson.
© 2017 John Wiley & Sons, Ltd. Published 2017 by John Wiley & Sons, Ltd.

1. The timely onset of labor and birth is a critical determinant of perinatal outcome. The mean duration of singleton pregnancy is 40 weeks (280 days) dated from the first day of the last menstrual period (LMP). "Term" is defined as two standard deviations from the mean or, more precisely, 37–42 weeks (266–294 days) of gestation. Both preterm birth (defined as delivery prior to 37 0/7 weeks of gestation) and post-term pregnancy (failure to deliver before 42 0/7 weeks) are associated with an increased risk of adverse pregnancy events. However, under certain conditions, earlier delivery may be appropriate for either maternal or fetal indications.

2. Contraindications to continued expectant management <34 weeks include intra-amniotic infection (chorioamnionitis), excessive vaginal bleeding, nonreassuring fetal testing, fetal demise, and select maternal complications (such as severe pulmonary or cardiac disease). Under such conditions, delivery may need to be expedited. Confirmation of fetal lung maturity by amniocentesis is not necessary.

3. Interventions to improve neonatal outcome in the event of impending delivery <34 weeks include: (i) transfer to a tertiary care center; (ii) a course of antenatal corticosteroids (either betamethasone or dexamethasone); and (iii) magnesium sulfate for neuroprotection (proven benefit in improving neurologic outcome if given for a minimum of 12 hours in women delivering <32 weeks).

4. Complications include oligohydramnios, abnormal Doppler studies, and/or co-morbid conditions in the mother (such as chronic hypertension or preeclampsia).

5. Complications may include suspected worsening fetal organ damage, potential for fetal intracranial hemorrhage (such as neonatal alloimmune thrombocytopenia), prior fetal surgery or urgent need for neonatal surgery, and/or potential for adverse maternal effects from fetal condition.

6. Pregnancy complications not deemed by ACOG to require preterm delivery include well-controlled pregestational or gestational diabetes (whether or not they are on medications), prior unexplained stillbirth, morbid obesity (BMI >40 kg/m^2) and advanced maternal age.

7. According to ACOG, elective induction of labor at or after 39-0/7 weeks is a reasonable option in a well-dated pregnancy without documenting fetal lung maturity by amniocentesis. In HIV-positive women and twins, elective delivery can be performed at 38-0/7 weeks. The risk of failed induction leading to cesarean delivery should be discussed. In nulliparous patients with an unfavorable cervical exam (Bishop score <6), the risk of cesarean is clearly increased. Whether this is true also in multiparous women or nulliparous women with a favorable cervical exam is not clear.

44 Obesity

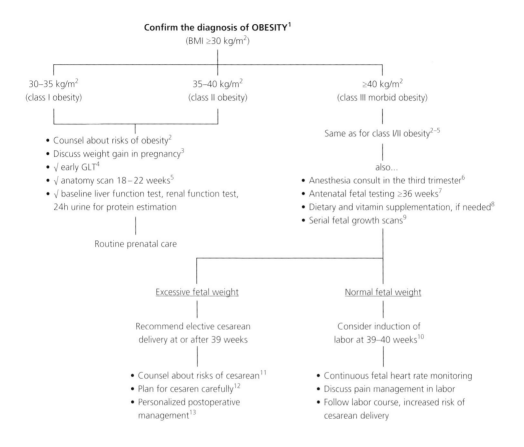

Confirm the diagnosis of OBESITY[1]
(BMI ≥30 kg/m²)

30–35 kg/m²	35–40 kg/m²	≥40 kg/m²
(class I obesity)	(class II obesity)	(class III morbid obesity)

- Counsel about risks of obesity[2]
- Discuss weight gain in pregnancy[3]
- √ early GLT[4]
- √ anatomy scan 18–22 weeks[5]
- √ baseline liver function test, renal function test, 24h urine for protein estimation

Routine prenatal care

Same as for class I/II obesity[2–5]

also...
- Anesthesia consult in the third trimester[6]
- Antenatal fetal testing ≥36 weeks[7]
- Dietary and vitamin supplementation, if needed[8]
- Serial fetal growth scans[9]

Excessive fetal weight

Recommend elective cesarean delivery at or after 39 weeks

- Counsel about risks of cesarean[11]
- Plan for cesaren carefully[12]
- Personalized postoperative management[13]

Normal fetal weight

Consider induction of labor at 39–40 weeks[10]

- Continuous fetal heart rate monitoring
- Discuss pain management in labor
- Follow labor course, increased risk of cesarean delivery

1. Body mass index (BMI) is the preferred method for reporting obesity. Normal weight is a BMI of 18.5–24.9 kg/m², overweight is 25–29.9 kg/m², and obesity is ≥30 kg/m². Obesity is further classified by BMI into class I (30–34.9 kg/m²), class II (35–39.9 kg/m²), and class III also known as morbid obesity (≥40 kg/m²). The prevalence of obesity in the USA has doubled in the last 25 years. In women of reproductive age, the prevalence of obesity now exceeds 30% and the prevalence of overweight is 55–60%. The problem of obesity is greatest among Hispanic and non-Hispanic black populations.

2. Maternal obesity is an independent risk factor for a number of long- and short-term pregnancy complications in both the mother and fetus (see table below).

3. Although both pre-pregnancy BMI and excessive weight gain during pregnancy are

Obstetric Clinical Algorithms, Second Edition. Errol R. Norwitz, George R. Saade, Hugh Miller and Christina M. Davidson.
© 2017 John Wiley & Sons, Ltd. Published 2017 by John Wiley & Sons, Ltd.

independent determinants of pregnancy outcome, pre-pregnancy BMI appears to be the more important factor. That said, the Institute of Medicine (IOM) recommends that obese women limit their weight gain in pregnancy to <15 lbs (<6.8 kg) versus 23–25 lbs (11.2–15.9 kg) in normal weight women and 15–25 lbs (6.8–11.2 kg) in overweight women. Nutrition counseling and introduction of a moderate exercise program may be helpful.

4. Given the increased risk of gestational diabetes (GDM), an early non-fasting 50-g glucose load test (GLT) should be performed at the first prenatal visit. If this early GLT is normal, it should be repeated at 24–28 weeks.

5. A detailed anatomic survey of the fetus is indicated in all obese women. Specific attention should be paid to evaluating the fetal brain, spine, and heart. Not only are obese women at increased risk of having a fetus with neural tube defect (NTD), but the ability to make this diagnosis is limited, because: (i) circulating MS-AFP levels are lower in obese than in lean women; and (ii) maternal obesity significantly impairs sonographic visualization of the fetal anatomy. Maternal obesity alone is not an indication for a fetal echocardiogram, but this should be considered if there is any uncertainty about cardiac anatomy.

6. Women with morbid obesity (BMI ≥40 kg/ m²) should have an anesthesia consultation in the third trimester. Both regional and general anesthesia are of concern in this population. Regional anesthesia is preferred, but placement of spinal or epidural anesthesia may be technically difficult requiring multiple attempts. On the other hand, the risks of general anesthesia in this population include difficult intubation and an inability to extubate in a timely fashion due to sleep apnea and obstruction. Early placement of an epidural catheter may be desired, although there is an increased risk of migration of the catheter out of the epidural space in such patients.

7. Because of the association between maternal obesity and stillbirth, weekly fetal testing with NST and/or BPP starting at 36 weeks should be considered in women with a BMI ≥40 kg/m², although proven benefit is lacking.

8. Bariatric surgery is becoming more common among obese women of reproductive age. This includes restrictive (banding), malabsorptive (surgical resection and bypass), and combination procedures (Roux-én-Y gastric bypass). Such patients are at increased risk of nutritional and vitamin deficiencies, and may require supplementation with iron, vitamin B12, folate, and calcium.

9. Consider serial fetal growth scans every 3–4 weeks after 24 weeks in morbidly obese women given the risk of fetal macrosomia. Recommend elective cesarean delivery at or after 39 weeks if the estimated fetal weight is excessive (defined as ≥5,000-g in a nondiabetic or ≥4,500-g in a diabetic) to minimize the risk of birth trauma, primarily shoulder dystocia and resultant brachial plexus injury.

10. Given the association between maternal obesity and stillbirth, consider induction of labor at or after 39 weeks in women with a BMI ≥40 kg/m² and no macrosomia. Induction of labor for the indication of "impending macrosomia" does not decrease the risk of cesarean delivery or birth trauma, and is therefore not routinely recommended.

11. Maternal obesity is associated with increased perioperative complications, including excessive blood loss, venous thromboembolism (VTE), surgical site infection (SSI), and postpartum endomyometritis.

12. A number of strategies should be considered in preparation for surgery in obese pregnant women to abrogate the risks of surgical complications, including: (i) preoperative cardiac

evaluation (EKG, maternal echo), especially if the patient has diabetes or chronic hypertension; (ii) preoperative high-dose broad-spectrum antibiotics given 20–60 minutes before skin incision to decrease SSI; (iii) use of a large operating table; (iv) taping the pannus out of the surgical field; (v) use of the appropriate skin incision; (vi) routine closure of the subcutaneous layer with/without a subcutaneous drain; and (vii) routine VTE prophylaxis, including pneumatic compression stockings with/without perioperative heparin prophylaxis.

13. Morbidly obese women are also at increased risk of postpartum/postoperative complications, including VTE and postpartum endomyometritis. Strategies to prevent these complications may include: (i) early ambulation and continued use of pneumatic compression stockings/heparin prophylaxis to prevent VTE; (ii) delayed removal of sutures/staples for a full week to allow the skin to heal completely; and (iii) possibly administration of broad-spectrum antibiotics for 24–48 hours to decrease the risk of SSI/postpartum endomyometritis, although without proven benefit.

Obstetric complications in obese pregnant women

Complication	OR (95% CI) or % versus normal weight
Early pregnancy	
• Spontaneous abortion (miscarriage)	1.8 (1.1–3.0)
• Recurrent miscarriage	3.5 (1.1–21.0)
• Congenital anomalies	2.6 (1.5–4.5)
– Neural tube defects	1.2 (1.1–1.3)
– Congenital heart disease	3.3 (1.0–10.3)
– Omphalocele	
Late pregnancy	
• Hypertensive disorder of pregnancy	3.2 (1.8–5.8)
• Gestational diabetes mellitus (GDM)	2.6 (2.1–3.4)
• Preterm birth	1.5 (1.1–2.1)
• Intrauterine fetal demise (stillbirth)	2.8 (1.9–4.7)
Peripartum	
• Cesarean delivery	48% vs 20%
• Decreased VBAC success	85% vs 66%
• Operative morbidity	34% vs 20%
Fetal/neonatal complications	
• Fetal macrosomia (estimated fetal weight ≥4,500 g)	2.2 (1.6–3.1)
• Shoulder dystocia	3.6 (2.1–6.3)
• Birth weight >4,500 g	2.0 (1.4–3.0)
• Childhood obesity	2.3 (2.0–2.6)

45 Oligohydramnios[1]

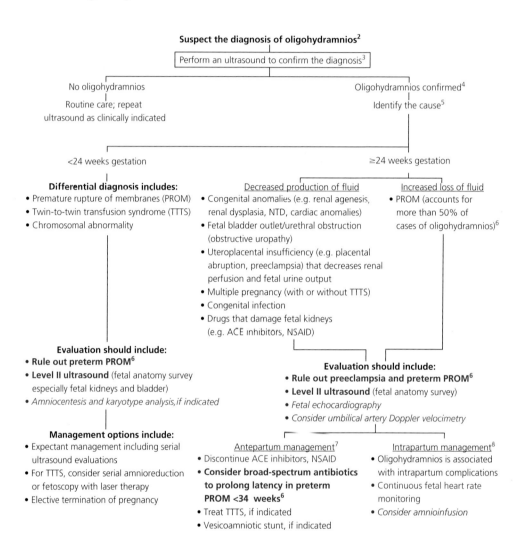

Suspect the diagnosis of oligohydramnios[2]

Perform an ultrasound to confirm the diagnosis[3]

No oligohydramnios
Routine care; repeat
ultrasound as clinically indicated

Oligohydramnios confirmed[4]
Identify the cause[5]

<24 weeks gestation

≥24 weeks gestation

Differential diagnosis includes:
- Premature rupture of membranes (PROM)
- Twin-to-twin transfusion syndrome (TTTS)
- Chromosomal abnormality

Decreased production of fluid
- Congenital anomalies (e.g. renal agenesis, renal dysplasia, NTD, cardiac anomalies)
- Fetal bladder outlet/urethral obstruction (obstructive uropathy)
- Uteroplacental insufficiency (e.g. placental abruption, preeclampsia) that decreases renal perfusion and fetal urine output
- Multiple pregnancy (with or without TTTS)
- Congenital infection
- Drugs that damage fetal kidneys (e.g. ACE inhibitors, NSAID)

Increased loss of fluid
- PROM (accounts for more than 50% of cases of oligohydramnios)[6]

Evaluation should include:
- **Rule out preterm PROM[6]**
- **Level II ultrasound** (fetal anatomy survey especially fetal kidneys and bladder)
- *Amniocentesis and karyotype analysis, if indicated*

Evaluation should include:
- **Rule out preeclampsia and preterm PROM[6]**
- **Level II ultrasound** (fetal anatomy survey)
- *Fetal echocardiography*
- *Consider umbilical artery Doppler velocimetry*

Management options include:
- Expectant management including serial ultrasound evaluations
- For TTTS, consider serial amnioreduction or fetoscopy with laser therapy
- Elective termination of pregnancy

Antepartum management[7]
- Discontinue ACE inhibitors, NSAID
- **Consider broad-spectrum antibiotics to prolong latency in preterm PROM <34 weeks[6]**
- Treat TTTS, if indicated
- Vesicoamniotic stunt, if indicated

Intrapartum management[8]
- Oligohydramnios is associated with intrapartum complications
- Continuous fetal heart rate monitoring
- *Consider amnioinfusion*

Obstetric Clinical Algorithms, Second Edition. Errol R. Norwitz, George R. Saade, Hugh Miller and Christina M. Davidson.
© 2017 John Wiley & Sons, Ltd. Published 2017 by John Wiley & Sons, Ltd.

1. The amnion is a thin fetal membrane that begins to form on the eighth day post conception as a small sac covering the dorsal surface of the embryonic disk. The amnion gradually encircles the growing embryo. It is filled with amniotic fluid, which has a number of critical functions: (i) it cushions the fetus from external trauma; (ii) it protects the umbilical cord from excessive compression; (iii) it allows unrestricted fetal movement, thereby promoting the development of the fetal musculoskeletal system; (iv) it contributes to fetal pulmonary development; (v) it lubricates the fetal skin; (vi) it prevents maternal chorioamnionitis and fetal infection through its bacteriostatic properties; and (vii) it assists in fetal temperature control. Amniotic fluid volume is maximal at 34 weeks (750–800 mL) and decreases thereafter to 600 mL at 40 weeks. The amount of fluid continues to decrease beyond 40 weeks. Amniotic fluid volume is a marker of fetal well-being. Normal amniotic fluid volume suggests that uteroplacental perfusion is adequate. Oligohydramnios is associated with increased perinatal morbidity and mortality at any gestational age.

2. Oligohydramnios refers to an abnormally small amount of amniotic fluid surrounding the fetus. It is seen in 5–8% of all pregnancies. It should be suspected if the fundal height is significantly less than expected for gestational age.

3. Ultrasonography is a more accurate method of estimating amniotic fluid than measurement of fundal height. Several ultrasound techniques are described, including: (i) subjective assessment of amniotic fluid volume; (ii) measurement of the single deepest pocket (free of umbilical cord); (iii) Amniotic Fluid Index (AFI), which is a semi-quantitative method for estimating amniotic fluid volume which minimizes inter- and intraobserver error. AFI refers to the sum of the maximum vertical pocket of amniotic fluid (in cm) in each of the four quadrants of the uterus. Normal AFI beyond 20 weeks' gestation ranges from 5 to 20 cm.

4. Oligohydramnios is an ultrasound diagnosis. It is defined sonographically in a singleton pregnancy as either a total amniotic fluid volume <300 mL, absence of a single vertical pocket ≥2 cm, or an AFI measurement <5th percentile for gestational age or <5 cm at term. In twins, absence of a single vertical pocket ≥2 cm is used to define oligohydramnios.

5. Maintenance of amniotic fluid volume is a dynamic process that reflects a balance between fluid production and absorption. Prior to 8 weeks' gestation, amniotic fluid is produced by passage of fluid across the amnion and fetal skin (transudation). At 8 weeks, the fetus begins to urinate into the amniotic cavity. Fetal urine quickly becomes the primary source of amniotic fluid production. Near term, 800–1000 mL of fetal urine is produced each day. The fetal lungs produce some fluid (300 mL per day at term), but much of it is swallowed before entering the amniotic space. Prior to 8 weeks' gestation, transudative amniotic fluid is passively reabsorbed. At 8 weeks' gestation, the fetus begins to swallow. Fetal swallowing quickly becomes the primary source of amniotic fluid absorption. Near term, 500–1000 mL of fluid is absorbed each day by fetal swallowing. A lesser amount of amniotic fluid is absorbed through the fetal membranes and enters the fetal bloodstream. Near term, 250 mL of amniotic fluid is absorbed by this route every day. Small quantities of amniotic fluid cross the amnion and enter the maternal bloodstream (10 mL per day near term). Every effort should be made to identify the cause of oligohydramnios. However, no cause will be found in approximately 30% of cases.

6. See Chapter 56, Preterm Premature Rupture of the Membranes.

7. The effect of oligohydramnios on the fetus depends on severity, gestational age, and underlying cause. Pulmonary hypoplasia, musculoskeletal deformities due to uterine compression (such as clubfoot), and/or amniotic band syndrome

(adhesions between amnion and fetus causing serious deformities, including limb amputation) may develop in some cases. Antepartum treatment options are limited, unless a structural defect (such as an obstructive posterior urethral valve) is identified and is amenable to *in utero* surgical repair or shunting.

8. The timing of delivery depends on gestational age, etiology, and fetal well-being. Oligohydramnios at term is an indication for delivery, regardless of the cause. During labor, oligohydramnios is associated with an increased risk of nonreassuring fetal testing and cesarean delivery. Infusion of crystalloid solution into the amniotic cavity (amnioinfusion) may improve abnormal fetal heart rate patterns, decrease cesarean delivery rate, and (possibly) minimize the risk of neonatal meconium aspiration syndrome.

46 Recurrent Pregnancy Loss

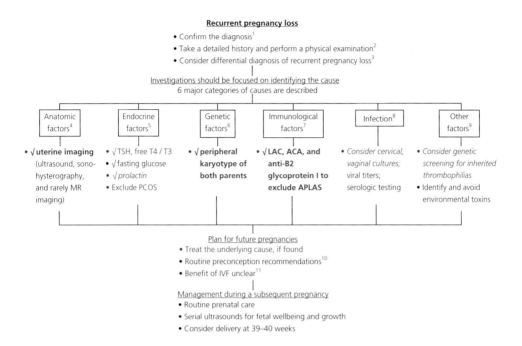

Recurrent pregnancy loss
- Confirm the diagnosis[1]
- Take a detailed history and perform a physical examination[2]
- Consider differential diagnosis of recurrent pregnancy loss[3]

Investigations should be focused on identifying the cause
6 major categories of causes are described

Anatomic factors[4]	Endocrine factors[5]	Genetic factors[6]	Immunological factors[7]	Infection[8]	Other factors[9]
• √ **uterine imaging** (ultrasound, sono-hysterography, and rarely MR imaging)	• √ TSH, free T4 / T3 • √ fasting glucose • √ *prolactin* • Exclude PCOS	• √ **peripheral karyotype of both parents**	• √ **LAC, ACA, and anti-B2 glycoprotein I to exclude APLAS**	• *Consider cervical, vaginal cultures; viral titers; serologic testing*	• *Consider genetic screening for inherited thrombophilias* • Identify and avoid environmental toxins

Plan for future pregnancies
- Treat the underlying cause, if found
- Routine preconception recommendations[10]
- Benefit of IVF unclear[11]

Management during a subsequent pregnancy
- Routine prenatal care
- Serial ultrasounds for fetal wellbeing and growth
- Consider delivery at 39–40 weeks

1. Recurrent pregnancy loss (RPL) is defined as the occurrence of three or more consecutive unexplained spontaneous early pregnancy losses before 10 weeks of gestation. This condition complicates approximately 1% of reproductive-age women.

2. Couples should ideally be seen prior to pregnancy. The pattern, trimester, and characteristics of the prior pregnancy losses should be reviewed. Exposure to environmental toxins/drugs, and prior gynecologic or obstetric infections should be specifically enquired about. A genetic pedigree should be developed and the possibility of consanguinity investigated. Physical examination may reveal evidence of maternal systemic disease or uterine anomalies. Laboratory tests and imaging studies should be individualized.

3. The differential diagnosis of RPL can be divided into six categories (discussed below). Unfortunately, many couples (>50%) will have no identifiable cause even after extensive investigation. Informative and supportive counseling serves an important role. Couples are often anxious, frustrated, and on the verge of despair. This can lead to anxious patients and/or physicians exploring empiric or alternative treatments that have dubious benefit. Fortunately, the prognosis of unexplained RPL is good, and 60–70% of couples will have a subsequent healthy pregnancy in the absence of obstetric intervention.

Obstetric Clinical Algorithms, Second Edition. Errol R. Norwitz, George R. Saade, Hugh Miller and Christina M. Davidson.
© 2017 John Wiley & Sons, Ltd. Published 2017 by John Wiley & Sons, Ltd.

4. <u>Anatomic factors</u> (account for 10–15% of cases of RPL). Congenital uterine anomalies resulting from Mullerian fusion abnormalities (such as didelphys or septate uterus) are most often associated with second trimester losses. Surgical revision may be helpful in some cases. Cervical insufficiency also accounts for second trimester losses, although this is regarded largely as a functional rather than a structural defect. Elective (prophylactic) cervical cerclage placement may be beneficial in selected patients.

5. <u>Endocrine factors</u> (10–15% of cases). Metabolic disorders (hypothyroidism, diabetes, polycyctic ovarian syndrome (PCOS)) require diagnosis and treatment of the underlying disease. Luteal phase deficiency is purported to result from insufficient progesterone secretion by the corpus luteum resulting in inadequate preparation of the endometrium for implantation and/or an inability to maintain early pregnancy, although the existence of such a diagnosis remains speculative. Two "out-of-phase" endometrial biopsies (in which histological dating lags behind menstrual dating by ≥2 days) in consecutive cycles are required for the diagnosis. Progesterone supplementation is commonly prescribed, but without proven benefit.

6. <u>Genetic factors</u> (5–10% of cases). Abnormal parental chromosomal abnormalities are the only proven cause of RPL. The most frequent karyotypic abnormality is a balanced translocation and is found most often in the female partner: 2/3 are reciprocal (exchange of chromatin between any two non-homologous chromosomes without loss of genetic material) and 1/3 are Robertsonian (fusion of chromosomes that have the centromere very near one end of a chromosome (typically 13, 14, 15, 21, or 22) with loss of one centromere and two short arms). The overall risk of spontaneous miscarriage in couples with a balanced translocation is >25%. Recurrent embryonic aneuploidy may represent non-random events in some predisposed couples.

Most aneuploid losses are the result of advanced maternal age. Prenatal diagnosis via amniocentesis or chorionic villus sampling may be useful in some situations to facilitate diagnosis, but no treatment is available.

7. <u>Immunological factors</u> (5–10% of cases). Antiphospholipid antibody syndrome (APLAS) is an autoimmune disorder characterized by circulating antibodies against membrane phospholipids and at least one specific clinical syndrome (RPL, unexplained thrombosis, autoimmune thrombocytopenia, or possibly unexplained IUGR and recurrent early preeclampsia). The diagnosis requires at least one confirmatory serologic test (lupus anticoagulant (LAC), anti-cardiolipin antibody (ACA), or anti-β2-glycoprotein I), which is positive on at least two occasions 8–12 weeks apart. The treatment is low-dose aspirin plus prophylactic heparin starting at the end of the first trimester. Alloimmunity (immunological differences between individuals) has been proposed as a factor between reproductive partners that may cause RPL. During normal pregnancy, the mother's immune system is thought to recognize semi-allogeneic (50% "non-self") fetal antigens and to produce "blocking" factors to protect the fetus. Failure to produce these blocking factors may play a role, but as yet the scientific evidence is limited and there is no specific diagnostic test. Immunotherapy has been used in an attempt to promote immune tolerance to paternal antigen, but has not been shown to be beneficial.

8. <u>Infection</u> (5% of cases). Listeria monocytogenes, mycoplasma hominis, Ureaplasma urealyticum, Toxoplasma gondii and viruses (herpes simplex, cytomegalovirus, rubella) have been variously associated with spontaneous abortion, but none have been proven to cause RPL. Diagnosis can be made using cervical cultures, viral titers, or serum antibodies. Directed antibiotic therapy may be useful if a causative agent is identified. Empiric treatment

prior to pregnancy with doxycycline or erythro-mycin is of unclear benefit.

9. <u>Other factors</u>. (i) Inherited thrombophilias may increase the risk of RPL (especially factor V Leiden mutations), but there is no consistent evidence that anticoagulation improves the chances of carrying a pregnancy to term. (ii) Environmental toxins such as smoking, alco-hol, and heavy coffee consumption have been associated with spontaneous miscarriage, but not RPL. Regardless, use should be curtailed if possible. (iii) Drugs such as folic acid antagonists, valproic acid, warfarin, anesthetic gases, tetrachloroethylene, and Isotretinoin (Accutane) have also been implicated.

10. Routine preconception counseling includes avoiding all alcohol and starting prenatal vita-mins with folic acid supplementation 1 mg daily.

11. *In vitro* fertilization (IVF) with or without preimplantation genetic diagnosis is often recommended for couples with RPL. With the possible exception of IVF with donor gametes in couples with documented genetic disorders (such as a parental balanced translocation), IVF is of unclear benefit in this setting.

47 Placenta Accreta

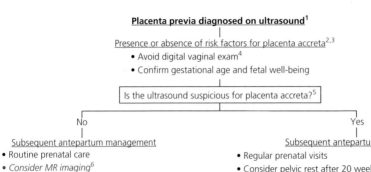

Placenta previa diagnosed on ultrasound[1]
|
Presence or absence of risk factors for placenta accreta[2,3]
- Avoid digital vaginal exam[4]
- Confirm gestational age and fetal well-being
|
Is the ultrasound suspicious for placenta accreta?[5]

No

Subsequent antepartum management
- Routine prenatal care
- *Consider MR imaging[6]*
- **Consider serial ultrasound examinations[7]**
|
Delivery management[8]
- √ CBC, T&S, coagulation screen
- Early anesthesia consultation
- When cesarean is performed for placenta previa, be prepared for intraoperative diagnosis of placenta accreta (may require hysterectomy, so consider dorsal lithotomy positioning)

Yes

Subsequent antepartum management
- Regular prenatal visits
- Consider pelvic rest after 20 weeks
- Consider early MFM and anesthesia consultation
- *Consider empiric antenatal steroids after 24 weeks*
- *Consider iron, dextran, erythropoietin to build up hematocrit*
- **Serial ultrasound examinations[7]**
- **Consent for cesarean and possible need for further surgery (hysterectomy) and blood transfusion[9]**
|
Consider elective cesarean-hysterectomy at 34–36 weeks[9,10]
|
Careful preoperative planning[11]
|
Intraoperative management
- **√ CBC, coagulation screen, T&S, large-bore iv access**
- *Consider preoperative internal iliac artery balloon catheters*
- Early and aggressive fluid and blood product resuscitation
- Consider midline vertical skin incision, high vertical ("classical") hysterotomy, immediate closure of hysterotomy (do not remove placenta!) and puerperal hysterectomy[12]

1. Placenta previa refers to a placenta that overlies or is proximate to the internal os of the cervix. It complicates 0.3–0.5% of pregnancies. The majority of cases of placenta previa are diagnosed during routine sonography in asymptomatic women, usually during the second trimester. Transvaginal ultrasound is superior to transabdominal ultrasound for this indication and, therefore, transvaginal ultrasound must be performed to confirm the diagnosis.

2. Placenta accreta is a general term used to describe the clinical condition when part of the placenta, or the entire placenta, invades and is inseparable from the uterine wall. Three grades of abnormal placental attachment are defined

Obstetric Clinical Algorithms, Second Edition. Errol R. Norwitz, George R. Saade, Hugh Miller and Christina M. Davidson.
© 2017 John Wiley & Sons, Ltd. Published 2017 by John Wiley & Sons, Ltd.

according to the depth of invasion: (i) accreta: chorionic villi attach to the myometrium, rather than being restricted within the decidua basalis (81.6%); (ii) increta: chorionic villi invade into the myometrium (11.8%); (iii) percreta: chorionic villi invade through the myometrium (6.6%). Of these, placenta accreta is the most common type and complicates 3 in 1000 deliveries.

3. Women at greatest risk of placenta accreta are those who have myometrial damage caused by a previous cesarean delivery with either anterior or posterior placenta previa overlying the uterine scar. Anterior or central placental location has been found to be a significant risk factor in the presence of a previous scar (28.6% vs. 1.9%, $p < .001$), but not in its absence (2.4% vs. 6.0%, $p = .239$). Additional risk factors include advanced maternal age, multiparity, hypertensive disorders of pregnancy, smoking, and any condition resulting in myometrial tissue damage followed by a secondary collagen repair (myomectomy, classical cesarean delivery, endometrial defects due to vigorous curettage resulting in Asherman syndrome, submucous leiomyomas, thermal ablation, uterine irradiation/radiation of lower abdomen, and uterine artery embolization). Placenta previa alone is associated with a 3.3% incidence of accreta, which increases to 11–24% with placenta previa and one prior cesarean, 40% with placenta previa and two prior cesareans, and >60% with placenta previa and three or more prior cesareans. An unexplained elevation in maternal serum a-fetoprotein (MS-AFP) at 15–20 weeks' gestation is also associated with abnormal placentation.

4. Most women with placenta previa and accreta do not develop symptoms during pregnancy. However, some women may present with acute onset of bright red vaginal bleeding, which is usually painless. Abdominal pain is rare. Other causes of antepartum hemorrhage include placenta previa alone (see Chapter 48, Placenta Previa), placental abruption (Chapter 49, Placental Abruption), vasa previa (Chapter 71,

Vasa previa), early labor, and genital tract lesions (cervical polyps or erosions). Bleeding is of maternal origin. If excessive, it can lead to hemodynamic instability and shock.

When a woman presents with antepartum hemorrhage, pelvic examination should be avoided until placenta previa is excluded on ultrasound (preferably by transvaginal approach). Digital vaginal examination with a placenta previa may provoke catastrophic hemorrhage and should not be performed. In the setting of placenta previa, fetal malpresentation is common.

5. The major sonographic features of placenta accreta include: (i) loss of normal hypoechoic retroplacental zone; (ii) multiple vascular lacunae (irregular vascular spaces) within placenta, giving a "Swiss cheese" or "moth-eaten" appearance; the presence of lacunae in the placenta at 15–20 weeks has been found to be the most predictive sonographic sign of placenta accreta, with a sensitivity of 79% and a positive predictive value of 92%; the risk of placenta accreta increases with an increased number of lacunae; (iii) blood vessels or placental tissue bridging uterine-placental margin, myometrial-bladder interface, or crossing uterine serosa; (iv) retroplacental myometrial thickness of <1 mm; (v) numerous coherent vessels visualized with 3D power Doppler in basal view; in the majority of cases, power and color Doppler do not significantly improve the diagnosis over that achieved by grayscale sonography alone; (vi) first trimester ultrasound findings of gestational sac in the lower uterine segment and gestational sac abnormally close to uterine scar.

6. If the ultrasound examination is equivocal, consider magnetic resonance (MR) imaging. Initial studies suggested that MR imaging was more sensitive than ultrasound in diagnosing placenta accreta, but recent studies have found no difference between the two modalities (with a sensitivity of approximately 50%). MR imaging may be particularly useful for posterior previa, a situation in which ultrasound is more limited.

7. Serial ultrasound examinations may be useful to follow placental location, fetal presentation, fetal growth, and sonographic markers of placenta accreta. As pregnancy progresses, >90% of low-lying placentas identified early in pregnancy will appear to move away from the cervix and out of the lower uterine segment. This is thought to be due to the placenta preferentially growing towards a better vascularized fundus, whereas the placenta overlying the less well-vascularized cervix may undergo atrophy. In some cases, this atrophy leaves vessels running through the membranes, unsupported by placental tissue or cord (vasa previa). In cases where the atrophy is incomplete, a succenturiate lobe may develop.

8. A placenta previa requires delivery by cesarean. In a stable patient, cesarean should be performed at 36 0/7–37 6/7 weeks of gestation. Controversy exists as to the mode of delivery when the placenta lies in proximity to the internal os. Three small retrospective studies suggest that women with placenta previa should have a transvaginal ultrasound in the late 3rd trimester and that those with a placenta-internal os distance of less than 2 cm should be delivered by cesarean. Another small retrospective study demonstrated that more than two-thirds of women with a placental edge to cervical os distance of >10 mm deliver vaginally without increased risk of hemorrhage.

9. The goal of antepartum management in the setting of placenta accreta is to maximize fetal maturation while minimizing risk to mother and fetus. Nonreassuring fetal testing ("fetal distress") and excessive maternal hemorrhage are contraindications to expectant management, and may necessitate immediate cesarean irrespective of gestational age. Contraindications to emergency cesarean include a previable fetus (<23–24 weeks), intrauterine fetal demise, maternal hemodynamic instability or uncontrolled coagulopathy, or failure to obtain maternal consent for surgery.

10. In the setting of placenta previa and suspected placenta accreta, the recommended management is planned preterm cesarean hysterectomy with the placenta left in situ because removal of the placenta is associated with significant hemorrhagic morbidity. The results of a recent decision analysis suggested that combined maternal and neonatal outcomes are optimized in stable patients with ultrasonographic evidence of placenta previa and placenta accreta with delivery at 34 weeks of gestation without amniocentesis. ACOG supports delivery at 34 0/7–35 6/7 weeks of gestation for placenta previa with suspected accreta, increta or percreta.

11. Preoperative consultation with anesthesiology and notification of the blood bank are indicated before scheduled surgery. Additional surgical services such as gynecologic oncology, urology, general surgery, neonatology, interventional radiology and/or vascular surgery may provide additional surgical expertise if needed. Use of a preoperative summary, or checklist may be helpful to confirm that needed preparations have been made and to identify the name and contact information for consultants in case they are needed for intraoperative or perioperative assistance. Consider mode of anesthesia (usually general endotracheal anesthesia and possible epidural for postoperative pain control), utility of central monitoring (arterial line, central venous line and/or Swan–Ganz catheter), preoperative cystoscopy and stenting of ureters, use of cell saver equipment and/or normovolemic hemodilution to minimize need for blood transfusion, adequate suction capacity, blood warmers, body warmers, and pneumatic compression stockings (for DVT prophylaxis).

12. The uterine incision should be located such that it avoids the placenta. A classical uterine incision, often transfundal, may be necessary to avoid the placenta and allow delivery of the infant. In some cases, a posterior uterine wall incision after exteriorization of the uterus may be desired.

48 Placenta Previa

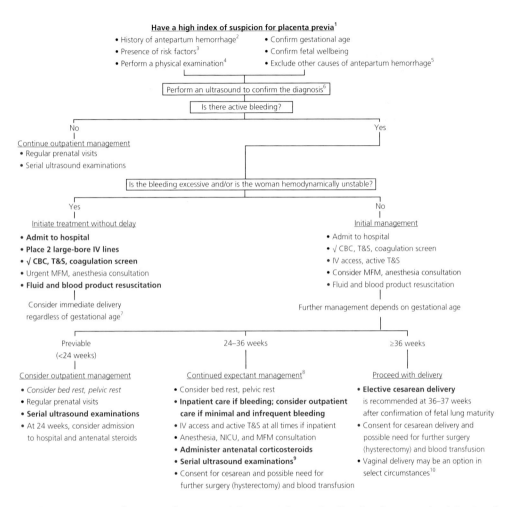

Have a high index of suspicion for placenta previa[1]

- History of antepartum hemorrhage[2]
- Presence of risk factors[3]
- Perform a physical examination[4]
- Confirm gestational age
- Confirm fetal wellbeing
- Exclude other causes of antepartum hemorrhage[5]

Perform an ultrasound to confirm the diagnosis[6]

Is there active bleeding?

No

Continue outpatient management
- Regular prenatal visits
- Serial ultrasound examinations

Yes

Is the bleeding excessive and/or is the woman hemodynamically unstable?

Yes

Initiate treatment without delay
- **Admit to hospital**
- **Place 2 large-bore IV lines**
- **√ CBC, T&S, coagulation screen**
- Urgent MFM, anesthesia consultation
- **Fluid and blood product resuscitation**

Consider immediate delivery regardless of gestational age[7]

No

Initial management
- Admit to hospital
- √ CBC, T&S, coagulation screen
- IV access, active T&S
- Consider MFM, anesthesia consultation
- Fluid and blood product resuscitation

Further management depends on gestational age

Previable (<24 weeks)

Consider outpatient management
- *Consider bed rest, pelvic rest*
- Regular prenatal visits
- **Serial ultrasound examinations**
- At 24 weeks, consider admission to hospital and antenatal steroids

24–36 weeks

Continued expectant management[8]
- Consider bed rest, pelvic rest
- **Inpatient care if bleeding; consider outpatient care if minimal and infrequent bleeding**
- IV access and active T&S at all times if inpatient
- Anesthesia, NICU, and MFM consultation
- **Administer antenatal corticosteroids**
- **Serial ultrasound examinations[9]**
- Consent for cesarean and possible need for further surgery (hysterectomy) and blood transfusion

≥36 weeks

Proceed with delivery
- **Elective cesarean delivery** is recommended at 36–37 weeks after confirmation of fetal lung maturity
- Consent for cesarean delivery and possible need for further surgery (hysterectomy) and blood transfusion
- Vaginal delivery may be an option in select circumstances[10]

1. Placenta previa refers to implantation of the placenta over the cervical os in advance of the fetal presenting part. It complicates 1 in 200 pregnancies, and accounts for 20% of all cases of antepartum hemorrhage.

2. Symptoms may include the acute onset of bright-red vaginal bleeding, which is usually painless. Bleeding is of maternal origin. Fetal malpresentation is common, because the placenta prevents engagement of the presenting part. It may be an incidental finding on routine ultrasound in an asymptomatic patient.

3. Risk factors for placenta previa include multiparity, advanced maternal age, prior

Obstetric Clinical Algorithms, Second Edition. Errol R. Norwitz, George R. Saade, Hugh Miller and Christina M. Davidson.
© 2017 John Wiley & Sons, Ltd. Published 2017 by John Wiley & Sons, Ltd.

placenta previa, prior cesarean delivery, and smoking.

4. When a woman presents with antepartum hemorrhage, bimanual pelvic examination should be avoided until placenta previa is excluded on ultrasound.

5. Other causes of antepartum hemorrhage include placental abruption (see Chapter 49), vasa previa (see Chapter 71), early labor, and genital tract lesions (cervical polyps or erosions).

6. Placenta previa is an ultrasound diagnosis. Transperineal and/or transvaginal ultrasound may be necessary to confirm the diagnosis, and is regarded as safe in this setting. Of note, only 5% of placenta previa identified by ultrasound at a routine second trimester fetal anatomy survey will persist to term. Placenta accreta (abnormal attachment of placental villi to the uterine wall) is rare (1 in 2,500 pregnancies), but complicates 3–5% of pregnancies with placenta previa, 10–25% with placenta previa and one prior cesarean, 40% with placenta previa and two prior cesareans, and >60% with placenta previa and three or more prior cesareans (see Chapter 47, Placenta Accreta).

7. Emergent cesarean delivery may be needed. Contraindications to emergent cesarean include a previable fetus (<23–24 weeks), intrauterine fetal demise, maternal hemodynamic instability or uncontrolled coagulopathy, or failure to obtain maternal consent for surgery.

8. The aim of antepartum management in the setting of placenta previa is to maximize fetal maturation while minimizing risk to mother and fetus. Non-reassuring fetal testing and excessive maternal hemorrhage are contraindications to expectant management, and may necessitate immediate cesarean, irrespective of gestational age. However, most episodes of bleeding are not life-threatening. With careful monitoring, delivery can be safely delayed in most cases. Outpatient management may be an option for women with a single small bleed if they can comply with restrictions on activity and maintain proximity to a hospital. Placenta previa may resolve with time, thereby permitting vaginal delivery.

9. Serial ultrasound examinations are useful to follow placental location, fetal presentation (malpresentation is common), and possibly fetal growth (although placenta previa is not associated with intrauterine growth restriction (IUGR)).

10. Vaginal delivery is rarely appropriate in the setting of placenta previa, but may be indicated in the setting of intrauterine fetal demise, fetal malformation(s) incompatible with life, advanced labor with engagement of the fetal head and minimal vaginal bleeding, or an indicated delivery with a previable fetus. A double set-up examination in labor may be appropriate when ultrasound cannot exclude placenta previa and the patient is strongly motivated for vaginal delivery. This procedure is performed in the operating room with surgical anesthesia and two surgical teams. One team is scrubbed and ready for immediate cesarean in the event of hemorrhage or nonreassuring fetal testing. The other team then performs a gentle bimanual examination initially of the vaginal fornices and then the cervical os. If a previa is present, immediate cesarean is indicated. If no placenta is palpated, amniotomy can be performed and labor induced.

49 Placental Abruption

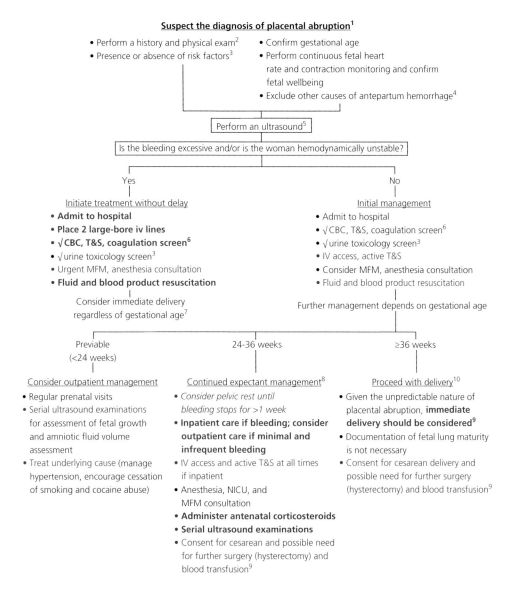

Suspect the diagnosis of placental abruption[1]

- Perform a history and physical exam[2]
- Presence or absence of risk factors[3]

- Confirm gestational age
- Perform continuous fetal heart rate and contraction monitoring and confirm fetal wellbeing
- Exclude other causes of antepartum hemorrhage[4]

Perform an ultrasound[5]

Is the bleeding excessive and/or is the woman hemodynamically unstable?

Yes

Initiate treatment without delay
- **Admit to hospital**
- **Place 2 large-bore iv lines**
- **√ CBC, T&S, coagulation screen[6]**
- √ urine toxicology screen[3]
- Urgent MFM, anesthesia consultation
- **Fluid and blood product resuscitation**

Consider immediate delivery regardless of gestational age[7]

No

Initial management
- Admit to hospital
- √ CBC, T&S, coagulation screen[6]
- √ urine toxicology screen[3]
- IV access, active T&S
- Consider MFM, anesthesia consultation
- Fluid and blood product resuscitation

Further management depends on gestational age

Previable (<24 weeks)

Consider outpatient management
- Regular prenatal visits
- Serial ultrasound examinations for assessment of fetal growth and amniotic fluid volume assessment
- Treat underlying cause (manage hypertension, encourage cessation of smoking and cocaine abuse)

24-36 weeks

Continued expectant management[8]
- *Consider pelvic rest until bleeding stops for >1 week*
- **Inpatient care if bleeding; consider outpatient care if minimal and infrequent bleeding**
- IV access and active T&S at all times if inpatient
- Anesthesia, NICU, and MFM consultation
- **Administer antenatal corticosteroids**
- **Serial ultrasound examinations**
- Consent for cesarean and possible need for further surgery (hysterectomy) and blood transfusion[9]

≥36 weeks

Proceed with delivery[10]
- Given the unpredictable nature of placental abruption, **immediate delivery should be considered[9]**
- Documentation of fetal lung maturity is not necessary
- Consent for cesarean delivery and possible need for further surgery (hysterectomy) and blood transfusion[9]

Obstetric Clinical Algorithms, Second Edition. Errol R. Norwitz, George R. Saade, Hugh Miller and Christina M. Davidson.
© 2017 John Wiley & Sons, Ltd. Published 2017 by John Wiley & Sons, Ltd.

1. Placental abruption refers to premature separation of a normally implanted placenta from the uterine wall. The bleeding that results may be revealed vaginally (in 80% of cases) or concealed within the uterus. Abruption that is clinically recognized complicates 1% of all pregnancies. Abruption that is severe enough to result in the death of the fetus occurs in 1 in 420 deliveries.

2. Signs and symptoms of placental abruption may include vaginal bleeding (80%), uterine tenderness or back pain (65%), and nonreassuring fetal heart rate monitoring (60%). Other findings include frequent, hypertonic contractions and preterm labor. Bleeding is of maternal origin. Uterine tenderness suggests extravasation of blood into the myometrium (Couvelaire uterus). The amount of vaginal bleeding may not be a reliable indicator of the severity of the hemorrhage since bleeding may be concealed. Serial measurements of fundal height and abdominal girth are useful to monitor large retroplacental blood collections. Rarely, placental abruption may be an incidental finding on routine ultrasound. When a woman presents with antepartum hemorrhage, pelvic examination should be avoided until placenta previa is excluded on ultrasound.

3. Preeclampsia is the most common risk factor and is found in 50% of women with placental abruption. Other risk factors for placental abruption include prior placental abruption (recurrence rate is 10% after one abruption, 25% after two abruptions), blunt trauma, smoking, cocaine, uterine anomaly or fibroids, multiparity, advanced maternal age, preterm premature rupture of the membranes, chorioamnionitis, possibly thrombophilias, and rapid decompression of an overdistended uterus (such as multiple pregnancy or polyhydramnios).

4. Other causes of antepartum hemorrhage include placenta previa (see Chapter 48, Placenta Previa), vasa previa (see Chapter 71, Vasa previa), early labor, and genital tract lesions (cervical polyps or erosions).

5. Placental abruption is a clinical diagnosis. An ultrasound should be performed to exclude placenta previa, confirm gestational age, document estimated fetal weight and amniotic fluid volume, and confirm a live fetus. Sonographic evaluation will fail to reveal >50% of placental abruptions; however, in cases in which bleeding is visualized sonographically, the likelihood of abruption is very high. The risk of stillbirth correlates with the extent of placental separation; stillbirth rates are high with >50% separation. Placental abruption is also associated with a twofold increase in fetal growth restriction and an increased rate of congenital anomalies. Portwine discoloration of the amniotic fluid at the time of amniocentesis or cesarean delivery is highly suggestive of placental abruption.

6. When abruption is severe enough to result in the death of the fetus, blood loss may be >50% of maternal blood volume and coagulation defects can develop rapidly. Up to 5 liters of blood may extravasate into the myometrium, with little or no revealed bleeding. The release of placental thromboplastin into the maternal circulation can trigger disseminated intravascular coagulation (DIC) and is also strongly uterotonic. Coagulopathy is uncommon with a surviving fetus.

7. Emergency cesarean delivery may be needed. Contraindications to emergency cesarean include a previable fetus (<23–24 weeks), intrauterine fetal demise, maternal hemodynamic instability or uncontrolled coagulopathy, or failure to obtain maternal consent for surgery. Even in the setting of fetal death or previability, however, cesarean may be indicated if hemorrhage is so extensive that the life of the mother is at risk.

8. The goal of antepartum management is to maximize fetal maturation while minimizing risk to mother and fetus. Hospitalization is

indicated to evaluate the maternal and fetal conditions. Nonreassuring fetal testing ("fetal distress") and excessive maternal hemorrhage are contraindications to expectant management, and may necessitate immediate cesarean irrespective of gestational age. However, most episodes of bleeding are not life-threatening. With careful monitoring, delivery can be safely delayed in most cases. Outpatient management may be an option if the bleeding is small and infrequent and if the woman can maintain proximity to a hospital. Placental abruption is a relative contraindication to tocolysis. Serial ultrasound examinations are useful to follow the appearance of the placenta, fetal presentation, amniotic fluid volume, and fetal growth. Women with a very early abruption can develop chronic abruption-oligohydramnios sequence (CAOS).

9. Postpartum hemorrhage should be anticipated following a severe placental abruption.

Uterine contractility is impaired by fibrin degradation products, thus uterine atony may occur. Persistent atony despite the administration of uterotonics may require a hysterectomy. Maternal deaths from abruption occur most often postpartum, when ongoing blood loss occurs in patients with inadequate correction of hemorrhagic shock and coagulopathy. Acute renal tubular and cortical necrosis may result in addition to renal ischemia from hypovolemia.

10. Mode and timing of delivery depend on the condition and gestational age of the fetus, the condition of the mother, the amount of associated hemorrhage and the state of the cervix. Labor with extensive placental abruption may be rapid due to the persistently hypertonic uterus. Early amniotomy may expedite delivery. Oxytocin can be initiated, if needed. If vaginal delivery does not appear imminent, cesarean delivery may be indicated.

50 Polyhydramnios[1]

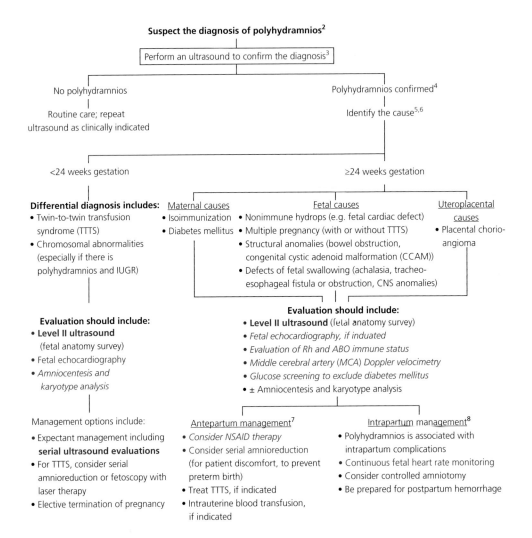

Suspect the diagnosis of polyhydramnios[2]

Perform an ultrasound to confirm the diagnosis[3]

No polyhydramnios

Routine care; repeat ultrasound as clinically indicated

Polyhydramnios confirmed[4]

Identify the cause[5,6]

<24 weeks gestation

≥24 weeks gestation

Differential diagnosis includes:
- Twin-to-twin transfusion syndrome (TTTS)
- Chromosomal abnormalities (especially if there is polyhydramnios and IUGR)

Maternal causes
- Isoimmunization
- Diabetes mellitus

Fetal causes
- Nonimmune hydrops (e.g. fetal cardiac defect)
- Multiple pregnancy (with or without TTTS)
- Structural anomalies (bowel obstruction, congenital cystic adenoid malformation (CCAM))
- Defects of fetal swallowing (achalasia, tracheo-esophageal fistula or obstruction, CNS anomalies)

Uteroplacental causes
- Placental chorio-angioma

Evaluation should include:
- **Level II ultrasound** (fetal anatomy survey)
- Fetal echocardiography
- *Amniocentesis and karyotype analysis*

Evaluation should include:
- **Level II ultrasound** (fetal anatomy survey)
- *Fetal echocardiography, if indicated*
- *Evaluation of Rh and ABO immune status*
- *Middle cerebral artery (MCA) Doppler velocimetry*
- *Glucose screening to exclude diabetes mellitus*
- ± Amniocentesis and karyotype analysis

Management options include:
- Expectant management including **serial ultrasound evaluations**
- For TTTS, consider serial amnioreduction or fetoscopy with laser therapy
- Elective termination of pregnancy

Antepartum management[7]
- *Consider NSAID therapy*
- Consider serial amnioreduction (for patient discomfort, to prevent preterm birth)
- Treat TTTS, if indicated
- Intrauterine blood transfusion, if indicated

Intrapartum management[8]
- Polyhydramnios is associated with intrapartum complications
- Continuous fetal heart rate monitoring
- Consider controlled amniotomy
- Be prepared for postpartum hemorrhage

1. The amnion is a thin fetal membrane that begins to form on the eighth day postconception as a small sac covering the dorsal surface of the embryonic disc. The amnion gradually encircles the growing embryo. It is filled with amniotic fluid which has a number of critical functions: (i) it cushions the fetus from external trauma; (ii) it protects the umbilical cord from excessive

Obstetric Clinical Algorithms, Second Edition. Errol R. Norwitz, George R. Saade, Hugh Miller and Christina M. Davidson.
© 2017 John Wiley & Sons, Ltd. Published 2017 by John Wiley & Sons, Ltd.

compression; (iii) it allows unrestricted fetal movement, thereby promoting the development of the fetal musculoskeletal system; (iv) it contributes to fetal pulmonary development; (v) it lubricates the fetal skin; (vi) it prevents maternal chorioamnionitis and fetal infection through its bacteriostatic properties; and (vii) it assists in fetal temperature control. Amniotic fluid volume is maximal at 34 weeks (750–800 mL) and decreases thereafter to 600 mL at 40 weeks. The amount of fluid continues to decrease beyond 40 weeks. Amniotic fluid volume is a marker of fetal well-being. Normal amniotic fluid volume suggests that uteroplacental perfusion is adequate. Abnormal amount of amniotic fluid volume is associated with an unfavorable perinatal outcome.

2. Polyhydramnios refers to an abnormally large amount of amniotic fluid surrounding the fetus. It is seen in 0.5–1.5% of all pregnancies. It should be suspected if the fundal height is significantly more than expected for gestational age.

3. Ultrasonography is a more accurate method of estimating amniotic fluid than measurement of fundal height. Several ultrasound techniques are described, including: (i) subjective assessment of amniotic fluid volume; (ii) measurement of the single deepest pocket (free of umbilical cord); (iii) Amniotic Fluid Index (AFI), which is a semi-quantitative method for estimating amniotic fluid volume which minimizes inter- and intra-observer error. AFI refers to the sum of the maximum vertical pocket of amniotic fluid (in cm) in each of the four quadrants of the uterus. Normal AFI beyond 20 weeks' gestation ranges from 5–20 cm.

4. Polyhydramnios is an ultrasound diagnosis. It is defined sonographically in a singleton pregnancy as either a total amniotic fluid volume >2 L, a single vertical pocket ≥10 cm, or an AFI measurement >95th percentile for gestational age or >20 cm at term. In twins, a single vertical pocket ≥10 cm is used to define polyhydramnios.

5. Maintenance of amniotic fluid volume is a dynamic process that reflects a balance between fluid production and absorption. Prior to 8 weeks' gestation, amniotic fluid is produced by the passage of fluid across the amnion and fetal skin (transudation). At 8 weeks, the fetus begins to urinate into the amniotic cavity. Fetal urine quickly becomes the primary source of amniotic fluid production. Near term, 800–1000 mL of fetal urine is produced each day. The fetal lungs produce some fluid (300 mL per day at term), but much of it is swallowed before entering the amniotic space. Prior to 8 weeks' gestation, transudative amniotic fluid is passively reabsorbed. At 8 weeks' gestation, the fetus begins to swallow. Fetal swallowing quickly becomes the primary source of amniotic fluid absorption. Near term, 500–1000 mL of fluid is absorbed each day by fetal swallowing. A lesser amount of amniotic fluid is absorbed through the fetal membranes and enters the fetal bloodstream. Near term, 250 mL of amniotic fluid is absorbed by this route every day. Small quantities of amniotic fluid cross the amnion and enter the maternal bloodstream (10 mL per day near term).

6. Every effort should be made to identify the cause. However, no cause will be found in 50–60% of cases of polyhydramnios.

7. Uterine overdistension may result in maternal dyspnea or refractory edema of the lower extremities and vulva. It can also lead to preterm PROM as well as premature labor and delivery. Antepartum treatment options are limited. Nonsteroidal anti-inflammatory drugs (NSAID) (such as indomethacin) can decrease fetal urine production, but may also cause premature closure of the ductus arteriosus *in utero* especially if given after 32 weeks' gestation, leading to persistent pulmonary hypertension. Removal of fluid by amniocentesis is

only transiently effective as fluid will typically reaccumulate within 24–72 hours. Treatment of the underlying disorder (such as laser therapy for TTTS or intrauterine transfusion for pregnancies complicated by isoimmunization and severe fetal anemia) may reverse the polyhydramnios.

8. During labor, polyhydramnios can result in fetal malpresentation, dysfunctional labor, and/or postpartum hemorrhage. Controlled amniotomy may reduce the incidence of complications resulting from rapid decompression of the uterus (such as placental abruption and cord prolapse).

51 Post-term Pregnancy[1]

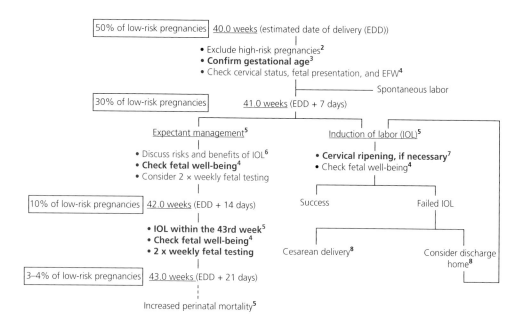

50% of low-risk pregnancies | 40.0 weeks (estimated date of delivery (EDD))

- Exclude high-risk pregnancies[2]
- **Confirm gestational age[3]**
- Check cervical status, fetal presentation, and EFW[4]

Spontaneous labor

30% of low-risk pregnancies | 41.0 weeks (EDD + 7 days)

Expectant management[5]

- Discuss risks and benefits of IOL[6]
- **Check fetal well-being[4]**
- Consider 2 × weekly fetal testing

Induction of labor (IOL)[5]

- **Cervical ripening, if necessary[7]**
- Check fetal well-being[4]

Success | Failed IOL

10% of low-risk pregnancies | 42.0 weeks (EDD + 14 days)

- **IOL within the 43rd week[5]**
- **Check fetal well-being[4]**
- **2 x weekly fetal testing**

Cesarean delivery[8] | Consider discharge home[8]

3–4% of low-risk pregnancies | 43.0 weeks (EDD + 21 days)

Increased perinatal mortality[5]

1. Post-term (prolonged) pregnancy refers to a pregnancy that has extended to or beyond a gestational age of 42.0 weeks (294 days) from the first day of the last normal menstrual period. The term "post dates" is poorly defined is best avoided. An alternative approach is to date the pregnancy relative to the estimated date of delivery (EDD); 42.0 weeks would therefore be EDD + 14 days.

2. Delivery is typically recommended when the risks to the fetus of continuing the pregnancy are greater than those faced by the neonate after birth. High-risk pregnancies should not be allowed to go post-term because, in these pregnancies, the balance appears to shift in favor of delivery at around 38–39 weeks of gestation. This is true also of twin pregnancies. These

guidelines therefore apply only to uncomplicated low-risk post-term pregnancies.

3. Accurate pregnancy dating is important in minimizing the false diagnosis of post-term pregnancy. The EDD is most reliably and accurately determined early in pregnancy. This may be based on a known LMP in women with regular, normal menstrual cycles. Other clinical data should be consistent with the EDD, including:

- The size of the uterus at early examination (in the first trimester) should be consistent with dates.
- The perception of fetal movement (quickening) usually occurs at 18–20 weeks in nulliparous women and 16–18 weeks in multiparous women.

Obstetric Clinical Algorithms, Second Edition. Errol R. Norwitz, George R. Saade, Hugh Miller and Christina M. Davidson.
© 2017 John Wiley & Sons, Ltd. Published 2017 by John Wiley & Sons, Ltd.

- The fetal heart can be heard with a nonelectronic fetal stethoscope by 18–20 weeks in most patients.
- At 20 weeks, the fundal height should be approximately 20 cm above the symphysis pubis, which usually corresponds with the umbilicus.

Inconsistencies or concern about the accuracy of the pregnancy dating require further assessment with ultrasonography. Useful measurements include the crown–rump length of the fetus during the first trimester and the biparietal diameter or head circumference and femur length during the second trimester. Because of the normal variations in size of fetuses in the third trimester, dating the pregnancy at that time is less reliable (±3 weeks).

4. Even though proven benefit is lacking, antenatal fetal surveillance for post-term pregnancies (>42 weeks) has become standard practice. Options for fetal surveillance include nonstress testing, biophysical profile (BPP) or modified BPP (amniotic fluid volume estimation), the oxytocin challenge test (OCT), or a combination of these modalities. No single method has been shown to be superior. Of note, Doppler velocimetry alone is not recommended for this indication. Although no firm recommendation can be made regarding the frequency of antenatal surveillance in post-term patients, many experts would advise twice-weekly testing with some evaluation of amniotic fluid volume performed at least weekly. Delivery should be affected immediately if there is evidence of fetal compromise or oligohydramnios. There is insufficient evidence to show that initiating antenatal surveillance at 40–42 weeks improves the pregnancy outcome or confers any additional benefit to the fetus.

5. At 41 weeks (EDD + 7 days), both expectant management and induction of labor are associated with low complication rates and good perinatal outcomes in low-risk post-term gravida. Since delivery cannot always be brought about readily, maternal risks and considerations are apt to confound this decision. Factors that need to be considered include gestational age, results of antepartum fetal testing, favorability of the cervix, and maternal preference after discussion of the risks and benefits of the management options. According to current obstetric practice, labor is generally induced at or after 41 weeks when the cervix is favorable, as the risk of failed induction and subsequent cesarean delivery is low. If the cervix is unfavorable, the optimal approach is less clear. Even if the cervix is unfavorable, there appears to be a small advantage to induction of labor at or after 41 weeks, regardless of parity or method of induction. However, expectant management is a reasonable alternative in this setting.

6. ACOG has no specific recommendations about the timing of delivery. However, most authorities would recommend induction of labor (IOL) for all low-risk pregnancies sometime during the 43rd week of gestation (EDD + 14 days to EDD + 21 days), because of the increased risk to the fetus of continuing the pregnancy. These include an increase in perinatal mortality (stillbirth), uteroplacental insufficiency (chronic IUGR leading to "fetal dysmaturity syndrome"), fetal macrosomia (which is associated with prolonged labor, cephalopelvic disproportion, and shoulder dystocia with resultant risks of orthopedic or neurologic injury), meconium aspiration syndrome, and birth asphyxia. In addition to the risks to the fetus, post-term pregnancy is also associated with risks to the mother including an increase in labor dystocia, severe perineal injury, and a doubling in the rate of cesarean delivery.

7. The introduction of preinduction cervical maturation has resulted in fewer failed and serial inductions, lower fetal and maternal morbidity, a shorter hospital stay, and possibly a lower rate of cesarean delivery in the general obstetric population. Both PGE_2 (dinoprostone) and PGE_1 (misoprostol) have been used for

induction of labor in post-term pregnancies. Although the dose, dosage interval, route of administration, and side effect profile vary slightly between the different preparations, these agents appear to be equally effective. Overall, these medications are well tolerated with few reported side effects. Higher doses of prostaglandins have been associated with an increased risk of uterine tachysystole and hyperstimulation leading to nonreassuring fetal testing. As such, lower doses are preferable.

Given the risk of uterine hyperstimulation, continuous fetal heart rate monitoring should be carried out routinely to ensure fetal well-being.

8. The decision of whether to proceed with cesarean delivery or discharge the patient home in the setting of failed induction of labor should be individualized. Factors that need to be considered include the precise gestational age, results of antepartum fetal testing, and maternal preference.

52 Pregnancy Termination

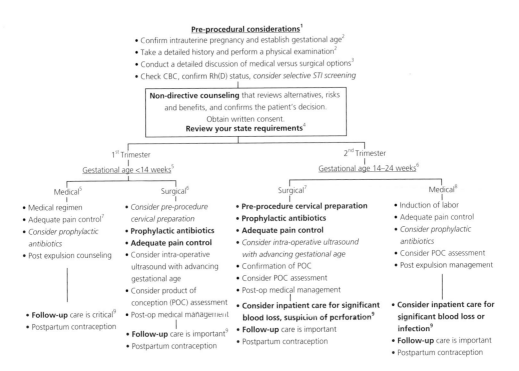

<u>**Pre-procedural considerations[1]**</u>
- Confirm intrauterine pregnancy and establish gestational age[2]
- Take a detailed history and perform a physical examination[2]
- Conduct a detailed discussion of medical versus surgical options[3]
- Check CBC, confirm Rh(D) status, *consider selective STI screening*

Non-directive counseling that reviews alternatives, risks and benefits, and confirms the patient's decision.
Obtain written consent.
Review your state requirements[4]

1ˢᵗ Trimester
<u>Gestational age <14 weeks[5]</u>

2ⁿᵈ Trimester
<u>Gestational age 14–24 weeks[6]</u>

Medical[5]
- Medical regimen
- Adequate pain control[7]
- *Consider prophylactic antibiotics*
- Post expulsion counseling

- **Follow-up** care is critical[9]
- Postpartum contraception

Surgical[6]
- *Consider pre-procedure cervical preparation*
- **Prophylactic antibiotics**
- **Adequate pain control**
- Consider intra-operative ultrasound with advancing gestational age
- Consider product of conception (POC) assessment
- Post-op medical management

- **Follow-up** care is important[9]
- Postpartum contraception

Surgical[7]
- **Pre-procedure cervical preparation**
- **Prophylactic antibiotics**
- **Adequate pain control**
- *Consider intra-operative ultrasound with advancing gestational age*
- Confirmation of POC
- Consider POC assessment
- Post-op medical management
- **Consider inpatient care for significant blood loss, suspicion of perforation[9]**
- **Follow-up** care is important
- Postpartum contraception

Medical[8]
- Induction of labor
- Adequate pain control
- *Consider prophylactic antibiotics*
- Consider POC assessment
- Post expulsion management

- **Consider inpatient care for significant blood loss or infection[9]**
- **Follow-up** care is important
- Postpartum contraception

1. Although rates of pregnancy termination are decreasing in the U.S., it remains an essential part of obstetric and gynecologic care as an elective procedure and for women whose medical and/or social circumstances make it the proper choice. Of increasing concern are the many cities and states in which this service is no longer available or only available in a limited capacity due to political influences rather than health concerns. Most pregnancy terminations are performed in the first trimester (90%), in unmarried women (85%), frequently in pregnancies that were unintended (50%), and in women of lower socio-economic status.

2. All patients considering termination should first have the location and gestational age of their pregnancy confirmed. While many providers chose to use ultrasound for this purpose, a firm LMP with a confirmatory pelvic examination is acceptable. Patients should also be assessed for any medical conditions that may affect the nature and location of the procedure performed (such as diabetes, hypertension, cardiac disease, or thrombophilia).

3. The approval by the FDA in 2000 of mifepristone (a progesterone receptor antagonist) with misoprostol (prostaglandin E1) for pregnancy

Obstetric Clinical Algorithms, Second Edition. Errol R. Norwitz, George R. Saade, Hugh Miller and Christina M. Davidson.
© 2017 John Wiley & Sons, Ltd. Published 2017 by John Wiley & Sons, Ltd.

termination provided a much-needed option to surgical termination. Medical termination now accounts for 25% of all procedures. While the original medical regimen included mifepristone 600 mg orally followed by misoprostol 400 mcg orally 24–48 hours later, there are now several other regimens that have gained acceptance with equal efficacy and lower cost (e.g. mifepristone 200 mg orally followed by misoprostol 600–800 mcg vaginally 6–8 hours later). Medical termination avoids an invasive procedure, need for anesthesia, and has a high success rate particularly at ≤9 weeks (95%). But it does result in moderate blood loss and requires careful follow-up to ensure complete expulsion. Around 5% of patients will ultimately need a surgical procedure. Surgical termination is invasive and requires pain management in a suitable facility. Advantages are that it requires less procedure time, has a slightly higher success rate (99%), and does not require follow-up.

4. Counseling should include education about the alternatives to termination and the risks and benefits of each procedure. Other issues that should be addressed include social support, domestic violence, STI risk, contraception, and pre-existing mental disorders that might be affected by the procedure. Because of the changing political landscape, many states now have mandatory wait times, requirements for ultrasound prior to any procedure, and elaborate documentation. Providers should consult their state professional organizations to determine how their local policies affect them and their patients.

5. First trimester termination is increasingly accomplished by medical intervention (25%), particularly at <63 days of gestation where the success rates are very high. Prophylactic antibiotics are not necessary, but may be considered in patients at high risk for STIs. Medical termination is also very successful beyond the first trimester, with success rates of 92–97% depending on the gestational age, therapeutic regimen,

and clinical setting. With advancing gestational age, there is a greater risk of retained POC and need for subsequent surgical intervention. Follow-up is essential to confirm successful termination, particularly in view of misoprostol teratogenic potential if the pregnancy were to continue. Traditional two-week follow-up visits can be replaced by various strategies (phone calls, serial hCG measurements, and follow-up ultrasound examination).

6. Surgical termination in the first trimester is easily accomplished in both outpatient and inpatient facilities. Pre-cervical preparation is generally recommended either in the form of rigid dilators (such as laminaria) or vaginal misoprostol (400 mcg) for 2–3 hours prior to the procedure. Vaginal misoprostol is often favored because it is equally effective, less painful, and cheaper. Prophylactic antibiotics have been shown to significantly reduce post-procedural infection. All patients require some degree of sedation for the procedure, usually anesthesia with or without a paracervical block. The recovered tissue should be evaluated to ensure that the procedure has been successfully completed. Some states require that the tissue be sent to pathology. Some patients with suspected fetal anomalies may request genetic analysis in anticipation of future pregnancies.

7. Second trimester termination follows many of same principles outlined for first trimester terminations. However, state regulations are generally more restrictive with advancing gestational age. Additional genetic testing (include micro-array analysis on amniotic fluid, fetal or placental tissue) or pathologic examination may be requested since many such procedures are performed due to concerns about an underlying chromosomal, genetic, or structural defect. The cost, expediency, and integrity of the fetus following the procedure are factors that may need to be considered when counseling such patients. The technique used for surgical termination is dependent on the providers' experience and

training. Ultrasound guidance can be used in an attempt to avoid uterine perforation, reduce procedure time, and ensure complete tissue evacuation.

8. Medical termination in the second trimester typically includes mifepristone 200 mg orally followed by a combination of vaginal and oral misoprostol, with high success rates within 24–48 hours. Doses of misoprostol used are often higher than that used in the first trimester (up to 800 mcg every 3–6 hours depending on the route of administration). Oxytocin is not effective at gestational ages <20 weeks, because of the absence of myometrial oxytocin receptors. There is no benefit to routine use of prophylactic antibiotics in low-risk women. There is often a greater need for analgesia or anesthesia for second trimester terminations, which is easily accomplished as these procedures are generally performed in a hospital setting. Fetal tissues should be carefully examined after delivery to ensure that there are no retained products, considering that 10–15% of these deliveries will require a surgical procedure to remove residual products of conception.

9. Follow-up visits are essential following medical termination and may drive patient selection. Such patients should be monitored for evidence of excessive blood loss and for infectious and surgical complications. Counseling should also include a discussion about contraception, lifestyle modifications (smoking cessation, weight loss), and optimization of comorbid conditions (such as diabetes and hypertension).

53 Prenatal Diagnosis

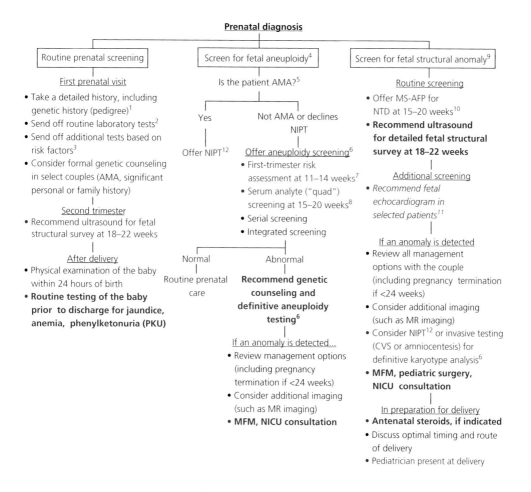

Prenatal diagnosis

Routine prenatal screening

First prenatal visit
- Take a detailed history, including genetic history (pedigree)[1]
- Send off routine laboratory tests[2]
- Send off additional tests based on risk factors[3]
- Consider formal genetic counseling in select couples (AMA, significant personal or family history)

Second trimester
- Recommend ultrasound for fetal structural survey at 18–22 weeks

After delivery
- Physical examination of the baby within 24 hours of birth
- **Routine testing of the baby prior to discharge for jaundice, anemia, phenylketonuria (PKU)**

Screen for fetal aneuploidy[4]

Is the patient AMA?[5]

Yes — Offer NIPT[12]

Not AMA or declines NIPT

Offer aneuploidy screening[6]
- First-trimester risk assessment at 11–14 weeks[7]
- Serum analyte ("quad") screening at 15–20 weeks[8]
- Serial screening
- Integrated screening

Normal
Routine prenatal care

Abnormal
Recommend genetic counseling and definitive aneuploidy testing[6]

If an anomaly is detected...
- Review management options (including pregnancy termination if <24 weeks)
- Consider additional imaging (such as MR imaging)
- **MFM, NICU consultation**

Screen for fetal structural anomaly[9]

Routine screening
- Offer MS-AFP for NTD at 15–20 weeks[10]
- **Recommend ultrasound for detailed fetal structural survey at 18–22 weeks**

Additional screening
- *Recommend fetal echocardiogram in selected patients[11]*

If an anomaly is detected
- Review all management options (including pregnancy termination if <24 weeks)
- Consider additional imaging (such as MR imaging)
- Consider NIPT[12] or invasive testing (CVS or amniocentesis) for definitive karyotype analysis[6]
- **MFM, pediatric surgery, NICU consultation**

In preparation for delivery
- **Antenatal steroids, if indicated**
- Discuss optimal timing and route of delivery
- Pediatrician present at delivery

1. Ask about prior pregnancies, underlying medical conditions, personal and family history, and medication/drug exposure. Patient history may identify a fetus at risk for aneuploidy (genetic anomalies) or structural anomalies.

2. Routine testing at the first prenatal visit should include: CBC, T&S, RPR, rubella serology, hepatitis B serology, HIV, PAP smear, PPD, cervical cultures (gonorrhoea, chlamydia), and urinalysis. Toxoplasmosis, varicella, CMV, urine toxicology, and TSH screening are not routinely recommended. All pregnant women should be offered genetic screening for cystic fibrosis carrier status (although the test is most reliable in Caucasian couples). In the late second trimester,

Obstetric Clinical Algorithms, Second Edition. Errol R. Norwitz, George R. Saade, Hugh Miller and Christina M. Davidson.
© 2017 John Wiley & Sons, Ltd. Published 2017 by John Wiley & Sons, Ltd.

additional screening tests are recommended: repeat CBC, T&S, RPR, and urinalysis. Consider repeat HIV in high-risk couples (Chapter 27, Human Immunodeficiency Virus). Screening for gestational diabetes at 24–28 weeks (Chapter 10, Gestational Diabetes Mellitus). Perineal culture for GBS carrier status at 35–36 weeks gestation (Chapter 24, Group B β-Hemolytic Streptococcus).

3. Additional genetic screening tests in patients at high-risk include: sickle cell disease (African ethnicity), β-thalassemia (Mediterranean women), and Tay–Sachs disease, Canavan disease, Niemann–Pick disease, Bloom syndrome, familial dysautonomia, Fanconi anemia, and Gaucher disease (in couples of Eastern European (Ashkenazi) Jewish extraction).

4. Major chromosomal abnormalities include trisomy 21 (Down syndrome, with an overall risk of 1/800 livebirths but strongly associated with maternal age), trisomy 18 (Edwards syndrome, 1/6000), trisomy 13 (Patau syndrome, 1/15000), and sex chromosomal disorders such as 47,XXY (Klinefelter syndrome, 1/500) and 45,X (Turner syndrome, 1/2500 livebirths but accounts for around 25% of early miscarriage). Many of these chromosomal disorders are due to nondisjunction events. Genetic abnormalities are classified according to the mode of genetic transmission: (i) autosomal dominant in 70% of cases (Huntington chorea, neurofibromatosis, achondroplasia, Marfan syndrome); (ii) autosomal recessive in 20% (sickle cell disease, cystic fibrosis, Tay–Sachs disease, β-thalassemia); (iii) X-linked recessive in 5% (Duchenne muscular dystrophy, hemophilia); (iv) X-linked dominant in <1% (vitamin D-resistant rickets); and (v) multifactorial inheritance in 3–5% (neural tube defect, club feet, hydrocephaly, cleft lip, cardiac anomalies).

5. Advanced maternal age (AMA) refers to women ≥35 years of age on her due date (see Chapter 32, Advanced Maternal Age). Such women account for 5–8% of deliveries and 20–30% of Down syndrome births.

6. Chorionic villous sampling (CVS) can be offered for karyotype analysis at 10–14 weeks. CVS involves sampling of placental tissue which can be used for DNA analysis, cytogenetic testing or enzyme assays. Advantages include earlier diagnosis. Disadvantages include potential for maternal cell contamination and sampling of cells destined to become placenta rather than fetus. CVS performed <9 weeks is associated with a threefold increase in limb reduction defects. After 15 weeks, ultrasound-guided amniocentesis can be performed and amniocytes isolated for karyotype analysis. The procedure-related pregnancy loss rate for both procedures is estimated at approximately 1/400. Early amniocentesis (<15 weeks) is associated with increased pregnancy loss and is thus not recommended.

7. Nuchal translucency (NT) measurements at 11–14 weeks correlate with fetal aneuploidy. A measurement of >2.5 mm is seen in 2–6% of fetuses of which 50–70% will have a chromosomal anomaly. However, it is not a sensitive enough test to use on its own. First-trimester risk assessment screening incorporates NT and the two maternal serum analyte markers, pregnancy-associated plasma protein-A (PAPP-A) and β-subunit of human chorionic gonadotropin (β-hCG).

8. Second-trimester maternal serum analyte screening uses a panel of biochemical markers to adjust the maternal age-related risk for fetal aneuploidy. The standard quadruple panel test ("quad test") at 15–20 weeks uses four maternal serum markers (AFP, β-hCG, estriol, and inhibin A). The most important variable is gestational age, which accounts for the majority of false-positive results. This test has detection rate for trisomy 21 of 75–85% with a false positive rate of 5%.

9. Congenital anomalies refer to structural defects present at birth. Major congenital

anomalies (those incompatible with life or requiring major surgery) occur in 2–3% of live-births, and 5% of livebirths have minor malformations. Some 30–40% of congenital anomalies have a known cause, including chromosomal abnormalities (0.5%), single gene defects (1%), multifactorial disorders, and teratogenic exposures. However, 60–70% have no known cause.

10. Elevated levels of maternal serum α-feto-protein (MS-AFP) at 15–20 weeks (defined variably as ≥2.0 or ≥2.5 multiples of the median (MoM)) are associated with open neural tube defect (NTD). A detailed sonographic exam of the fetal spine and head (for hydrocephalus, "lemon sign" and "banana sign") is indicated. If the spine and head are normal, consider other causes of elevated MS-AFP, including wrong dates, twins, IUFD, IUGR, placental abruption, abnormal placentation, and other fetal anomalies (anterior abdominal wall defects, renal defects).

11. Fetal echocardiogram at 20–22 weeks is indicated in women at risk of having a fetus with a cardiac defect, including couples with a personal or family history of congenital heart disease, women with pregestational diabetes, an abnormal four-chamber and/or outflow tract view of the fetal heart on routine second-trimester ultrasound, select medication exposure in pregnancy (lithium, paroxetine), low PAPP-A (<0.4 MoM) at 11–14 weeks' gestation, and IVF conception.

12. Noninvasive prenatal testing (NIPT) refers to the analysis of cell-free fetal DNA in the maternal circulation to screen for fetal aneuploidy. This maternal blood test, which can be sent as early as 9 weeks, has a sensitivity of >99% for trisomy 21 with a false positive rate of 0.2%. But it is a screening test, and the diagnosis should always be confirmed by a diagnostic test (CVS or amniocentesis).

54 Preterm Labor

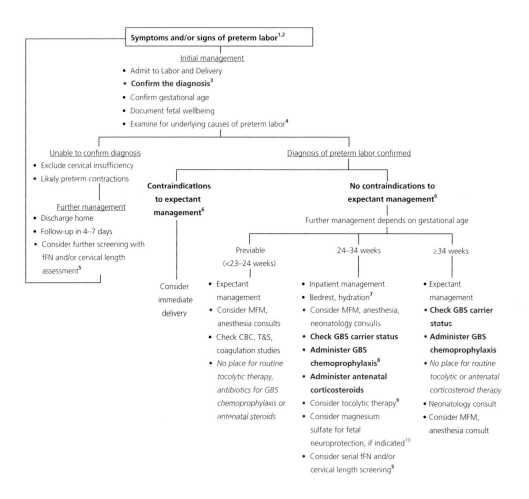

1. Labor is defined as an increase in myometrial activity resulting in effacement and dilation of the uterine cervix and delivery of the products of conception. Preterm labor refers to the onset of labor prior to 37 weeks of gestation. It occurs in 8–12% of deliveries, but accounts for >85% of perinatal mortality.

2. Several risk factors for preterm birth have been identified (see Chapter 55, Screening for

---

Obstetric Clinical Algorithms, Second Edition. Errol R. Norwitz, George R. Saade, Hugh Miller and Christina M. Davidson.
© 2017 John Wiley & Sons, Ltd. Published 2017 by John Wiley & Sons, Ltd.

Preterm Birth). However, >50% of spontaneous preterm births occur in women with no apparent risk factors. Moreover, although obstetric care providers are getting better at identifying women at risk of preterm birth, it is not clear that this outcome can be prevented.

3. A definitive diagnosis of preterm labor is necessary before further treatment options are considered. Diagnosis requires the presence of both uterine contractions and cervical change (or, in nulliparous patients, an initial cervical exam >2 cm and/or >80% effacement in the setting of uterine contractions of increasing intensity and frequency). Uterine activity in the absence of cervical change should be regarded as preterm contractions, and does not require further treatment.

4. Preterm labor probably represents a syndrome rather than a diagnosis since the etiologies are varied. Of all preterm births, 20% are iatrogenic and performed for maternal or fetal indications, such as diabetes, placenta previa or intrauterine growth restriction (IUGR). A further 20–30% result from intra-amniotic infection/inflammation, 20–25% occur in the setting of preterm premature rupture of membranes (pPROM), and the remaining 25–30% are the result of spontaneous preterm labor.

5. Fetal fibronectin (fFN) testing and cervical length assessment to identify patients at risk of preterm birth are discussed further in Chapter 55, Screening for Preterm Birth.

6. Contraindications to expectant management include intrauterine infection, nonreassuring fetal testing ("fetal distress"), unexplained vaginal bleeding, and intrauterine fetal demise or a lethal fetal anomaly.

7. Bedrest and hydration are commonly recommended in the setting of preterm labor, but without proven efficacy.

8. Screening for GBS carrier status and GBS chemoprophylaxis are discussed further in Chapter 24, Group B β-hemolytic streptococcus.

9. Pharmacologic therapy remains the cornerstone of modern management of preterm labor. Although a number of alternative agents are now available (see table below), there are no reliable data to suggest that any of these agents is able to delay premature delivery for longer than a few days. No single agent has a clear therapeutic advantage; as such, the side-effect profile of each of the drugs will often determine which to use in a given clinical setting. The only agent approved by the FDA in the United States for the treatment of preterm labor is ritodrine hydrochloride (which is no longer on formulary in the USA). Maintenance tocolytic therapy beyond 48 hours has not been shown to confer any therapeutic benefit, but does pose a significant risk of adverse side effects. The concurrent use of two or more tocolytic agents has not been shown to be more effective than a single agent alone, and the additive risk of side effects generally precludes this course of management. However, the use of sequential therapy (discontinuation of one agent followed by initiation of an alternative) may be beneficial.

10. Recent data suggest that very low birth weight infants (<1500 g, typically <32 weeks) exposed to IV magnesium sulfate 12–24 hours prior to delivery may be partially protected against neurologic injury, including cerebral palsy.

Common options for short-term tocolytic therapy			
Route of administration	Tocolytic agent (dosage)	Major maternal side-effects	Major fetal side-effects
Magnesium sulfate	IV (4–6 g bolus, then 2–3 g/h infusion)	Nausea, ileus, headache, weakness, hypotension, pulmonary edema, cardiorespiratory arrest	Decreased beat-to-beat variability, neonatal drowsiness, hypotonia, ?congenital ricketic syndrome
β-Adrenergic agonists			
Terbutaline sulfate	IV (2 ug/min infusion, max 80 ug/min) SC (0.25 mg q 20 min)	Jitteriness, anxiety, restlessness, nausea, vomiting, rash, cardiac dysrhythmias, myocardial ischemia, palpitations, chest pain, hypotension, tachycardia, pulmonary edema, paralytic ileus, hypokalemia, hyperglycemia, acidosis	Fetal tachycardia, hypotension, ileus, hyperinsulinemia, hypoglycemia, hyperbilirubinemia, hypocalcemia, ?hydrops fetalis
Prostaglandin inhibitors			
Indometacin	Oral (25–50 mg q 4–6 h) Rectal (100 mg q 12 h)	Gastrointestinal effects (nausea, heartburn), rash, headache, interstitial nephritis, ?increased bleeding time	Transient oliguria, oligohydramnios, ?necrotizing enterocolitis, ?intraventricular hemorrhage Premature closure of neonatal ductus arteriosus and persistent pulmonary hypertension
Calcium channel blockers			
Nifedipine	Oral (20–30 mg q 4–8 h)	Hypotension, reflex tachycardia, headache, nausea, flushing, potentiates the cardiac depressive effect of magnesium sulfate, hepatotoxicity	

55 Screening for Preterm Birth

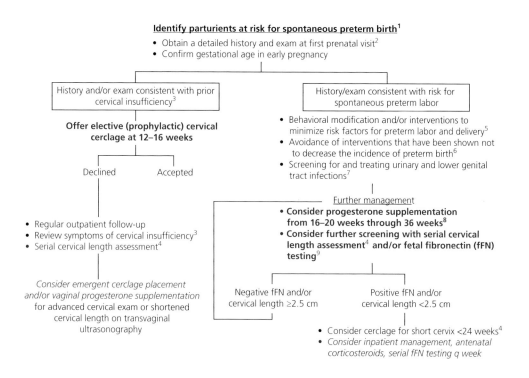

Identify parturients at risk for spontaneous preterm birth[1]
- Obtain a detailed history and exam at first prenatal visit[2]
- Confirm gestational age in early pregnancy

History and/or exam consistent with prior cervical insufficiency[3]

Offer elective (prophylactic) cervical cerclage at 12–16 weeks

Declined   Accepted

- Regular outpatient follow-up
- Review symptoms of cervical insufficiency[3]
- Serial cervical length assessment[4]

Consider emergent cerclage placement and/or vaginal progesterone supplementation for advanced cervical exam or shortened cervical length on transvaginal ultrasonography

---

History/exam consistent with risk for spontaneous preterm labor

- Behavioral modification and/or interventions to minimize risk factors for preterm labor and delivery[5]
- Avoidance of interventions that have been shown not to decrease the incidence of preterm birth[6]
- Screening for and treating urinary and lower genital tract infections[7]

Further management
- **Consider progesterone supplementation from 16–20 weeks through 36 weeks[8]**
- **Consider further screening with serial cervical length assessment[4] and/or fetal fibronectin (fFN) testing[9]**

Negative fFN and/or cervical length ≥2.5 cm

Positive fFN and/or cervical length <2.5 cm

- Consider cerclage for short cervix <24 weeks[4]
- *Consider inpatient management, antenatal corticosteroids, serial fFN testing q week*

---

1. Twenty percent of preterm births are indication (iatrogenic) and performed for either maternal or fetal indications. A further 20–30% result from intra-amniotic infection/inflammation, 20–25% occur in the setting of preterm PROM (pPROM), and 25–30% are the result of spontaneous preterm labor. This algorithm deals only with the prevention of spontaneous preterm labor and delivery.

2. Risk factors associated with spontaneous preterm labor and delivery may be nonmodifiable or modifiable factors (see table below). In theory, identification of risk factors for preterm

delivery before conception or early in pregnancy will facilitate interventions that may help prevent this complication. However, causality is difficult to assess and most preterm births occur among women with no risk factors. Furthermore, the number of effective interventions is limited.

3. See Chapter 35, Cervical Insufficiency.

4. The relative risk of preterm birth increases as cervical length decreases. However, routine use of cervical ultrasonography for prediction of preterm birth in asymptomatic women is not

---

Obstetric Clinical Algorithms, Second Edition. Errol R. Norwitz, George R. Saade, Hugh Miller and Christina M. Davidson.
© 2017 John Wiley & Sons, Ltd. Published 2017 by John Wiley & Sons, Ltd.

currently recommended due to lack of effective interventions and low specificity. Data regarding the use of cervical cerclage for asymptomatic women with a shortened cervix (<2.5 cm) are conflicting; as such, this procedure cannot be routinely recommended.

5. Interventions that may decrease the risk of spontaneous preterm birth include smoking cessation, avoidance of illicit substance use (especially cocaine), avoidance of multiple pregnancies at ART, reduced occupational fatigue, and treatment of symptomatic genital infections. Interventions that may be recommended but are less likely to have a beneficial effect include an improvement in overall maternal nutrition (although there are no specific nutritional supplements which have been shown to decrease preterm birth) and regular antenatal care.

6. Several interventions have been shown in well-designed studies not to decrease the incidence of preterm birth and, as such, cannot routinely be recommended. These include home uterine activity monitoring, bed rest, broad-spectrum antibiotic therapy (in the absence of pPROM), and maintenance tocolytic therapy (such as long-term outpatient oral or intravenous β-agonist therapy; see Chapter 54, Preterm Labor).

7. All parturients should have a first-trimester urine culture to exclude asymptomatic bacteriuria. Regular screening is recommended also in the 2nd and 3rd trimesters in women at high risk for asymptomatic bacteriuria, including women with sickle cell trait, recurrent urinary tract infections, diabetes, and renal disease. Lower genital tract infections (such as BV, gonorrhea, chlamydia, ureaplasma, and trichomoniasis) have been associated with preterm birth.

Symptomatic infections should be treated. Screening for chlamydia is recommended for all pregnant women, while screening for gonorrhea is recommended only for women at high risk. Routine screening of asymptomatic women for other lower genital tract infections cannot be recommended at this time.

8. Progesterone supplementation (17α-hydroxyprogesterone caproate) from 16–20 weeks through 36 weeks may reduce the rate of preterm birth in high-risk women. Further investigations are needed to evaluate the effectiveness of progesterone supplementation to decrease the incidence of preterm delivery in other high- and low-risk populations and to better understand its mechanism of action.

9. The fetal fibronectin (fFN) assay is likely the best predictor of preterm birth because of the low prevalence of positive results in asymptomatic low-risk women. However, sensitivity and positive predictive value are also low. Disadvantages are its cost and the need to collect cervicovaginal secretions from the posterior fornix using a speculum. According to ACOG, candidates for fFN testing include *symptomatic* women between 24–0/7 and 34–6/7 weeks of gestation with intact amniotic membranes and cervical dilation <3 cm. Under these conditions, 80% of women will be fFN negative (<50 ng/mL). A negative fFN effectively excludes imminent preterm delivery: <1% of women will deliver within 14 days. A positive fFN test will predict delivery within the next 14 days in only 16% (1 in 6) of symptomatic women. As such, the value of the fFN test lies primarily in its negative predictive value (124 of 125 symptomatic women with a negative fFN test will not deliver within 14 days). If the fFN test is negative and clinical concern persists, consider repeating the test in 1–2 weeks.

Risk factors for preterm birth

Nonmodifiable risk factors

Prior preterm birth
African-American race
Maternal age <18 or >40 years
Low pre-pregnancy weight
Low socio-economic status
Chronic hypertension
Intra-amniotic infection
Diethylstilbestrol (DES) exposure
Cervical injury or anomaly
Uterine anomaly or fibroid
Premature cervical dilation (>2 cm) or effacement (>80%)
Overdistended uterus (multiple pregnancy, polyhydramnios)
Vaginal bleeding
? Excessive uterine activity

Modifiable risk factors

Smoking (≥10 cigarettes per day)
Illicit drug use (especially cocaine)
Absent prenatal care
Short interpregnancy interval
Anemia
Bacteriuria/urinary tract infection
Lower genital/gingival infection
? Strenuous work during pregnancy
? High personal stress

---

56 Preterm Premature Rupture of the Membranes[1]

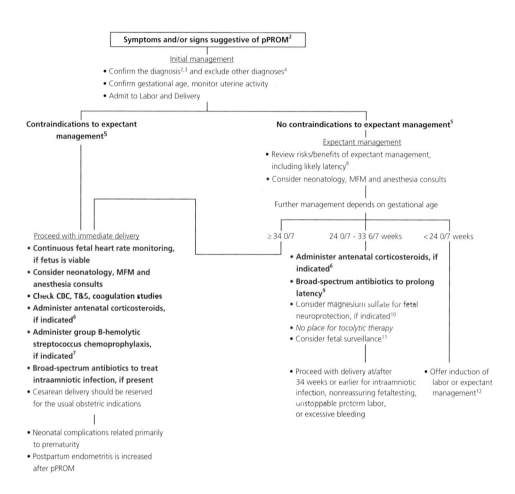

Symptoms and/or signs suggestive of pPROM[2]

Initial management
- Confirm the diagnosis[2,3] and exclude other diagnoses[4]
- Confirm gestational age, monitor uterine activity
- Admit to Labor and Delivery

Contraindications to expectant management[5]

No contraindications to expectant management[5]

Expectant management
- Review risks/benefits of expectant management, including likely latency[8]
- Consider neonatology, MFM and anesthesia consults

Further management depends on gestational age

Proceed with immediate delivery
- **Continuous fetal heart rate monitoring, if fetus is viable**
- **Consider neonatology, MFM and anesthesia consults**
- **Check CBC, T&S, coagulation studies**
- **Administer antenatal corticosteroids, if indicated[6]**
- **Administer group B-hemolytic streptococcus chemoprophylaxis, if indicated[7]**
- **Broad-spectrum antibiotics to treat intraamniotic infection, if present**
- Cesarean delivery should be reserved for the usual obstetric indications

- Neonatal complications related primarily to prematurity
- Postpartum endometritis is increased after pPROM

≥ 34 0/7   24 0/7 - 33 6/7 weeks   < 24 0/7 weeks

- **Administer antenatal corticosteroids, if indicated[6]**
- **Broad-spectrum antibiotics to prolong latency[9]**
- Consider magnesium sulfate for fetal neuroprotection, if indicated[10]
- *No place for tocolytic therapy*
- Consider fetal surveillance[11]

- Proceed with delivery at/after 34 weeks or earlier for intraamniotic infection, nonreassuring fetal testing, unstoppable preterm labor, or excessive bleeding

- Offer induction of labor or expectant management[12]

1. Premature rupture of the membranes (PROM) refers to rupture of the fetal membranes prior to the onset of labor. It can occur at term or preterm. Preterm PROM (pPROM) refers to PROM prior to 37 0/7 weeks of gestation. pPROM complicates 3% of pregnancies and is responsible for approximately one third of all preterm births. Risk factors for pPROM include prior pPROM, vaginal bleeding in the second or third trimester, short cervical length, chorioamnionitis, amniocentesis, low body mass index, cigarette smoking, illicit drug use, and low

Obstetric Clinical Algorithms, Second Edition. Errol R. Norwitz, George R. Saade, Hugh Miller and Christina M. Davidson.
© 2017 John Wiley & Sons, Ltd. Published 2017 by John Wiley & Sons, Ltd.

socio-economic status. Factors which are <u>not</u> associated with pPROM include coitus, cervical examinations, maternal exercise, and parity.

2. Preterm PROM is largely a <u>clinical</u> diagnosis. It is usually suggested by a history of watery vaginal discharge, and confirmed on sterile speculum examination by finding a pool of vaginal fluid or fluid passing through the cervical os with valsalva which has an alkaline pH (it turns yellow nitrazine paper blue) and demonstrates microscopic ferning on drying. Findings of diminished amniotic fluid volume on ultrasound may further suggest the diagnosis.

3. If the diagnosis is equivocal, ultrasound guided transabdominal instillation of dye into the amniotic cavity (indigo carmine rather than methylene blue because of the association of methylene blue with methemoglobinemia) and documentation of leakage of dye into the vagina (by staining of a tampon or pad within 20–30 min) will confirm the diagnosis.

4. Differential diagnosis of PROM includes urinary incontinence, excessive vaginal discharge, and cervical mucus ("show").

5. The management of pPROM is largely based on gestational age. Contraindications to expectant management include intra-amniotic infection (chorioamnionitis), nonreassuring fetal testing, clinically significant placental abruption or active labor. The optimal gestational age for delivery is unclear and controversial, however, current recommendations favor delivery at or beyond 34 0/7 weeks of gestation. Prior to 34 0/7 weeks, pPROM should be managed expectantly in the absence of contraindications. If expectant management is undertaken beyond 34 0/7 weeks of gestation, it should only be done after the care provider and patient have carefully considered the risks and benefits and should not extend beyond 37 0/7 weeks of gestation.

6. Administration of antenatal glucocorticoids has been shown to reduce neonatal mortality and decrease the incidence of respiratory distress syndrome, intraventricular hemorrhage, and necrotizing enterocolitis if administered to pregnancies threatening to deliver prior to 34 weeks of gestation, regardless of membrane status. A single course should be administered to women with pPROM between 24 0/7 and 34 0/7 weeks of gestation. There is no proven benefit to antenatal corticosteroids after 34 weeks and multiple courses of steroids are not recommended. A single repeat ("rescue") course has been shown to be beneficial in the setting of intact membranes. While a second dose is not associated with an increased rate of neonatal sepsis in women with pPROM, there is also no benefit identified.

7. Intrapartum (not antepartum) group B β-hemolytic streptococcus chemoprophylaxis is indicated for all women with pPROM, unless a negative perineal culture for group B β-hemolytic streptococcus has been documented within the prior 5 weeks. Intravenous penicillin is the antibiotic of choice.

8. Latency refers to the interval between rupture of the membranes and delivery and is inversely related to gestational age at membrane rupture. Severe oligohydramnios is associated with shortened latency. In general, 50% of pregnancies complicated by pPROM will deliver within one week of membrane rupture. The benefit of expectant management of pPROM is fetal maturity from pregnancy prolongation. Risks include clinically evident intraamniotic infection (15–25%), postpartum infection (15–20%), abruptio placentae (2–5%) and a 1-2% risk of antenatal fetal demise that is primarily attributed to infection and umbilical cord accident.

9. Prophylactic broad-spectrum antibiotics have been shown to prolong latency in the setting of pPROM, reduce maternal and neonatal

infections, and reduce gestational age-dependent morbidity. There is currently no evidence to recommend one regimen over another, however, the use of amoxicillin-clavulanic acid has been associated with increased rates of necrotizing enterocolitis and is no longer recommended. The most common regimen is Ampicillin 2 gm/erythromycin 250 mg IV q6h for 48 h followed by amoxicillin 250 mg/erythromycin 333 mg po q8h for 5 days. Substitution of a single dose of azithromycin for erythromycin has recently been shown not to affect latency or any other measured maternal or fetal outcomes.

10. Fetuses in pregnancies complicated by pPROM are at risk for infection, cord accident, placental abruption, and (possibly) uteroplacental insufficiency. While it is generally accepted that some form of fetal monitoring is necessary, the type and frequency of this monitoring are controversial. Options include weekly or daily nonstress testing and/or biophysical profile, as well as periodic ultrasound evaluation of amniotic fluid volume and fetal growth. Indeed, complications such as placental abruption, cord accident, and intra-amniotic infection cannot be predicted or reliably detected by such antenatal fetal testing.

11. Randomized controlled trials have demonstrated that maternal administration of magnesium sulfate used for fetal neuroprotection when birth is anticipated before 32 0/7 weeks of gestation reduces the risk of cerebral palsy in surviving infants. In the largest of these trials, 85% of the women enrolled had pPROM between 24 and 32 weeks of gestation. Women with pPROM before 32 0/7 weeks of gestation should be considered candidates for fetal neuroprotective treatment with magnesium sulfate.

12. Previable pPROM occurs in less than 1% of pregnancies. Women presenting with PROM before neonatal viability should be offered immediate delivery. Counseling should include a discussion of the maternal risks of chorioamnionitis/endometritis, placental abruption, retained placenta, sepsis (1%) and death (rare) as well as fetal risks of lethal pulmonary hypoplasia (especially with oligohydramnios prior to 26 weeks of gestation) and perinatal survival rates of only 14.4% in the setting of pPROM before 22 weeks of gestation compared to 57.7% after 22 weeks. If the patient opts for and has no contraindications to expectant management, outpatient surveillance can be considered after an initial 24–48 hour period of inpatient observation. Women are then readmitted to the hospital either for delivery if a contraindication to expectant management arises or once viability has been reached. If admitted at viability, latency antibiotics, antenatal corticosteroids, and magnesium sulfate should be administered.

57 Vaginal Birth after Cesarean (VBAC)

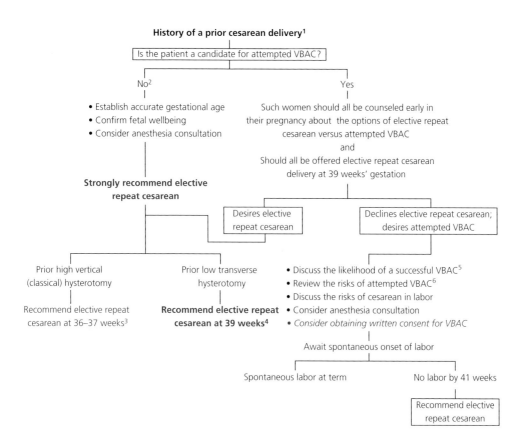

History of a prior cesarean delivery[1]

Is the patient a candidate for attempted VBAC?

No[2]

- Establish accurate gestational age
- Confirm fetal wellbeing
- Consider anesthesia consultation

Strongly recommend elective repeat cesarean

Yes

Such women should all be counseled early in their pregnancy about the options of elective repeat cesarean versus attempted VBAC
and
Should all be offered elective repeat cesarean delivery at 39 weeks' gestation

Desires elective repeat cesarean

Declines elective repeat cesarean; desires attempted VBAC

Prior high vertical (classical) hysterotomy

Recommend elective repeat cesarean at 36–37 weeks[3]

Prior low transverse hysterotomy

Recommend elective repeat cesarean at 39 weeks[4]

- Discuss the likelihood of a successful VBAC[5]
- Review the risks of attempted VBAC[6]
- Discuss the risks of cesarean in labor
- Consider anesthesia consultation
- *Consider obtaining written consent for VBAC*

Await spontaneous onset of labor

Spontaneous labor at term

No labor by 41 weeks

Recommend elective repeat cesarean

1. Cesarean delivery refers to delivery of a fetus via the abdominal route (laparotomy) requiring an incision into the uterus (hysterotomy). It is now the second most common surgical procedure (behind male circumcision) accounting for around 20–25% of all deliveries in the United Kingdom and 30–35% of deliveries in the United States. Approximately one-third of cesarean deliveries are elective repeat procedures.

2. Absolute contraindications for attempted VBAC include one or more prior high vertical ("classical") cesarean deliveries, two or more prior lower uterine segment transverse cesarean deliveries, non-reassuring fetal testing (previously referred to as "fetal distress"), transverse lie, placenta previa, or delivery in a setting that is unable to offer immediate access to anesthesia services or unable to perform an

Obstetric Clinical Algorithms, Second Edition. Errol R. Norwitz, George R. Saade, Hugh Miller and Christina M. Davidson.
© 2017 John Wiley & Sons, Ltd. Published 2017 by John Wiley & Sons, Ltd.

emergent cesarean. <u>Relative contraindications</u> include breech presentation, prior full-thickness myomectomy, or a prior uterine rupture.

3. In women who have had one or more prior high vertical ("classical") cesarean deliveries, an elective repeat cesarean should be performed at 36–37 weeks' gestation prior to the onset of labor. This is because of the high risk of uterine rupture in such women (4–8%) and the knowledge that 50% of such uterine ruptures occur prior to labor. Confirmation of fetal lung maturity by amniocentesis is not necessary.

4. According to ACOG, elective repeat cesarean can be performed after 39 0/7 weeks in a well-dated pregnancy without documenting fetal lung maturity by amniocentesis. In HIV-positive women and twins, an elective cesarean can be performed after 38 0/7 weeks.

5. A successful VBAC can be achieved in 65–80% of women. Factors associated with successful VBAC include one or more prior vaginal deliveries, estimated fetal weight <4,000 g, and a non-recurrent indication for the prior cesarean (breech, placenta previa) rather than a potentially recurrent indication (such as cephalopelvic disproportion).

6. Attempted VBAC is associated with a number of risks, including:
- Failed VBAC leading to <u>cesarean delivery</u> with an associated increased risk of maternal mortality (approximately 0.01%; 2- to 10-fold higher than for vaginal birth and elective cesarean prior to labor) and maternal morbidity (infection, thromboembolic events, wound dehiscence).
- Uterine rupture, which may be life-threatening. Symptoms and signs of uterine rupture include acute onset of fetal bradycardia (70%), abdominal pain (10%), vaginal bleeding (5%), hemodynamic instability (5–10%), and/or loss of the presenting part (<5%).

Epidural anesthesia may mask some of these features. Risk factors for uterine rupture include the type of prior uterine incision (<1% for lower uterine segment transverse incision, 2–3% for lower segment vertical, and 4–8% for high vertical), two or more prior cesareans (4%), prior uterine rupture, "excessive" use of oxytocin (although the term "excessive" is poorly defined), dysfunctional labor pattern (especially prolonged second stage or arrest of dilatation), and induction of labor (especially with the use of prostaglandins). Factors not associated with uterine rupture include epidural anesthesia, unknown uterine scar, fetal macrosomia, and indication for prior cesarean. Uterine rupture is associated with significant maternal mortality and morbidity (including the need for emergent cesarean and possible blood transfusion) as well as a fivefold increased risk of fetal morbidity (hypoxic ischemic brain injury) and death. NOTE: Uterine rupture should be distinguished from uterine dehiscence, which refers to subclinical separation of the prior uterine incision that is often detected only by manual exploration of the scar following vaginal delivery or at the time of elective cesarean. It occurs in 2–3% of women with a prior cesarean delivery. In the absence of vaginal bleeding, no further treatment is necessary.
- Increased risk of <u>puerperal (cesarean) hysterectomy</u>. This is a rare event (1 in 6,000 deliveries) that is performed primarily as an emergency when the mother's life is at risk due to uncontrolled hemorrhage. It is a highly morbid procedure and is therefore performed only as a last resort. Warming blanket, three-way Foley catheter, and blood products should be available. Blood loss is often excessive (2–4 L) and blood transfusions are usually required (90%). Despite a high morbidity, overall maternal mortality is low (0.3%). Although women will be subsequently be amenorrheic and sterile, menopausal symptoms will not develop if the ovaries are left.

58 Teratology

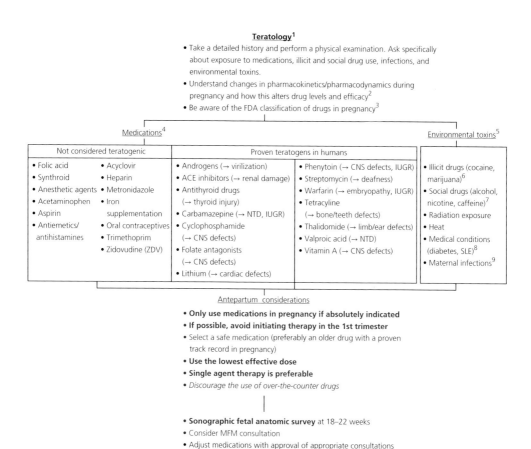

Teratology[1]
- Take a detailed history and perform a physical examination. Ask specifically about exposure to medications, illicit and social drug use, infections, and environmental toxins.
- Understand changes in pharmacokinetics/pharmacodynamics during pregnancy and how this alters drug levels and efficacy[2]
- Be aware of the FDA classification of drugs in pregnancy[3]

Medications[4]

Not considered teratogenic		Proven teratogens in humans		Environmental toxins[5]
• Folic acid • Synthroid • Anesthetic agents • Acetaminophen • Aspirin • Antiemetics/ antihistamines	• Acyclovir • Heparin • Metronidazole • Iron supplementation • Oral contraceptives • Trimethoprim • Zidovudine (ZDV)	• Androgens (→ virilization) • ACE inhibitors (→ renal damage) • Antithyroid drugs (→ thyroid injury) • Carbamazepine (→ NTD, IUGR) • Cyclophosphamide (→ CNS defects) • Folate antagonists (→ CNS defects) • Lithium (→ cardiac defects)	• Phenytoin (→ CNS defects, IUGR) • Streptomycin (→ deafness) • Warfarin (→ embryopathy, IUGR) • Tetracyline (→ bone/teeth defects) • Thalidomide (→ limb/ear defects) • Valproic acid (→ NTD) • Vitamin A (→ CNS defects)	• Illicit drugs (cocaine, marijuana)[6] • Social drugs (alcohol, nicotine, caffeine)[7] • Radiation exposure • Heat • Medical conditions (diabetes, SLE)[8] • Maternal infections[9]

Antepartum considerations
- **Only use medications in pregnancy if absolutely indicated**
- **If possible, avoid initiating therapy in the 1st trimester**
- Select a safe medication (preferably an older drug with a proven track record in pregnancy)
- **Use the lowest effective dose**
- **Single agent therapy is preferable**
- *Discourage the use of over-the-counter drugs*

- **Sonographic fetal anatomic survey** at 18–22 weeks
- Consider MFM consultation
- Adjust medications with approval of appropriate consultations

1. Teratology refers to the study of abnormal development, both in utero and postnatally. We refer here to human teratology, which includes both structural and functional abnormalities.

2. Pharmacokinetics is the study of how a drug moves through the body. Drug absorption is altered in pregnancy because gastric emptying and intestinal motility are decreased. Pulmonary tidal volume is increased which affects the absorption of inhaled drugs. The volume of distribution changes in pregnancy with a 40% increase in plasma volume, 7–8 L increase in total body water, and 20–40% increase in body fat. Despite these changes (which decrease drug levels), albumin declines and free fatty acid and lipoprotein levels rise. As a result, the protein binding of many drugs is decreased in pregnancy

Obstetric Clinical Algorithms, Second Edition. Errol R. Norwitz, George R. Saade, Hugh Miller and Christina M. Davidson. © 2017 John Wiley & Sons, Ltd. Published 2017 by John Wiley & Sons, Ltd.

leading to an increase in circulating free (biologically active) drug levels. Drug metabolism and elimination also change in pregnancy. High steroid hormone levels affect hepatic metabolism and prolong the half-life of some drugs. Glomerular filtration rate increases 50–60%, thereby increasing the renal clearance of other drugs.

3. The FDA has defined five risk categories for drug use in pregnancy (see table below). Individual agents are assigned to a risk category according to their risk/benefit ratio (e.g., oral contraceptives are not teratogenic, but are classified as category X because there is no benefit to being on the pill once you are pregnant). The FDA will eliminate these categories and replace them with three subsections, **Pregnancy**, **Lactation,** and **Females and Males of Reproductive Potential** that will provide more relevant risk-benefit information in a consistent manor.

4. Some 20–25% of women report using medications on a regular basis throughout pregnancy. Major congenital anomalies occur in 3–4% of live births, and 70% of such anomalies have no known cause. It is estimated that 2–3% are due to medications and 1% to environmental toxins. With the exception of large molecules (such as heparin), all drugs given to the mother cross the placenta to some degree. The effect of a given drug on a fetus depends on dose, time and duration of exposure as well as poorly-defined genetic and environmental factors. A fetus is at highest risk for injury during embryogenesis (days 17–54 post-conception). Paternal exposure has never been shown to be teratogenic. Drug trials are difficult to carry out in pregnancy because of concern over the fetus. As such, many drugs have not been validated for use or safety in human pregnancy. Recommendations often rely on data from animal models. The occurrence of thalidomide-associated embryopathy has led to the belief that human teratogenicity cannot be predicted by animal studies. However, every drug that has since been found to be teratogenic in humans has caused similar effects in animals.

5. A number of environmental toxins have been implicated in fetal injury: (i) Ionizing radiation has been associated with spontaneous abortion, microcephaly, mental retardation, and (possibly) malignancy in later life. Fetal

The Food and Drug Administration (FDA) in the United States Classification of Drugs in Pregnancy		
Category	Criteria	Examples
A	Well-controlled studies in pregnant women have not shown an increased risk of fetal abnormalities	Vitamin C, folic acid, L-thyroxine
B	Animal studies have shown no evidence of harm to the fetus or have confirmed an adverse effect in the fetus, but there are no adequate and well-controlled studies in pregnant women	Benadryl, xylocaine, α-methyldopa, ampicillin, hydrochlorothiazide
C	No adequate or well-controlled studies in pregnant women have been conducted	Theophylline, nifedipine, β-blockers, digoxin, acyclovir, zidovudine (ZDV)
D	Studies in pregnant women have demonstrated a risk to the fetus. However, the benefits of therapy may outweigh the potential risk	Cytoxan, ACE inhibitors, phenytoin, spironolactone, methotrexate
X	Studies in animals or pregnant women have shown evidence of fetal abnormalities. The use of the product is contraindicated in women who are or may become pregnant.	Radioisotopes, isotretinoin (vitamin A), oral contraceptives

exposure of at least >5 Rad is required for any adverse effect, which is a 1,000-fold higher than most imaging studies (estimated fetal exposure from common radiological procedures is 1–3 mRad). (ii) <u>Heat</u> has been weakly associated with spontaneous abortion and neural tube defects. (iii) <u>Electromagnetic field exposure</u> has not consistently been shown to be injurious to the fetus.

6. The illicit drug which has been most commonly implicated in fetal injury is <u>cocaine</u>, which has been associated with IUGR, cerebral infarction, and placental abruption. Reported congenital anomalies (limb reduction defects, porencephalic cysts, microcephaly, bowel atresia, necrotizing enterocolitis, and long-term behavioral effects) may be secondary to cocaine-induced vasospasm. <u>Marijuana</u> has no clear teratogenic effects, but a weak and inconsistent association between marijuana and preterm birth, IUGR, and neurodevelopmental delay has been proposed.

7. A number of social drugs have been implicated in fetal injury: (i) <u>Alcohol</u> causes fetal alcohol syndrome, which is characterized by facial abnormalities (midfacial hypoplasia), central nervous system dysfunction (microcephaly, mental retardation), and IUGR. Renal and cardiac defects may also occur. The risk of anomalies is related to the extent of alcohol use: 10% with rare use, 15% with moderate use, and 30–40% with heavy use (>6 drinks per day). There is no safe level of alcohol use in pregnancy. (ii) <u>Cigarette smoking</u> is associated with subfertility, spontaneous abortion, preterm birth, perinatal mortality, and low-birth-weight infants. Neonatal exposure is associated with SIDS, asthma, respiratory infections, and attention deficit disorder.

20–30% of women continue to smoke during pregnancy. (iii) <u>Caffeine</u> has no clear teratogenic effects, but has been weakly associated with spontaneous abortion.

8. Certain medical conditions can cause birth defects. Diabetes, for example, can cause congenital heart disease, neural tube defects, and caudal regression. The risk is directly related to the degree of glycemic control around the time of conception. Some patients with systemic lupus erythematosus (SLE) will produce anti-Ro/SSA and/or anti-La/SSB antibodies that cause congenital heart block and result in neonatal lupus. Maternal phenylketonuria (PKU) can cause microcephaly, intellectual disability, and congenital heart disease.

9. In utero infection with Toxoplasmosis, Rubella, Cytomegalovirus, Herpes (TORCH infections) and syphilis can cause major congenital malformations (microcephaly), short- and long-term disability (blindness, hearing loss, developmental delay), and death. More recently the Zika virus has been shown to be associated with microcephaly. Diagnostic and therapeutic recommendations for Zika are still being developed, but the current recommendations include women and their partners avoiding the Caribbean and South American countries where the virus is endemic or delaying childbirth (refer to the CDC for the latest recommendations). The Zika virus illustrates the importance of a detailed history of a patient's recent travel, past infections and immunizations, which are essential in preventing adverse outcomes, especially in patients at high risk (such as women who are immunosuppressed, have cats, or engage in an occupation that would increase their risk of exposure).

59 Term Premature Rupture of the Membranes[1]

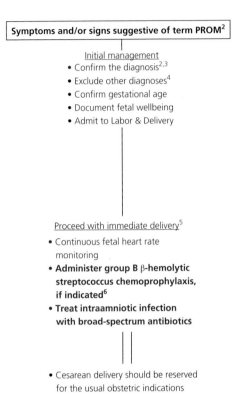

Symptoms and/or signs suggestive of term PROM[2]

Initial management
- Confirm the diagnosis[2,3]
- Exclude other diagnoses[4]
- Confirm gestational age
- Document fetal wellbeing
- Admit to Labor & Delivery

Proceed with immediate delivery[5]
- Continuous fetal heart rate monitoring
- **Administer group B β-hemolytic streptococcus chemoprophylaxis, if indicated[6]**
- **Treat intraamniotic infection with broad-spectrum antibiotics**

- Cesarean delivery should be reserved for the usual obstetric indications

1. Premature rupture of the membranes (PROM) refers to rupture of the fetal membranes prior to the onset of labor. It can occur at term or preterm. Term PROM (tPROM) refers to PROM occurring at or after 37 0/7 weeks of gestation. tPROM complicates 8% of all term pregnancies.

2. Term PROM is largely a clinical diagnosis. It is usually suggested by a history of watery vaginal discharge and confirmed on sterile speculum examination by finding a pool of vaginal fluid or fluid passing through the cervical os with valsalva which has an alkaline pH (it turns yellow nitrazine paper blue) and demonstrates microscopic ferning on drying. Findings of diminished amniotic fluid volume on ultrasound may further suggest the diagnosis.

3. Differential diagnosis of tPROM includes urinary incontinence, excessive vaginal discharge, and cervical mucus ("show").

Obstetric Clinical Algorithms, Second Edition. Errol R. Norwitz, George R. Saade, Hugh Miller and Christina M. Davidson.
© 2017 John Wiley & Sons, Ltd. Published 2017 by John Wiley & Sons, Ltd.

4. Generally, 50% of women with tPROM managed expectantly give birth within 5 hours and 95% give birth within 28 hours of membrane rupture. The most significant maternal consequence of tPROM is intrauterine infection, the risk of which increases with the duration of membrane rupture. Induction of labor is associated with a reduced time to delivery and lower rates of chorioamnionitis, endometritis, and admission to the neonatal intensive care unit without increasing the rates of cesarean delivery or operative vaginal delivery. Induction of labor with prostaglandins may be associated with higher rates of chorioamnionitis than induction with oxytocin. There are insufficient data on which to base a recommendation for mechanical methods of cervical ripening in the setting of tPROM.

5. If spontaneous labor does not occur near the time of presentation and cesarean delivery is not indicated, labor should be induced. Oxytocin infusion is generally preferred.

6. Intrapartum (not antepartum) group B β-hemolytic streptococcus (GBS) chemoprophylaxis is indicated for all women who have been identified as being GBS carriers by routine perineal culture at 35–36 weeks of gestation. If the patient's GBS carrier status is unknown, she should be given chemoprophylaxis if any risk factors are present (including GBS bacteriuria during pregnancy, amniotic membrane rupture ≥ 18 hours, fever in labor ($\geq 100.4\,°F$ or $>38.0\,°C$), or prior GBS-infected infant). Intravenous penicillin is the antibiotic of choice.

60 Twin Pregnancy

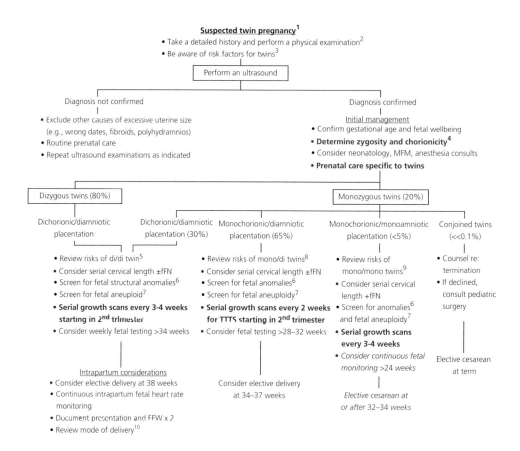

<u>**Suspected twin pregnancy**[1]</u>
- Take a detailed history and perform a physical examination[2]
- Be aware of risk factors for twins[3]

Perform an ultrasound

Diagnosis not confirmed
- Exclude other causes of excessive uterine size (e.g., wrong dates, fibroids, polyhydramnios)
- Routine prenatal care
- Repeat ultrasound examinations as indicated

Diagnosis confirmed

<u>Initial management</u>
- Confirm gestational age and fetal wellbeing
- **Determine zygosity and chorionicity**[4]
- Consider neonatology, MFM, anesthesia consults
- **Prenatal care specific to twins**

Dizygous twins (80%)

Monozygous twins (20%)

Dichorionic/diamniotic placentation
- Review risks of di/di twin[5]
- Consider serial cervical length ±fFN
- Screen for fetal structural anomalies[6]
- Screen for fetal aneuploid[7]
- **Serial growth scans every 3-4 weeks starting in 2nd trimester**
- Consider weekly fetal testing >34 weeks

Dichorionic/diamniotic placentation (30%)
- Review risks of mono/di twins[8]
- Consider serial cervical length ±fFN
- Screen for fetal anomalies[6]
- Screen for fetal aneuploidy[7]
- **Serial growth scans every 2 weeks for TTTS starting in 2nd trimester**
- Consider fetal testing >28–32 weeks

Monochorionic/diamniotic placentation (65%)

Monochorionic/monoamniotic placentation (<5%)
- Review risks of mono/mono twins[9]
- Consider serial cervical length +fFN
- Screen for anomalies[6] and fetal aneuploidy[7]
- **Serial growth scans every 3-4 weeks**
- *Consider continuous fetal monitoring >24 weeks*

Conjoined twins (<<0.1%)
- Counsel re: termination
- If declined, consult pediatric surgery

Elective cesarean at term

Elective cesarean at or after 32–34 weeks

<u>Intrapartum considerations</u>
- Consider elective delivery at 38 weeks
- Continuous intrapartum fetal heart rate monitoring
- Document presentation and EFW x 2
- Review mode of delivery[10]

Consider elective delivery at 34–37 weeks

1. Twin pregnancies comprise an increasing number of deliveries (3.3% of all births in 2011), primarily as a result of assisted reproductive technology (ART) and advancing maternal age at conception. The vast majority (96%) of multiple gestations are twin pregnancies arising from two fertilized oocytes (dizygous or "fraternal" twins). Identical (monozygous) twins account for approximately 20% of all twins, but the vast majority of pregnancy complications.

2. Suspect twins in women with excessive symptoms of pregnancy (e.g., nausea and vomiting) or uterine size larger than expected for gestational age.

3. Risk factors for twins include a family or personal history of dizygous twins (derived from two separate embryos), advanced maternal age, multiparity, African-American race, and ART. A history of monozygous twins is not a risk factor

---

Obstetric Clinical Algorithms, Second Edition. Errol R. Norwitz, George R. Saade, Hugh Miller and Christina M. Davidson.
© 2017 John Wiley & Sons, Ltd. Published 2017 by John Wiley & Sons, Ltd.

since it is a random event that occurs in 1 in 300 pregnancies.

4. Ultrasound will confirm the diagnosis, gestational age, fetal wellbeing, and chorionicity. Zygosity refers to the genetic makeup of the twins. Chorionicity refers to the timing of cell division, which establishes the arrangement of the fetal membranes. All dizygous twins have dichorionic/diamniotic (di/di) placentation. In monozygous (mono) twins, the timing of the cell division determines the chorionicity. If the zygote divides within 3 days of fertilization, the result is di/di placentation; if the division occurs on day 3–8, the result is mono/di placentation; day 8–13, mono/mono placentation; and after day 13, incomplete separation (conjoined twins). Determining chorionicity is of paramount importance to the management of all multiple gestations because it directly correlates with perinatal mortality. Ultrasound in early pregnancy can determine if the placentation is dichorionic ("twin peak" or lamda sign), or monochorionic (no peak and a thin filmy membrane). Identification of separate sex fetuses or two separate placentae confirm di/di placentation. Chorionicity can be confirmed by placental examination after delivery. Prenatal care should address the specific nutritional supplementation that includes an increase in dietary intake of 300 kcal, vitamins and minerals required of twin pregnancies.

5. Antepartum complications develop in 80% of twins versus 20–30% of singleton pregnancies. Preterm birth is the most common complication and should be managed similarly to singleton preterm labor with corticosteroid administration, magnesium for neuroprotection, and special attention to fluid management because of the increased risk of pulmonary edema. Fetal growth discordance (defined as ≥20–25% difference in estimated fetal weight (EFW)) occurs in 5–15% of twins, and is associated with a 6-fold increase in perinatal mortality. Maternal complications include an increased

risk of gestational diabetes, preeclampsia, preterm premature rupture of membranes, anemia, cholestasis of pregnancy, cesarean delivery (due primarily to malpresentation), and postpartum hemorrhage. Other fetal complications include an increased risk of fetal structural anomalies, IUFD of one or both twins (see Chapter 39, Intrauterine Fetal Demise), twin-to-twin transfusion syndrome (TTTS), twin reverse arterial perfusion (TRAP) sequence, and cord entanglement.

6. Twins are at increased risk of fetal structural anomalies compared with singletons. A detailed fetal anatomic survey of both fetuses is indicated at 18–22 weeks. Fetal echocardiography is not routinely recommended in twins.

7. Maternal serum alpha-fetoprotein (MS-AFP) and "quad panel" screening (MS-AFP, estriol, hCG, and inhibin A) has been standardized for twins as it is for singletons at 15–20 weeks. First trimester risk assessment (nuchal translucency + serum PAPP-A and β-hCG) at 11–14 weeks is rapidly becoming the preferred aneuploidy screening test for multiple pregnancies. In dizygous pregnancies, the risk of aneuploidy is independent for each fetus which changes the AMA-related risk from >35 to >33-years-old. For patients seeking noninvasive prenatal diagnostic testing (NIPT), cell-free DNA testing is available for twin gestations from some laboratories. Because the chance of one or both fetuses having a karyotypic abnormality is greater than for a singleton, some patients may chose amniocentesis as the definitive diagnostic test. It has been historically recommended when the probability of aneuploidy is equal to or greater than the procedure-related pregnancy loss rate (estimated at 1 in 400).

8. Di/di twins do not share a blood supply. On the other hand, vascular communications can be demonstrated in almost 100% of mono/di twins. TTTS results from an imbalance in blood flow from the "donor" twin to the "recipient"

and is seen in 15% of mono/di twin pregnancies. Both twins are at risk for adverse events. Following delivery, a difference in birth weight of ≥20% or a difference in hematocrit of ≥5 g/dL confirms the diagnosis. Prognosis depends on gestational age, severity, and underlying etiology. Overall perinatal mortality is 40–80%. Because the treatment options are complex and dependent on such factors as stage of disease and gestational age, an MFM specialist should be consulted. For many mono/di pregnancies complicated by TTTS at <26 weeks, fetoscopic laser photocoagulation of the placental vascular anastomoses has become the treatment of choice. Other options include expectant management, serial amniocentesis of the polyhydramniotic sac, indomethacin (to decrease fetal urine output), or selective fetal reduction. Most experts agree that delivery should occur between 34–37 weeks.

9. Perinatal mortality is high with mono/mono twins (65–70%), due primarily to cord entanglement. As such, delivery should occur by cesarean at 32–34 weeks' gestation.

10. Route of delivery of twins depends on gestational age, EFW, presentation, and maternal and fetal status. There is no inherent benefit of cesarean delivery for the sole indication of twin gestation, but some women may prefer it to the small risk of a combined vaginal and cesarean delivery (see Chapter 66, Intrapartum Management of Twin Pregnancy).

SECTION 5

Intrapartum/ Postpartum Complications

61 Breech Presentation

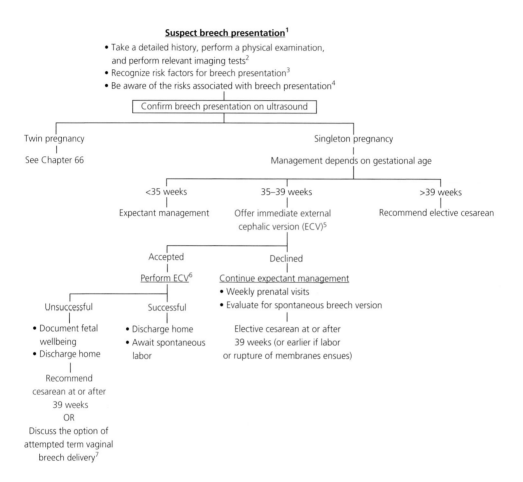

<u>Suspect breech presentation[1]</u>
- Take a detailed history, perform a physical examination, and perform relevant imaging tests[2]
- Recognize risk factors for breech presentation[3]
- Be aware of the risks associated with breech presentation[4]

Confirm breech presentation on ultrasound

Twin pregnancy

See Chapter 66

Singleton pregnancy

Management depends on gestational age

<35 weeks

Expectant management

35–39 weeks

Offer immediate external cephalic version (ECV)[5]

>39 weeks

Recommend elective cesarean

Accepted

Perform ECV[6]

Declined

<u>Continue expectant management</u>
- Weekly prenatal visits
- Evaluate for spontaneous breech version

Unsuccessful
- Document fetal wellbeing
- Discharge home

Recommend cesarean at or after 39 weeks
OR
Discuss the option of attempted term vaginal breech delivery[7]

Successful
- Discharge home
- Await spontaneous labor

Elective cesarean at or after 39 weeks (or earlier if labor or rupture of membranes ensues)

1. Breech presentation refers to presentation of the fetal buttocks and/or lower extremities at the pelvic inlet. The incidence depends on gestational age: 30% at 28 weeks, 15% at 32 weeks, and 3–4% at term.

2. The diagnosis of breech presentation can be made by physical examination (Leopold's maneuvers), vaginal examination or ultrasound. Ultrasound will also determine the type of breech: frank (where legs are flexed at the hips and extended at the knees), complete (where one or both knees are flexed) or incomplete/footling breech (where a foot extends below the buttocks). Fetal presentation should be assessed and documented beginning at 36 0/7 weeks of

Obstetric Clinical Algorithms, Second Edition. Errol R. Norwitz, George R. Saade, Hugh Miller and Christina M. Davidson.
© 2017 John Wiley & Sons, Ltd. Published 2017 by John Wiley & Sons, Ltd.

gestation to allow for external cephalic version to be offered.

3. Risk factors for breech presentation include prematurity, uterine anomaly (such as uterine septum), polyhydramnios, prior term breech presentation, multiple pregnancy, placenta previa, and fetal anomalies (such as anencephaly or hydrocephalus).

4. Breech presentation is associated with a two- to three-fold increased risk of fetal structural anomalies as compared to those in cephalic presentation. Persistent breech presentation also may be a predictor of a neurologically abnormal fetus.

5. *External cephalic version* (ECV) refers to the attempted conversion of breech to vertex by manual manipulation through the maternal abdomen. It is best performed at 35–37 weeks of gestation. Absolute contraindications to ECV are conditions that warrant delivery by cesarean, such as placenta previa or prior classical cesarean delivery. Rupture of the membranes is also considered a contraindication to ECV. Fetal heart rate changes during attempted ECVs are not uncommon and usually stabilize when the procedure is discontinued. Serious adverse effects associated with ECV are uncommon, but there have been a few reported cases of placental abruption and preterm labor. Additional risks include uterine rupture, fetomaternal hemorrhage and alloimmunization, and (rarely) fetal death. Most patients with a successful external cephalic version will give birth vaginally.

6. Prior to performing ECV, the obstetric care provider should confirm breech presentation on ultrasound and evaluate for any anomalies that would complicate a vaginal delivery, document gestational age and fetal well-being (reactive NST), ensure that no contraindications are present (such as placenta previa), and obtain written consent. Anti-Rh(D) immunoglobulin should be administered to prevent Rh alloimmunization,

if indicated. ECV should be performed under ultrasound guidance. A short-acting tocolytic agent (such as the β-adrenergic agonist terbutaline) and/or epidural analgesia have been shown in some studies to improve the success rate of ECV, and can be used in selected cases. The overall success rate of ECV ranges from 35% to 86%, with an average success rate of 58%. Predictors of success include multiparity and an oblique or transverse fetal lie. Nulliparity, advanced dilatation, fetal weight of less than 2,500 gm, anterior placenta, and low station are less likely to be associated with success. Non-stress testing (NST) should be performed after ECV to document fetal wellbeing regardless of whether or not the ECV was successful. Since an emergent cesarean delivery may be indicated during the procedure, ECV should be performed in a facility that is equipped for this; ECV performed in an ambulatory setting is discouraged.

7. Preterm singleton breech fetuses are best delivered by cesarean, in large part, due to the risk of entrapment of the aftercoming head. Management of the breech-presenting second twin is reviewed in Chapter 66, Intrapartum Management of Twin Pregnancy. Although controversial, the weight of evidence suggests that singleton term breech fetuses are most safely delivered by cesarean, because of the attendant risks of vaginal breech delivery including cord prolapse, birth trauma, entrapment of the aftercoming head, birth asphyxia, and death. That said, the American College of Obstetricians and Gynecologists recommends that the decision regarding mode of delivery should depend on the experience of the health care provider and that planned vaginal delivery of a term singleton breech fetus may be reasonable under hospital-specific protocol guidelines for both eligibility and labor management. Vaginal breech delivery may be a safe alternative to elective cesarean under certain circumstances: (i) gestational age greater than 37 weeks; (ii) frank or complete breech; (iii) no fetal anomalies noted on ultrasound exam; (iv) adequate

maternal pelvis; (v) estimated fetal weight 2500–4000 gm; (vi) no hyperextension ("star gazing") of the fetal head; (vii) adequate amniotic fluid volume (viii) immediate availability of emergency cesarean, if needed; (ix) an experienced operator; (x) adequate analgesia; and (xi) continuous fetal heart rate monitoring. While nulliparity is not a contraindication to a trial of vaginal delivery, significantly fewer nulliparas (37%) delivered vaginally as compared to multiparas (63%) in one study that examined a protocol for prelabor patient selection and intrapartum management criteria. The use of oxytocin for induction or augmentation of labor is controversial. Labor augmentation (but not induction) with oxytocin, duration of time from start of pushing in the second stage to delivery of ≥60 minutes, birth weight <2800 g, and no experienced clinician at delivery have been found to be significantly associated with adverse perinatal outcome. Before a vaginal breech delivery is planned, women should be informed that the risk of perinatal or neonatal mortality or short-term serious neonatal morbidity may be higher than if a cesarean delivery is planned. Informed consent should be documented.

62 Intrapartum Fetal Testing[1]

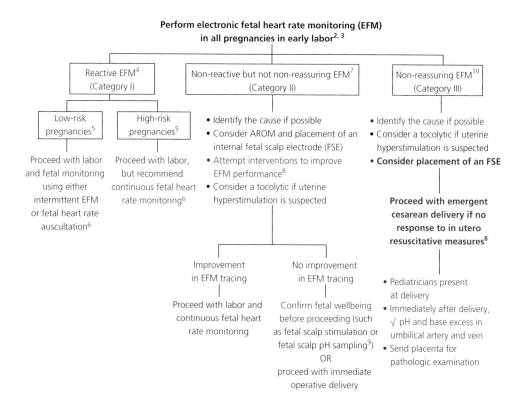

Perform electronic fetal heart rate monitoring (EFM) in all pregnancies in early labor[2, 3]

- **Reactive EFM[4] (Category I)**
  - **Low-risk pregnancies[5]** — Proceed with labor and fetal monitoring using either intermittent EFM or fetal heart rate auscultation[6]
  - **High-risk pregnancies[5]** — Proceed with labor, but recommend continuous fetal heart rate monitoring[6]

- **Non-reactive but not non-reassuring EFM[7] (Category II)**
  - Identify the cause if possible
  - Consider AROM and placement of an internal fetal scalp electrode (FSE)
  - Attempt interventions to improve EFM performance[8]
  - Consider a tocolytic if uterine hyperstimulation is suspected
  - **Improvement in EFM tracing** — Proceed with labor and continuous fetal heart rate monitoring
  - **No improvement in EFM tracing** — Confirm fetal wellbeing before proceeding (such as fetal scalp stimulation or fetal scalp pH sampling[9]) OR proceed with immediate operative delivery

- **Non-reassuring EFM[10] (Category III)**
  - Identify the cause if possible
  - Consider a tocolytic if uterine hyperstimulation is suspected
  - **Consider placement of an FSE**
  - **Proceed with emergent cesarean delivery if no response to in utero resuscitative measures[8]**
  - Pediatricians present at delivery
  - Immediately after delivery, √ pH and base excess in umbilical artery and vein
  - Send placenta for pathologic examination

1. Fetal morbidity and mortality can occur as a consequence of labor. A number of tests have therefore been developed to assess fetus wellbeing in labor. Attention has focused on hypoxic ischemic encephalopathy (HIE) as a marker of birth asphyxia and a predictor of long-term outcome. HIE is a clinical condition that develops within the first hours or days of life. It is characterized by abnormalities of tone and feeding, alterations in consciousness, and convulsions. In order to attribute such a state to birth asphyxia, the following four criteria must all be fulfilled: (i) profound metabolic or mixed acidemia (pH < 7.00) on an umbilical cord arterial blood sample, if obtained; (ii) Apgar score of 0–3 for longer than 5 min; (iii) neonatal neurological manifestations (seizures, coma); and (iv) multisystem organ dysfunction. At most, only 15% of cerebral palsy and mental retardation can be attributed to HIE.

2. <u>Electronic fetal heart rate monitoring</u> (EFM) – also known as cardiotocography (CTG) – refers to changes in the fetal heart rate

Obstetric Clinical Algorithms, Second Edition. Errol R. Norwitz, George R. Saade, Hugh Miller and Christina M. Davidson.
© 2017 John Wiley & Sons, Ltd. Published 2017 by John Wiley & Sons, Ltd.

pattern over time. It reflects maturity and integrity of the fetal autonomic nervous system as measured indirectly through patterns in the fetal heart rate. External EFM is non-invasive, simple to perform, readily available, and inexpensive. EFM interpretation is largely subjective and should always take into account gestational age, the presence or absence of congenital anomalies, and underlying clinical risk factors. Fetuses who are premature or growth-restricted are less likely to tolerate episodes of decreased placental perfusion and, as such, may be more prone to hypoxia and acidosis during labor. Drugs can also affect heart rate and variability.

3. Biophysical profile (BPP), umbilical artery Doppler velocimetry, and contraction stress test (CST) have not been well validated for use in labor. As such, they should not be used to document fetal well-being in labor. The addition of fetal pulse oximetry to EFM does not reduce the overall cesarean delivery rate or the incidence of neonatal encephalopathy and, as such, is not generally recommended.

4. A "reactive" EFM – defined as a normal baseline heart rate (110–160 bpm), moderate variability (which refers to peak-to-trough excursions of 5–25 bpm around the baseline), and at least two accelerations in 20 min each lasting ≥15 sec and peaking at ≥15 bpm above baseline (or ≥10 bpm for ≥10 sec if <32 weeks) – is reassuring and is associated with normal neurologic outcome. According to the 2008 NICHD Workshop Report on electronic fetal monitoring, this is referred to as a "Category I" tracing.

5. The designation "low-risk" and "high-risk" pregnancies refer to whether or not pregnancies are at risk of uteroplacental insufficiency (see Chapter 33, Antepartum Fetal Testing).

6. When compared with intermittent fetal heart rate auscultation, continuous fetal heart rate monitoring during labor is associated with a decrease in the incidence of seizures in the first 28 days of life, but no difference in other measures of short-term perinatal morbidity or mortality. Moreover, the increase in neonatal seizures does not translate into differences in long-term morbidity (cerebral palsy, mental retardation, or seizures after 28 days of life). However, continuous fetal heart rate monitoring is associated with a significant increase in obstetric intervention, including operative vaginal and cesarean delivery.

7. According to the 2008 NICHD Workshop Report on EFM, a "Category II" fetal heart rate tracing is one that falls between "Category I" and "Category III." It is an EFM tracing that is not formally reactive, but is not non-reassuring. It is also referred to as suspicious, equivocal, or indeterminate. It is the most common type of tracing, and can be seen in up to 60% of labors, suggesting that it is not specific to fetal hypoxia. A "Category II" tracing at term is associated with poor perinatal outcome in only 20% of cases. The significance of such a tracing depends on the clinical end-point. If the end-point is a 5-min Apgar score <7, then it has a sensitivity of 50–60% and positive predictive value of 10–15% (assuming a prevalence of 4%). If the end-point of interest is permanent cerebral injury, then it has a 99.9% false-positive rate.

8. Interventions to improve EFM performance include: discontinuation of oxytocin infusion, repositioning the patient (in an effort to improve venous return), oxygen supplementation by facemask, and intravenous fluid infusion.

9. Fetal scalp sampling refers to sampling of capillary blood from the fetal scalp during labor to measure pH. Capillary pH lies between that of arterial and venous blood. This technique was introduced by Saling in 1962, and is most useful in labor when alternative non-invasive tests are unable to confirm fetal well-being. Suggested management based on fetal scalp pH is as follows: (i) pH >7.25, continue expectant management;

(ii) pH 7.20–7.25, repeat at 20–30 min intervals until delivery; and (iii) pH <7.20, proceed with immediate and urgent delivery.

10. According to the 2008 NICHD Workshop Report on EFM, a "Category III" fetal heart rate tracing is one that is ominous and requires immediate action. It is also referred to as non-reassuring. It occurs in only 0.3% of intrapartum fetal heart rate tracings, but is associated with adverse events in over 50% of cases. It is characterized by absent fetal heart rate variability (defined as peak-to-trough excursions of 0 bpm around the baseline), absence of accelerations, and repetitive late or severe variable decelerations. Decelerations are regarded as "repetitive" if they occur with more than 50% of contractions.

63 Cesarean Delivery

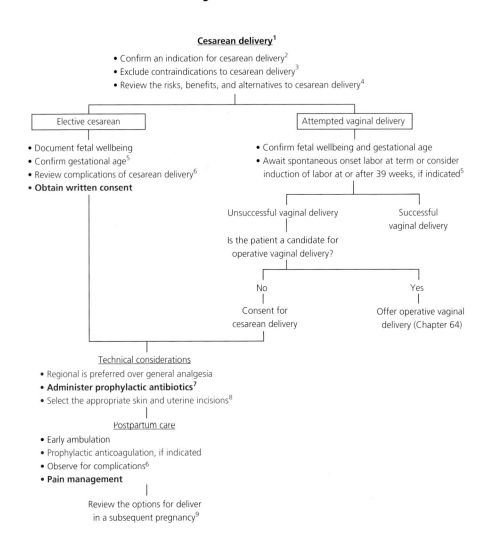

Cesarean delivery[1]
- Confirm an indication for cesarean delivery[2]
- Exclude contraindications to cesarean delivery[3]
- Review the risks, benefits, and alternatives to cesarean delivery[4]

Elective cesarean
- Document fetal wellbeing
- Confirm gestational age[5]
- Review complications of cesarean delivery[6]
- **Obtain written consent**

Attempted vaginal delivery
- Confirm fetal wellbeing and gestational age
- Await spontaneous onset labor at term or consider induction of labor at or after 39 weeks, if indicated[5]

Unsuccessful vaginal delivery

Is the patient a candidate for operative vaginal delivery?

No
Consent for cesarean delivery

Yes
Offer operative vaginal delivery (Chapter 64)

Successful vaginal delivery

Technical considerations
- Regional is preferred over general analgesia
- **Administer prophylactic antibiotics[7]**
- Select the appropriate skin and uterine incisions[8]

Postpartum care
- Early ambulation
- Prophylactic anticoagulation, if indicated
- Observe for complications[6]
- **Pain management**

Review the options for deliver in a subsequent pregnancy[9]

1. Cesarean delivery refers to delivery of a fetus via the abdominal route (laparotomy) requiring an incision into the uterus (hysterotomy). It is the second most common surgical procedure (behind male circumcision) accounting for 30–35% of all deliveries in the United States.

2. Most indications for cesarean are relative and rely on the judgment of the obstetric care

---

Obstetric Clinical Algorithms, Second Edition. Errol R. Norwitz, George R. Saade, Hugh Miller and Christina M. Davidson.
© 2017 John Wiley & Sons, Ltd. Published 2017 by John Wiley & Sons, Ltd.

provider. <u>Absolute indications</u> for cesarean include a prior high vertical ("classical") cesarean, complete placenta previa, absolute cephalopelvic disproportion (where the disparity between the size of the bony pelvis and the fetal head precludes vaginal delivery even under optimal conditions (CPD)), prior full-thickness myomectomy, prior uterine rupture, malpresentation (transverse lie), cord prolapse (Chapter 77, Cord Prolapse), active genital HSV infection in labor, and non-reassuring fetal testing (previously referred to as "fetal distress") prior to labor. <u>Relative indications</u> include a prior low transverse hysterotomy, labor dystocia (failure to progress in labor), breech presentation, relative CPD, multiple pregnancy, women with certain cardiac or cerebrovascular disease, select fetal anomalies (such as hydrocephalus), maternal request, and excessive hemorrhage at delivery. Puerperal hysterectomy is a highly morbid procedure and should only be performed as a last resort to save the life of the mother. A desire for permanent sterilization (bilateral tubal ligation) is not an adequate indication for cesarean delivery.

3. Contraindications to cesarean delivery include uncontrolled maternal coagulopathy and failure to obtain maternal consent.

4. The most common indication for a primary cesarean is failure to progress in labor, which is defined as abnormal or inadequate progress in labor. Causes include the 3 "P"s: inadequate "powers" (uterine contractions), inadequate "passage" (bony pelvis), or abnormalities of the "passenger"(fetal macrosomia, hydrocephalus, malpresentation). If contractions are "adequate," one of two events will occur: dilatation and effacement of the cervix with descent of the head, or worsening caput succedaneum (scalp edema) and molding (overlapping of the skull bones). If contractions are inadequate, consider augmentation with pitocin infusion with or without an intrauterine pressure catheter (IUPC).

5. Elective cesarean delivery should only be performed at or after 39 weeks, with the exception of HIV and twins where it can be performed at or after 38 weeks. Elective delivery prior to these gestational ages is best avoided, even after documentation of fetal lung maturity.

6. Complications of cesarean include excessive bleeding, infection, venous thromboembolic disease, injury to adjacent organs (bladder, bowel, ureters), and (rarely) injury to the fetus.

7. Routine use of broad-spectrum prophylactic antibiotics given within 60 minutes of surgery (and not after clamping of the cord after delivery) will decrease the incidence of postoperative febrile morbidity and surgical site infection. Penicillin for GBS chemoprophylaxis is not sufficient to prevent wound infection.

8. Skin incision may be either Pfannenstiel (low transverse incision, muscle separating, strong, but limited exposure) or midline vertical (offers the best exposure, but is weaker). Pfannenstiel skin incisions may be modified to improve exposure, if needed, by dividing the rectus muscles horizontally (Maylard incision) or lifting the rectus off the pubic bone (Cherney incision). Pfannenstiel should be the incision of choice. Similarly, a low transverse hysterotomy should be performed, if possible. Indications for high vertical ("classical") hysterotomy include extreme prematurity, malpresentation, multiple pregnancy, and failure to gain access to the lower uterine segment due, for example, to excessive adhesions. Elective surgery (such as myomectomy) should not be performed at the time of cesarean, because of the risk of bleeding.

9. A prior high vertical ("classical") cesarean, a prior low vertical cesarean, and two or more low transverse hysterotomies should be regarded as an absolute contraindication to attempted vaginal delivery, because of the risk of uterine dehiscence and rupture. Uterine rupture may be life-threatening. Symptoms and

signs include acute onset of fetal bradycardia (70%), abdominal pain (10%), vaginal bleeding (5%), hemodynamic instability (5–10%), and/or loss of the presenting part (<5%). In such women, repeat cesarean is best performed at 36–37 weeks. Vaginal birth after caesarean (VBAC) may be a reasonable alternative for elective repeat cesarean delivery in select patients so long as certain criteria are fulfilled, including: no induction of labor with prostaglandins, continuous fetal heart rate monitoring, adequate analgesia, carefully monitoring of the progress of labor to facilitate the early diagnosis of CPD, and immediate access to emergency cesarean. A successful VBAC can be achieved in 65–80% of women.

64 Operative Vaginal Delivery[1]

- **Confirm an indication for operative vaginal delivery[2]**
- **Exclude contraindications to operative vaginal delivery[3]**
- Be aware of the type of operative vaginal delivery you will be performing[4]
- Review the risks, benefits, and alternatives to operative vaginal delivery
- Discuss potential complications to the mother and fetus[5]

Ensure that all prerequisites for operative vaginal delivery have been fulfilled			
Maternal criteria	Fetal criteria	Uteroplacental criteria	Other criteria
• Adequate analgesia • Lithotomy position • Bladder empty • Clinical pelvimetry must be adequate in dimension and size to facilitate an atraumatic delivery • Verbal or written consent	• Vertex presentation • Fetal head must be engaged in pelvis • Position of fetal head must be known • Station of fetal head must be ≥+2 • Attitude of fetal head and presence of caput succedaneum and/or molding should be noted	• Cervix fully dilated • Membranes ruptured • No placenta previa	• Experienced operator who is fully acquainted with the use of the instrument • The capability to perform an emergency cesarean delivery if required

≥45° rotation required
Use rotational forceps (Kiellands, Barton forceps)

Vertex presentation, no rotation or rotation <45° required
Use "classic" forceps (Simpson, Tucker-McLane, Elliot forceps) OR vacuum extractor (Ventouse)[6]

Aftercoming head in a vaginal breech delivery
Use forceps designed to assist in breech deliveries (Piper forceps)

Technical considerations
- **Ensure correct placement of the forceps[7] or vacuum[8]**
- Apply traction in concert with maternal expulsive efforts

Successful operative vaginal delivery
Examine the fetus and maternal perineum, vagina and cervix

Unsuccessful operative vaginal delivery[9]
Proceed with cesarean delivery (no place for combined forceps and vacuum delivery)

1. Operative vaginal delivery refers to any operative procedure designed to expedite vaginal delivery, including forceps delivery and vacuum extraction.

2. Indications for operative vaginal delivery include: (i) *maternal indications* such as maternal exhaustion, inadequate maternal expulsive efforts (women with spinal cord injuries or neuromuscular diseases), need to avoid maternal expulsive efforts (women with certain cardiac or cerebrovascular disease); (ii) *fetal indications* such as non-reassuring fetal testing ("fetal distress"); and (iii) *other indications* such as prolonged second stage of labor (nullipara: ≥3 hours without regional analgesia, ≥4 hours

Obstetric Clinical Algorithms, Second Edition. Errol R. Norwitz, George R. Saade, Hugh Miller and Christina M. Davidson.
© 2017 John Wiley & Sons, Ltd. Published 2017 by John Wiley & Sons, Ltd.

with regional analgesia; multipara: ≥2 hours without regional analgesia, ≥3 hours with regional analgesia), elective shortening of the second stage of labor using outlet forceps.

3. Contraindications to operative vaginal delivery include placenta previa, absolute cephalopelvic disproportion or any other contraindication to vaginal delivery; prematurity (gestational age <34 weeks is an absolute contraindication for vacuum but not forceps delivery); suspected fetal skeletal dysplasia; suspected fetal coagulation disorder; fetal macrosomia (a relative contraindication); or failure to fulfill the prerequisites listed in the table below (such as station ≥2+, intact membranes, cervix not fully dilated or failure to obtain consent).

4. The 1988 ACOG classification of forceps deliveries is outlined in the table below. The old category of "high forceps" (in which forceps were placed with the fetal head floating and ballottable above the brim of the true pelvis) has been abandoned due to excessive fetal risk. Midforceps deliveries should be performed only by competent operators, and after careful consideration of alternative approaches (oxytocin administration, cesarean or continued expectant management) and of the potential fetal risks. Indications for vacuum extraction-assisted delivery are similar to those for forceps delivery.

5. Potential complications of operative vaginal delivery include maternal perineal injury (especially with rotational forceps delivery) and fetal complications such as facial bruising, laceration, and cephalhematoma (more common with vacuum extraction). Facial nerve palsy, skull fractures, cervical spine injuries, and intracranial hemorrhage are rare. Failed operative vaginal delivery is more common with vacuum than with forceps, and more common with the soft cup vacuum extractor that with the rigid "M" cup.

6. The choice of which instrument to use depends largely on clinician preference and experience. In some circumstances, one

instrument may be preferred over another. For example, vacuum extraction can be accomplished with minimal maternal analgesia. A vaginal birth is more likely to be achieved with forceps than with vacuum extractors, though.

7. Exact knowledge of fetal position, station, and degree of asynclitism (lateral flexion) is essential to proper forceps application. After performing a "phantom application," the posterior blade is placed first in order to prevent loss of station of the fetal head. When the sagittal suture is the anterior-posterior diameter or the head position is left occiput anterior, the left blade is inserted first. This facilitates locking the handles after application. Proper application is determined by assessing the position of the forceps relative to three landmarks on the fetal skull: the posterior fontanelle, sagittal suture, and parietal bones. Three checks for proper application include ensuring that: (i) the sagittal suture is perpendicular to the plane of the shanks throughout its length; (ii) the posterior fontanelle is one fingerbreadth away from the plane of the shanks and equidistant from the sides of the blades directly in front of the locked point of the articulated forceps; and (iii) if fenestrated blades are used, the amount of fenestration in front of the fetal head should not admit more than the tip of one finger. The purpose of these checks is to prevent asymmetric compression of the fetal head. If rotation is required, it should be performed at this time. Delivery is then accomplished by traction applied along the pelvic curve in concert with uterine contractions.

8. To promote flexion of the fetal head with descent, the suction cup of the vacuum should be placed over the "median flexing point" (i.e. symmetrically astride the sagittal suture with the posterior margin of the cup anterior to the posterior fontanelle and the opposite edge situated about 3 cm from the anterior fontanelle). Low suction (100 mmHg) should be applied. After ensuring that no maternal soft tissue is trapped between the cup and fetal head, suction should be increased to 500–600 mmHg and sustained downward

traction applied along the pelvic curve in concert with uterine contractions. Suction is released between contractions. Ideally, episiotomy should be avoided as pressure of the perineum on the vacuum cup will help to keep it applied to the fetal head and assist in flexion and rotation.

9. For vacuum-assisted vaginal delivery, the procedure should be abandoned if the vacuum cup detaches three times, if there is any evidence of fetal scalp trauma, if delivery is not effected within 20 minutes, or if there is no descent of the fetal head.

ACOG classification of forceps deliveries

Type of procedure	Criteria
Outlet forceps	1. Scalp is visible at the introitus without separating the labia
	2. Fetal skull has reached the level of the pelvic floor
	3. Sagittal suture is in the direction anteroposterior diameter or in the right or left occiput anterior or posterior position
	4. Fetal head is at or on the perineum
Low forceps	Leading point of the fetal skull (station) is station +2 or more but has not yet reached the pelvic floor
Mid-forceps	The head is engaged in the pelvis but the presenting part is above +2 station
High forceps	(Not included in this classification)

65 Severe Perineal Lacerations[1]

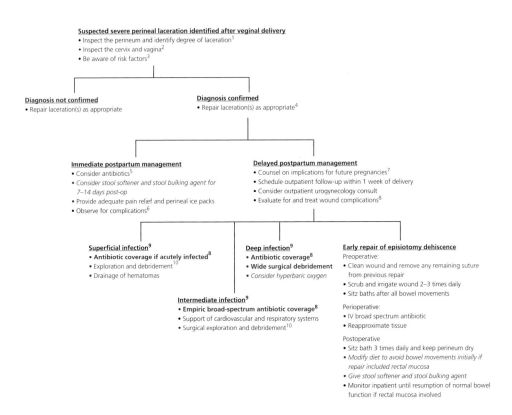

Suspected severe perineal laceration identified after vaginal delivery
- Inspect the perineum and identify degree of laceration[1]
- Inspect the cervix and vagina[2]
- Be aware of risk factors[3]

Diagnosis not confirmed
- Repair laceration(s) as appropriate

Diagnosis confirmed
- Repair laceration(s) as appropriate[4]

Immediate postpartum management
- Consider antibiotics[5]
- *Consider stool softener and stool bulking agent for 7–14 days post-op*
- Provide adequate pain relief and perineal ice packs
- Observe for complications[6]

Delayed postpartum management
- Counsel on implications for future pregnancies[7]
- Schedule outpatient follow-up within 1 week of delivery
- Consider outpatient urogynecology consult
- Evaluate for and treat wound complications[8]

Superficial infection[9]
- **Antibiotic coverage if acutely infected[8]**
- Exploration and debridement[10]
- Drainage of hematomas

Intermediate infection[9]
- **Empiric broad-spectrum antibiotic coverage[8]**
- Support of cardiovascular and respiratory systems
- Surgical exploration and debridement[10]

Deep infection[9]
- **Antibiotic coverage[8]**
- **Wide surgical debridement**
- *Consider hyperbaric oxygen*

Early repair of episiotomy dehiscence
Preoperative:
- Clean wound and remove any remaining suture from previous repair
- Scrub and irrigate wound 2–3 times daily
- Sitz baths after all bowel movements

Perioperative:
- IV broad spectrum antibiotic
- Reapproximate tissue

Postoperative:
- Sitz bath 3 times daily and keep perineum dry
- *Modify diet to avoid bowel movements initially if repair included rectal mucosa*
- *Give stool softener and stool bulking agent*
- Monitor inpatient until resumption of normal bowel function if rectal mucosa involved

1. Lower genital tract lacerations may involve the cervix, vagina or perineum. Perineal tears may follow any vaginal delivery and are classified by their depth. A first-degree tear is a superficial laceration of the vaginal mucosa, which may extend into the skin at the introitus. It does not involve deeper tissues and may not require repair. A second-degree tear involves the vaginal mucosa and perineal body. It may extend to the transverse perineal muscles and usually requires a suture repair. A third-degree tear extends into the muscle of the perineum and may involve both the transverse perineal muscles as well as the anal sphincter. It does not involve the rectal mucosa. A fourth-degree tear involves the anal sphincter and rectal mucosa. Third- and fourth-degree lacerations are considered severe perineal lacerations and may occur with or without an episiotomy. Midline episiotomies are associated with a greater risk of extension to a third- or fourth-degree tear as compared to a mediolateral episiotomy.

Obstetric Clinical Algorithms, Second Edition. Errol R. Norwitz, George R. Saade, Hugh Miller and Christina M. Davidson.
© 2017 John Wiley & Sons, Ltd. Published 2017 by John Wiley & Sons, Ltd.

2. Bleeding despite a firmly contracted uterus should prompt a thorough inspection of the upper vagina and cervix to exclude a genital tract laceration. Superficial cervical lacerations up to 1–2 cm are not uncommon and do not require repair unless they are bleeding. Deep cervical tears usually require surgical repair. Extensive vaginal or cervical tears should prompt a careful search for evidence of bleeding into the retroperitoneum or even into the peritoneum.

3. The frequency of third- or fourth-degree perineal lacerations is 5–6% in nulliparas and 0.5% in multiparas. Risk factors include nulliparity (7-fold risk), increasing birth weight and gestational age, operative vaginal delivery, occiput posterior position, episiotomy (2.5-fold increase in nulliparous women and 4.5-fold in multiparous women), and a prolonged second stage of labor. Cervical lacerations occur in 1% of nullipara and 0.5 % of multipara. Risk factors include young maternal age, operative vaginal delivery, and cerclage.

4. The surgical repair is performed in layers beginning with a running closure of the anal mucosa. The standard suture material is chromic catgut, but synthetic material may also be used, such as 3–0 polyglycolic acid (Vicryl) suture. The needle should be small and tapered for the mucosa (SH1 needle). The first suture should be placed approximately 1 cm above the apex and extend through the submucosa. The mucosa is then closed in a running or locking fashion and should not penetrate the mucosal layer, but rather bring the submucosa together to the level of the anal sphincter and perineal body. The anal sphincter should then be identified. This may require Allis clamp(s) to retrieve the cut edges, incorporating both the muscle and its capsule, which may have retracted laterally. It is important to suture the fascial sheath and not just the muscle when repairing the anal sphincter, since it is the sheath that

gives strength to the repair. Consider using a 2-0 suture for capsule repair because it will give support for a longer time. Two methods have been described to repair a laceration of the anal sphincter: end-to-end and overlapping. Both appear to have similar long-term outcomes.

5. There is no proven benefit from perioperative antibiotics administration at the time of repair. If antibiotics are given, a single IV dose of a second-generation cephalosporin (cefotetan or cefoxitin) or clindamycin in penicillin-allergic patients is recommended.

6. Short-term complications include greater blood loss, puerperal pain, infection, and wound disruption. If pain is severe or persistent, a physical exam should be performed to evaluate for the presence of a hematoma or infection. Up to 1 in 5 women who sustain an obstetric anal sphincter injury will develop a wound breakdown or infection.

7. Prior anal sphincter laceration does not appear to be a significant risk factor for recurrence of laceration, and most patients will go on to deliver vaginally for subsequent deliveries.

8. Should a wound infection be identified, it should be treated with strict perineal hygiene and oral antibiotics for 7 days (875 mg amoxicillin-clavulanate and 500 mg metronidazole twice daily). Women with wound breakdown can be offered immediate operative repair or conservative management with wound packing and perineal care. The wound can be surgically repaired when its surface is free of exudate and is covered by healthy granulation tissue. In rare cases, inadequately repaired episiotomies may lead to rectovaginal fistula formation. Long-term complications of third- and fourth-degree tears include higher rates of anal incontinence and dyspareunia.

9. Lower genital tract infections can be classified according to the depth of infection. A superficial infection is limited to the skin and subcutaneous tissues or to the superficial fascia along the episiotomy incision without necrosis. An intermediate infection includes superficial fascial necrosis (necrotizing fasciitis) and is diagnosed when the following criteria are present: (i) extensive necrosis with widespread undermining of surrounding tissue; (ii) moderate-to-severe systemic reaction with altered mental status; (iii) absence of muscle involvement; (iv) failure to demonstrate clostridia in wound and blood cultures; (v) absence of major vascular occlusion; (vi) pathologic examination of debrided tissue showing intense leukocytic infiltration, focal necrosis of fascia and surrounding tissues, and thrombosis of microvasculature.

Necrotizing fasciitis is a severe, superficial infection in which both layers of the superficial perineal fascia become necrotic as the infection spreads along fascial planes. It has an acute onset and a rapid course with prominent systemic manifestations and a high fatality rate (20–80%). A deep infection is myonecrosis, which is an infection beneath the deep fascia involving the muscles. It is most commonly caused by *Clostridium perfringens*.

10. An acutely infected episiotomy should not be repaired. Surgical exploration should be performed if there is skin edema or erythema beyond the immediate area of the episiotomy, if severe systemic manifestations are present, or if the infection does not resolve after 24–48 hours of IV antibiotic therapy.

66 Intrapartum Management of Twin Pregnancy

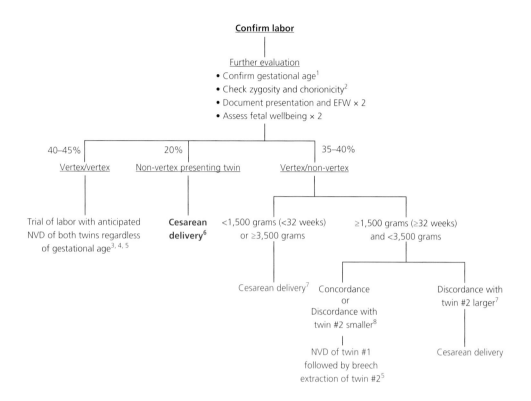

Confirm labor

Further evaluation
- Confirm gestational age[1]
- Check zygosity and chorionicity[2]
- Document presentation and EFW × 2
- Assess fetal wellbeing × 2

40–45%   20%   35–40%

Vertex/vertex   Non-vertex presenting twin   Vertex/non-vertex

Trial of labor with anticipated   **Cesarean**   <1,500 grams (<32 weeks)   ≥1,500 grams (≥32 weeks)
NVD of both twins regardless   **delivery[6]**   or ≥3,500 grams   and <3,500 grams
of gestational age[3, 4, 5]

Cesarean delivery[7]   Concordance   Discordance with
or   twin #2 larger[7]
Discordance with
twin #2 smaller[8]

NVD of twin #1   Cesarean delivery
followed by breech
extraction of twin #2[5]

1. Delivery of uncomplicated diamniotic/dichorionic twin pregnancies with a vertex presenting first twin can safely be offered a vaginal delivery based on a large well-designed randomized clinical trials. The optimal route of delivery ultimately has to consider gestational age (32–38 weeks), experience of the provider, and capabilities of the facility (which would include pediatric availability). It is generally recommended that diamniotic/dichorionic twin pregnancies be delivered at 38 weeks. If delivery is planned prior to 38 weeks, ACOG requires that there be a maternal or fetal indication. In rare cases where an amniocentesis is used to determine fetal lung maturity, it is acceptable to obtain amniotic fluid from only one sac (traditionally the non-presenting twin) for assessment of fetal pulmonary maturity. However, if there is discordant growth between the fetuses, it is recommended that both sacs be sampled.

2. Monoamniotic twin pregnancies should be delivered by elective cesarean at 32–34 weeks, because of the risk of fetal demise secondary to cord entanglement. Monochorionic/diamniotic twin pregnancies should be delivered between

Obstetric Clinical Algorithms, Second Edition. Errol R. Norwitz, George R. Saade, Hugh Miller and Christina M. Davidson.
© 2017 John Wiley & Sons, Ltd. Published 2017 by John Wiley & Sons, Ltd.

34–37 weeks, and can be delivered vaginally if presentation and fetal status are reassuring.

3. Continuous electronic fetal monitoring of both fetuses is required throughout labor and delivery. Intravenous access should be attained and blood readily available, if needed. Anesthesiology should be notified and regional anesthesia recommended. Cesarean delivery is indicated for the usual obstetric indications (such as non-reassuring fetal testing, placenta previa, or elective repeat cesarean after prior cesarean delivery). It is generally recommended that a neonatologist be present at delivery, because a second twin is more likely to require resuscitation. If a vaginal delivery is to be attempted, ultrasound equipment should be available throughout labor and delivery to document the fetal heart rate of the second twin, if necessary, and to confirm presentation (note that presentation of the second twin may change in up to 20% of cases after delivery of twin #1). With the possible exception of concordant, vertex/vertex, diamniotic twin pregnancies in labor at term, one should consider delivering twin pregnancies in the operating room with the availability of urgent cesarean delivery.

4. Internal podalic version and breech extraction of twin #2 are an acceptable option. An obstetrician skilled in operative vaginal delivery and vaginal breech delivery is a prerequisite for any such delivery.

5. In the setting of reassuring intrapartum fetal heart rate monitoring, there is no urgency to deliver twin #2, since delivery interval per se does <u>not</u> appear to affect perinatal outcome. However, a delivery interval of >15 min is associated with an increased risk of cesarean delivery. For this reason, active rather than expectant management of the second twin (artificial rupture of membranes, oxytocin augmentation, and/or breech extraction) is generally recommended.

6. There is no place for external cephalic version of twin #1.

7. Cesarean delivery is commonly recommended in this setting to avoid breech vaginal delivery of twin #2 (although several studies have suggested that vaginal breech delivery of fetuses <1,500 g may be safe).

8. Discordance is best defined as ≥20% difference between twins (= EFW of larger fetus - smaller fetus/EFW of larger fetus x 100, expressed as a %). When this level of discordance is met in twins, there is a significant increased risk of adverse perinatal outcome.

67 Postpartum Hemorrhage[1]

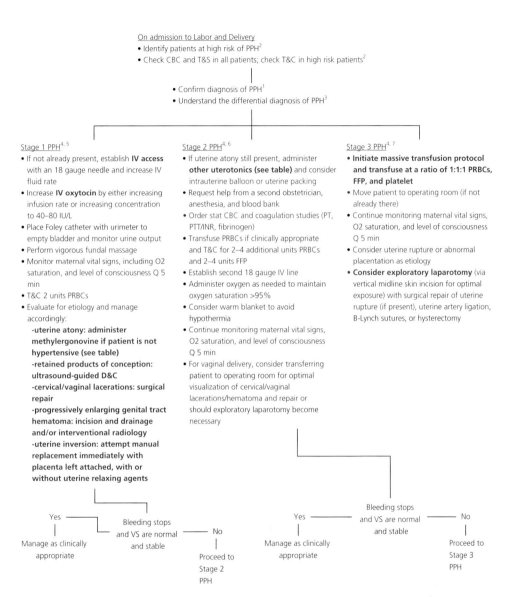

On admission to Labor and Delivery
- Identify patients at high risk of PPH[2]
- Check CBC and T&S in all patients; check T&C in high risk patients[2]

- Confirm diagnosis of PPH[1]
- Understand the differential diagnosis of PPH[3]

Stage 1 PPH[4, 5]
- If not already present, establish **IV access with an 18 gauge needle** and increase IV fluid rate
- Increase **IV oxytocin** by either increasing infusion rate or increasing concentration to 40–80 IU/L
- Place Foley catheter with urimeter to empty bladder and monitor urine output
- Perform vigorous fundal massage
- Monitor maternal vital signs, including O2 saturation, and level of consciousness Q 5 min
- T&C 2 units PRBCs
- Evaluate for etiology and manage accordingly:
  -uterine atony: administer **methylergonovine if patient is not hypertensive (see table)**
  -retained products of conception: **ultrasound-guided D&C**
  -cervical/vaginal lacerations: surgical **repair**
  -progressively enlarging genital tract **hematoma: incision and drainage and/or interventional radiology**
  -uterine inversion: attempt manual **replacement immediately with placenta left attached, with or without uterine relaxing agents**

Stage 2 PPH[4, 6]
- If uterine atony still present, administer **other uterotonics (see table)** and consider intrauterine balloon or uterine packing
- Request help from a second obstetrician, anesthesia, and blood bank
- Order stat CBC and coagulation studies (PT, PTT/INR, fibrinogen)
- Transfuse PRBCs if clinically appropriate and T&C for 2–4 additional units PRBCs and 2–4 units FFP
- Establish second 18 gauge IV line
- Administer oxygen as needed to maintain oxygen saturation >95%
- Consider warm blanket to avoid hypothermia
- Continue monitoring maternal vital signs, O2 saturation, and level of consciousness Q 5 min
- For vaginal delivery, consider transferring patient to operating room for optimal visualization of cervical/vaginal lacerations/hematoma and repair or should exploratory laparotomy become necessary

Stage 3 PPH[4, 7]
- **Initiate massive transfusion protocol and transfuse at a ratio of 1:1:1 PRBCs, FFP, and platelet**
- Move patient to operating room (if not already there)
- Continue monitoring maternal vital signs, O2 saturation, and level of consciousness Q 5 min
- Consider uterine rupture or abnormal placentation as etiology
- **Consider exploratory laparotomy** (via vertical midline skin incision for optimal exposure) with surgical repair of uterine rupture (if present), uterine artery ligation, B-Lynch sutures, or hysterectomy

Yes — Bleeding stops and VS are normal and stable — No

Manage as clinically appropriate

Proceed to Stage 2 PPH

Yes — Bleeding stops and VS are normal and stable — No

Manage as clinically appropriate

Proceed to Stage 3 PPH

Obstetric Clinical Algorithms, Second Edition. Errol R. Norwitz, George R. Saade, Hugh Miller and Christina M. Davidson.
© 2017 John Wiley & Sons, Ltd. Published 2017 by John Wiley & Sons, Ltd.

1. Hemorrhage is the single most significant cause of maternal death worldwide. In addition to death, serious morbidity may follow postpartum hemorrhage (PPH). Sequelae include adult respiratory distress syndrome, coagulopathy, shock, loss of fertility, and pituitary necrosis (Sheehan syndrome). PPH has traditionally been defined as an estimated blood loss (EBL) >500 mL at vaginal delivery or >1,000 mL following cesarean delivery. However, clinicians typically underestimate blood loss by 30–50%, and the average blood loss following vaginal and caesarean delivery approximates the definitions of PPH. More recently, PPH has been defined as a 10% drop in hematocrit from admission or bleeding requiring blood transfusion. Using this definition, PPH complicates 4% of vaginal deliveries and 6% of cesarean deliveries.

2. Risk factors for PPH include prolonged, augmented or rapid labor; history of PPH; episiotomy; preeclampsia; overdistended uterus (macrosomia, multiple pregnancy, polyhydramnios); operative delivery; prior cesarean delivery or uterine surgery (e.g., extensive myomectomy); large uterine fibroids; Asian or Hispanic ethnicity; chorioamnionitis; grandmultiparity; known coagulopathy; placenta previa; and abnormal placental adherence (placenta accreta, increta, percreta). In patients at high risk of PPH (e.g., placenta previa and accreta, known coagulopathy, active bleeding on admission, platelets <100,000/mL, hematocrit <30%), consider type and cross-blood products and early anesthesia consultation.

3. PPH is classified as primary or secondary. Primary PPH occurs within 24 hours of delivery; secondary PPH occurs between 24 hours and 6 weeks postpartum. Primary PPH is caused by uterine atony in ≥80% of cases. Even if atony is present, other etiologies should be considered if bleeding persists, such as genital tract lacerations and retained products of conception. Consider also coagulation defects and uterine inversion. Secondary PPH is caused most commonly by retained products of conception, infection, *inherited* coagulation defects, and subinvolution of the placental site.

4. In the healthy pregnant woman with physiologic hypervolemia of pregnancy, the usual signs of hemorrhage may not become evident until 15–20% (approximately 1200 mL) of total blood volume has been lost. Blood loss of 20–25% of blood volume (1200–1500 mL) produces tachycardia, vasoconstriction (cold, pale extremities), and a drop in mean arterial pressure (MAP) by 10–15% (to 70–75 mmHg). Blood loss of 25–35% of blood volume (1500–2000 mL) results in tissue hypoxia, tachycardia, restlessness, MAP drop of 25–30% (to 50–60 mmHg), and oliguria (<0.5 mL/kg per hour). When blood loss is severe, with loss of >30% of blood volume (>2000 mL), hemorrhagic shock occurs with tissue hypoxia, tachycardia (>120 bpm), hypotension (MAP <50 mmHg), altered consciousness, anuria, and disseminated intravascular coagulation (DIC). ACOG and the California Maternal Quality Care Collaborative divide PPH into three stages based on the amount of blood loss and the changes in vital signs, with each stage having goal-directed management.

5. In Stage 1 hemorrhage, the cumulative blood loss is >500 ml from a vaginal birth or >1000 ml from cesarean delivery with continued bleeding; or >15% change in vital signs or HR ≥110, blood pressure (BP) ≤85/45, O2 sat <95%; or increased bleeding during recovery or postpartum. This stage involves activation of a hemorrhage protocol and checklist. The ACOG patient safety checklist can be used as a guide. Since the most common cause of PPH is uterine atony, initial management is generally directed at this etiology. Medical management of uterine atony is outlined in the table below. While there is no established first line uterotonic agent after oxytocin administration, methylergonivine can be considered next in the non-hypertensive patient since it is only administered every 2-4 hours. Therefore, if uterine atony is still present after its

administration, the practitioner knows to immediately switch to a different uterotonic agent

6. In <u>Stage 2 hemorrhage</u>, there is continued bleeding or vital sign instability, but <1500 mL cumulative blood loss. Management during this stage focuses on sequentially advancing through medications and procedures if there has been no response to the management of Stage 1, including mobilizing help and Blood Bank support, keeping ahead with volume and blood products. There is continued focus on identifying and correcting the underlying etiology, with consideration for transferring the patient to the operating room, for possible surgical management.

7. In <u>Stage 3 hemorrhage,</u> the cumulative blood loss is now >1500 mL or >2 units packed red blood cells (PRBCs) have been given, vital signs are unstable, or there is suspicion of DIC. This stage involves activation of the Massive Transfusion protocol and invasive surgical approaches for control of bleeding.

Massive transfusion is defined as the replacement of one or more blood volumes (generally 8–10 or more RBC units) within 24 hours. Most protocols recommend a transfusion ratio of PRBCs, fresh frozen plasma (FFP) and platelets at 1:1:1. Hypocalcemia is one of the most clinically significant electrolyte disturbances noted in massive transfusion. Calcium is necessary for adequate clotting and myocardial contraction, thus ionized calcium should be frequently monitored and replaced to keep levels within a normal physiologic range. Acidosis and hypothermia are associated with increased morbidity and mortality in trauma patients. During massive transfusion resuscitation, the patient's arterial blood gas, electrolytes, and core temperature should be monitored to guide clinical management, all transfused fluids should be warmed, and direct warming of the patient should be initiated as needed to maintain euthermia.

If uterine rupture is clinically suspected, treatment is explorative laparotomy with surgical repair or hysterectomy. The main risk factor is prior uterine surgery (cesarean or extensive myomectomy).

Abnormal placentation includes abnormal attachment of placental villi to the myometrium (accreta), invasion into the myometrium (increta) or penetration through the myometrium (percreta). Risk factors include prior uterine surgery (cesarean), placenta previa, smoking, and multiparity. Placenta previa alone is associated with a 3% incidence of accreta, which increases to 10–25% with placenta previa and one prior cesarean, and >40% with placenta previa and two or more prior cesareans. If this is clinically suspected, management is D&C or explorative laparotomy with surgical repair or hysterectomy.

Medical management of postpartum hemorrhage

Drug	Dose	Route	Frequency	Pharmacokinetics	Side Effects	Contraindications
Pitocin® (Oxytocin)	10-40 units per 1000 ml (adjust according to response)	IV infusion	Continuous	IV administration • onset of action = immediate • $t_{1/2}$ = 3 min • plateau concentration reached after 30 min • oxytocin-induced desensitization is homologous & the uterus should remain responsive to other uterotonic agents (e.g., prostaglandins) IM administration • onset of action = 3-7 min • clinical effect = 30-60 min	• Hypotension with rapid IV infusion • "Water intoxication" (headache, vomiting, drowsiness, convulsions) if given in large volumes of electrolyte-free solution	Hypersensitivity to drug
Methergine® (Methylergonivine)	0.2 mg	IM (NOT given IV)	Q 2-4 hrs	• Onset of action = 2-5 min • $t_{1/2}$ = 30 min • clinical action sustained for ≥3 hrs	• Nausea & vomiting • ↑ central venous pressure and blood pressure → pulmonary edema, stroke, myocardial infarction	Heart disease, autoimmune conditions associated with Raynaud's phenomenon, peripheral vascular disease, AV shunts, HTN
Hemabate® (15-methyl-PG F2α)	250 mcg	IM or IMM (when tissue hypoperfusion may compromise absorption following IM injection, such as in shock pts) (NOT given IV)	Q 15-20 min up to 8 doses max (2 mg)		Nausea, vomiting, diarrhea, fever, bronchospasm	Cardiac or pulmonary disease

Cytotec® (Misoprostol)	400 mcg	Rectal or oral (sublingual or buccal)	One time	• Doses >400 mcg are associated with greater side effects and are no more effective than 400 mcg dose
				• Onset of action
				  • Oral tablets = 6 min
				  • Rectal = 11 min
				  • Vaginal = 20 min
					Fever, shivering	Hypersensitivity to drug

68 Retained Placenta

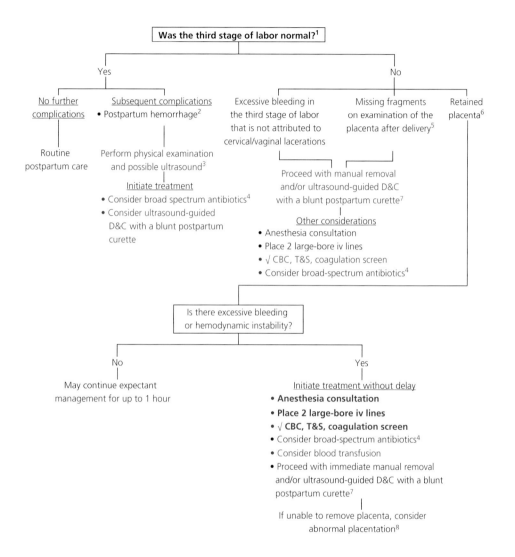

Was the third stage of labor normal?[1]

Yes

No further complications
→ Routine postpartum care

Subsequent complications
• Postpartum hemorrhage[2]
→ Perform physical examination and possible ultrasound[3]
Initiate treatment
• Consider broad spectrum antibiotics[4]
• Consider ultrasound-guided D&C with a blunt postpartum curette

No

Excessive bleeding in the third stage of labor that is not attributed to cervical/vaginal lacerations

Missing fragments on examination of the placenta after delivery[5]

Retained placenta[6]

Proceed with manual removal and/or ultrasound-guided D&C with a blunt postpartum curette[7]
Other considerations
• Anesthesia consultation
• Place 2 large-bore iv lines
• √ CBC, T&S, coagulation screen
• Consider broad-spectrum antibiotics[4]

Is there excessive bleeding or hemodynamic instability?

No
May continue expectant management for up to 1 hour

Yes
Initiate treatment without delay
• **Anesthesia consultation**
• **Place 2 large-bore iv lines**
• **√ CBC, T&S, coagulation screen**
• Consider broad-spectrum antibiotics[4]
• Consider blood transfusion
• Proceed with immediate manual removal and/or ultrasound-guided D&C with a blunt postpartum curette[7]

If unable to remove placenta, consider abnormal placentation[8]

1. The third stage of labor begins with delivery of the fetus and ends with delivery of the placenta and fetal membranes. It is usually managed expectantly. Uterine contractions result in cleavage of the placenta between the zona basalis and zona spongiosum. The three clinical signs of placental separation are: (i) a gush of blood ("separation bleed"); (ii) apparent lengthening

Obstetric Clinical Algorithms, Second Edition. Errol R. Norwitz, George R. Saade, Hugh Miller and Christina M. Davidson.
© 2017 John Wiley & Sons, Ltd. Published 2017 by John Wiley & Sons, Ltd.

of the umbilical cord; and (iii) elevation and contraction of the uterine fundus. Placental separation can be encouraged by gentle (not vigorous) uterine massage. Once signs of placental separation are apparent, delivery can be facilitated by use of "controlled cord traction" while simultaneously applying pressure between the symphysis pubis and the uterine fundus to avoid uterine inversion. There is no data to document an ideal duration of the third stage of labor prior to manual removal, however, no increase in hemorrhage has been noted until the third stage exceeds 30 minutes.

2. Postpartum hemorrhage (PPH) has traditionally been defined as an estimated blood loss (EBL) of >500 mL at vaginal delivery or >1000 mL following cesarean delivery. Clinicians typically underestimate blood loss by 30–50%. More recently, PPH has been defined as a 10% drop in hematocrit from admission or bleeding requiring blood transfusion (see Chapter 67, Postpartum Hemorrhage). Retained placental fragments are one cause of PPH.

3. A careful physical examination (including a bimanual examination) should be performed in all such women. Evidence of vaginal bleeding with an open cervical os suggests retained placental fragments and/or blood clots. Although an ultrasound examination is often performed in such women, management should be based primarily on their clinical presentation. Indeed, the definition of what constitutes a normal postpartum ultrasound is not clear.

4. Manual removal of the placenta following either vaginal or cesarean delivery carries with it an increased risk of endometritis. According to ACOG, it is common practice to administer prophylactic antibiotics to patients who give birth vaginally and in whom a manual removal of the placenta has been performed; however, there is no reliable data to support this practice.

5. The placenta and fetal membranes should be carefully examined after every delivery. Such an examination may identify defects suggestive of retained placental fragments, including retention of a cotyledon or succenturiate lobe.

6. Retained placenta is defined as failure of the placenta and fetal membranes to deliver within 30 minutes of delivery of the baby, which complicates up to 3.5% of vaginal births. If there is excessive bleeding, manual removal and/or D&C may be required earlier.

Three types of retained placenta have been described: (i) placenta adherens (failure of the myometrium to contract and detach the placenta); (ii) trapped placenta (a detached placenta trapped behind a closed cervix); and (iii) partial accreta (a small area of morbidly adherent placenta preventing detachment). Ultrasound studies of the third stage of labor have demonstrated that a retroplacental myometrial contraction is mandatory to cause the placenta to detach from the myometrium. A trapped placenta should be suspected clinically if the fundus feels small and contracted, or if the edge of the placenta is palpable through a tight cervical os. By contrast, the fundus is usually soft and wide with a placenta adherens. Ultrasound can be used to make this distinction. With a trapped placenta, the myometrium is seen to be thickened all around the uterus with a clear demarcation between the placenta and the myometrium; with an adherent placenta, the myometrium will be thickened in all areas except where the placenta is attached, where it will be thin. Placenta accreta is less common, and will usually be discovered only at the time of attempted manual removal.

7. Oxytocin has been shown to reduce bleeding in the third stage of labor. However, once the diagnosis of retained placenta is made, pharmacologic treatment is no longer effective. One exception may be in the setting of a trapped placenta, which may respond to

nitroglycerine (500 mcg sublingually) to help relax the cervix.

Retained placenta can be treated by manual removal, which should be carried out at 30–60 minutes postpartum or earlier if bleeding is excessive. The surgeon should identify the interface between the uterus and maternal surface of the placenta by following the umbilical cord through the vagina. Once the rough, velvety interface between the uterus and placenta is identified, the plane is gently dissected using a side-to-side motion of the fingers. The other hand is used to steady the fundus of the uterus through the woman's abdomen.

8. See Chapter 47, Placenta Accreta.

69 Postpartum Endomyometritis[1]

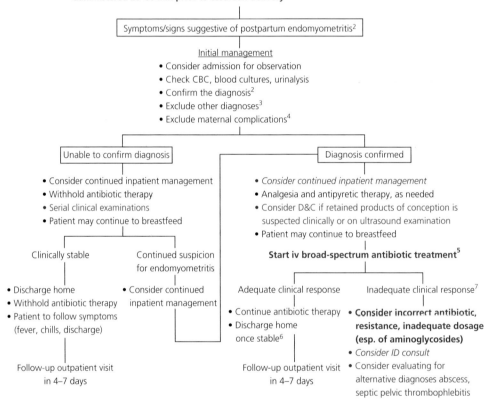

Routine implementation of practices to prevent postpartum endomyometritis

- Avoidance of frequent vaginal exams and unnecessary uterine instrumentation during delivery (including avoidance of manual removal of placenta at cesarean)
- **Routine antibiotic chemoprophylaxis (cephalosporin or clindamycin/gentamicin) administered 20–60 min prior to cesarean delivery**

Symptoms/signs suggestive of postpartum endomyometritis[2]

Initial management
- Consider admission for observation
- Check CBC, blood cultures, urinalysis
- Confirm the diagnosis[2]
- Exclude other diagnoses[3]
- Exclude maternal complications[4]

Unable to confirm diagnosis
- Consider continued inpatient management
- Withhold antibiotic therapy
- Serial clinical examinations
- Patient may continue to breastfeed

Diagnosis confirmed
- *Consider continued inpatient management*
- Analgesia and antipyretic therapy, as needed
- Consider D&C if retained products of conception is suspected clinically or on ultrasound examination
- Patient may continue to breastfeed

Start iv broad-spectrum antibiotic treatment[5]

Clinically stable
- Discharge home
- Withhold antibiotic therapy
- Patient to follow symptoms (fever, chills, discharge)

Follow-up outpatient visit in 4–7 days

Continued suspicion for endomyometritis
- Consider continued inpatient management

Adequate clinical response
- Continue antibiotic therapy
- Discharge home once stable[6]

Follow-up outpatient visit in 4–7 days

Inadequate clinical response[7]
- **Consider incorrect antibiotic, resistance, inadequate dosage (esp. of aminoglycosides)**
- *Consider ID consult*
- Consider evaluating for alternative diagnoses abscess, septic pelvic thrombophlebitis

1. Postpartum endomyometritis refers to a polymicrobial infection of the uterine cavity following delivery. It complicates approximately 6–8% of all deliveries. Risk factors for postpartum endomyometritis include cesarean delivery, prolonged rupture of the fetal membranes (>24 h), low socio-economic status, diabetes, multiple vaginal examinations, manual removal of the placenta, and internal fetal monitoring.

2. Postpartum endomyometritis is a <u>clinical</u> diagnosis characterized by fever, uterine tenderness,

Obstetric Clinical Algorithms, Second Edition. Errol R. Norwitz, George R. Saade, Hugh Miller and Christina M. Davidson.
© 2017 John Wiley & Sons, Ltd. Published 2017 by John Wiley & Sons, Ltd.

a foul purulent vaginal discharge, and/or an increase in vaginal bleeding during the puerperium. It occurs most commonly 5–10 days after delivery. Constitutional symptoms (chills, malaise) and an elevated white cell count are common findings, but are not required for the diagnosis. There is no place for radiologic imaging studies or culture of the endometrial cavity to confirm the diagnosis; however, imaging studies may be useful to exclude other possible diagnoses (such as retained placental tissue or septic pelvic thrombophlebitis).

3. The differential diagnosis of postpartum endomyometritis includes retained products of conception, mastitis, septic pelvic thrombophlebitis, pelvic/bladder flap hematoma or abscess, surgical site (wound) infection, infected episiotomy, and other infections (such as appendicitis, pyelonephritis, and pneumonia).

4. Maternal complications include necrotizing fasciitis, pulmonary edema, sepsis, adult respiratory distress syndrome (ARDS), and subsequent Asherman syndrome (especially following uterine instrumentation).

5. Prompt administration of intravenous broad-spectrum antibiotics will reduce maternal febrile morbidity and duration of hospitalization. Intravenous ampicillin 2 g q 6 h plus gentamicin 1.5 mg/kg q 8 h (after confirmation of normal renal function) are the antibiotics of choice following vaginal delivery. After cesarean delivery, clindamycin 900 mg iIV q 8 h should be added. If an abscess is suspected or renal impairment develops, aztreonam can be substituted for gentamicin.

6. Intravenous antibiotics should be continued until the patient is 24–48 hours afebrile and asymptomatic. There is no role for oral antibiotics once the patient is discharged (aside from patients with positive blood cultures who likely require antibiotics for a total of 10–14 days).

7. Ten percent of patients with symptomatic postpartum endomyometritis will fail to respond to intravenous antibiotics within 48–72 hours; 20% will be due to resistant organisms. Consider evaluating for other sources of infection such as pyelonephritis, an intra-abdominal abscess, or septic pelvic thrombophlebitis.

70 Mastitis

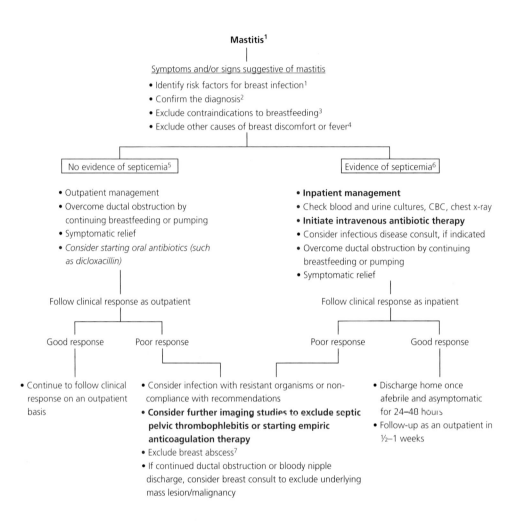

Mastitis[1]

Symptoms and/or signs suggestive of mastitis
- Identify risk factors for breast infection[1]
- Confirm the diagnosis[2]
- Exclude contraindications to breastfeeding[3]
- Exclude other causes of breast discomfort or fever[4]

No evidence of septicemia[5]	Evidence of septicemia[6]
• Outpatient management	• **Inpatient management**
• Overcome ductal obstruction by continuing breastfeeding or pumping	• Check blood and urine cultures, CBC, chest x-ray
• Symptomatic relief	• **Initiate intravenous antibiotic therapy**
• *Consider starting oral antibiotics (such as dicloxacillin)*	• Consider infectious disease consult, if indicated
	• Overcome ductal obstruction by continuing breastfeeding or pumping
	• Symptomatic relief

Follow clinical response as outpatient

Follow clinical response as inpatient

Good response — Poor response

Poor response — Good response

- Continue to follow clinical response on an outpatient basis

- Consider infection with resistant organisms or non-compliance with recommendations
- **Consider further imaging studies to exclude septic pelvic thrombophlebitis or starting empiric anticoagulation therapy**
- Exclude breast abscess[7]
- If continued ductal obstruction or bloody nipple discharge, consider breast consult to exclude underlying mass lesion/malignancy

- Discharge home once afebrile and asymptomatic for 24–48 hours
- Follow-up as an outpatient in ½–1 weeks

1. Mastitis refers to a regional infection of the breast parenchyma, usually by *Staphylococcus aureus*. Women at greatest risk are those who have experienced mastitis in a prior pregnancy, unilateral breast engorgement, and those with excoriation or injury of the nipple.

2. Mastitis is a clinical diagnosis with fever ≥100.4F (38.0C), chills, and focal unilateral breast erythema, edema, and tenderness with or without an elevated white blood cell count. It is more common in primiparous patients (>50%) and usually occurs during the third or forth week postpartum.

Obstetric Clinical Algorithms, Second Edition. Errol R. Norwitz, George R. Saade, Hugh Miller and Christina M. Davidson.
© 2017 John Wiley & Sons, Ltd. Published 2017 by John Wiley & Sons, Ltd.

3. Whenever possible, breastfeeding should be encouraged. Breastfed infants have a lower incidence of allergies, gastrointestinal infections, ear infections, respiratory infections, and (possibly) higher intelligence quotient (IQ) scores. Women who breastfeed appear to have a lower incidence of breast cancer, ovarian cancer, and osteoporosis. Breastfeeding is also a bonding experience between infant and mother. Under certain conditions, however, breastfeeding may be detrimental to the fetus. Contraindications to breastfeeding include infection with HIV, cytomegalovirus, and/or chronic hepatitis B or C. Breastfeeding is also contraindicated if the mother is on certain drugs, such as radioisotopes and certain cytotoxic agents.

4. Mastitis should be distinguished from breast engorgement, which typically occurs on days two to four postpartum in women who are not nursing or at any time if breastfeeding is interrupted. Conservative measures (pressure, ice packs, analgesics) are usually effective for the management of breast engorgement. Bromocriptine should not be used because of reports of serious adverse events (including seizures, strokes, and other cardiovascular events). Other causes of fever that should be excluded in the puerperium include endometritis, urinary tract infection/pyelonephritis, ear and throat infections, pneumonia, and (rarely) septic pelvic thrombophlebitis.

5. Mild mastitis without evidence of septicemia can be treated as an outpatient with oral antibiotics (dicloxicillin or cephalexin) for coverage of *staphylococcus aureus*, the most likely organism. Continuing breastfeeding or pumping is very important as well as managing engorgement and improving breastfeeding techniques. Finally, analgesia and local treatment of any nipple excoriations will provide symptomatic relief.

6. Severe mastitis with evidence of septicemia or mastitis that has been refractory to outpatient management should prompt admission and treatment with intravenous antibiotic therapy. Cultures from the affected nipple should be considered in view of the rising prevalence of MSRA mastitis. These patients need to be screened for a concurrent abscess, which will require parenteral treatment with vancomycin.

7. Approximately 5–10% of women will develop a breast abscess. Diagnosis can be made clinically and confirmed by ultrasonography, if indicated. Although surgical drainage was the historical approach, ultrasound-guided percutaneous drainage is now the standard of care with greater efficacy and lower recurrence rates. Smoking cessation should be encouraged to avoid recurrence. Patients >35 years old should also be evaluated for occult malignancy.

71 Vasa Previa

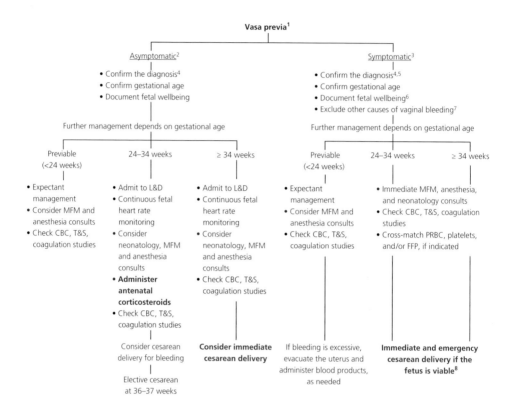

1. Vasa previa refers to the presence of fetal vessels coursing through the membranes overlying the internal os ahead of the presenting part of the fetus.

2. Vasa previa may be an incidental finding on routine ultrasound.

3. Most patients are asymptomatic. Symptoms may include the acute onset of bright-red vaginal bleeding, which is usually painless. It is often accompanied by decreased fetal movement. Risks for bleeding from fetal blood vessels include rupture of the fetal membranes, funic (cord) presentation, multiple pregnancy, placental abnormalities (such as an accessory or succenturiate lobe of placenta, velamentous cord insertion).

4. Vasa previa is an ultrasonographic diagnosis. Ultrasound may confirm funic presentation with or without velamentous cord insertion.

Obstetric Clinical Algorithms, Second Edition. Errol R. Norwitz, George R. Saade, Hugh Miller and Christina M. Davidson.
© 2017 John Wiley & Sons, Ltd. Published 2017 by John Wiley & Sons, Ltd.

5. In the setting of acute bleeding, consider performing a bedside Apt test (hemoglobin alkaline denaturation test). This involves the addition of 2–3 drops of a concentrated alkaline solution (sodium or potassium hydroxide) to 1 mL of blood collected from a vaginal pool. If the blood is maternal in origin, the erythrocytes rupture and the mixture turns brown. However, fetal erythrocytes are more resistant to rupture. If the blood is fetal in origin, the erythrocytes will not rupture and the mixture remains red. Certain maternal conditions (hemoglobinopathies) may give a false-positive test result.

6. Maternal complications are rare since the bleeding is fetal in origin. However, fetal mortality exceeds 75% due primarily to fetal exsanguination. Perinatal outcome depends primarily on the extent of the fetal bleeding, the gestational age, and the ability of the obstetric care provider to make the diagnosis and expedite delivery (which typically involves emergent caesarean delivery).

7. Other causes of vaginal bleeding include placenta previa, placental abruption, early labor, and genital tract lesions (cervical polyps or erosions).

8. Contraindications to emergency cesarean include a previable fetus (<23–24 weeks), intrauterine fetal demise, maternal hemodynamic instability or coagulopathy, or failure to obtain maternal consent for surgery.

72 Postpartum Psychiatric Disorders

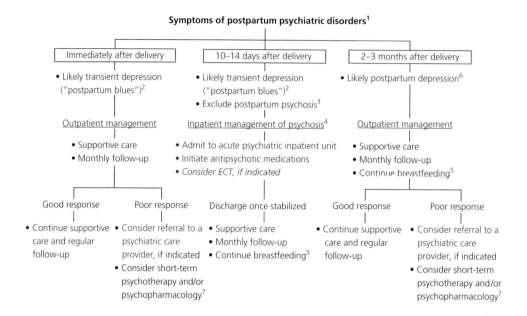

1. Pregnancy is generally thought of as a time of universal well-being. However, in women with established psychiatric disorders, pregnancy may exacerbate their symptoms. A patient's underlying psychiatric diagnosis as well as her social, cultural, and educational background will often determine her emotional adjustment to being pregnant. In general, pregnancies that are planned and/or desired create fewer conflicts within the individual and as such are better accepted. The puerperium has long been identified as a time of increased risk for mental illness. This is due in part to discontinuation of medications during pregnancy because of concern over the safety of the fetus.

2. A mild transient depression ("postpartum blues" or "maternity blues") is common immediately after delivery, occurring in >50% of all postpartum women. The etiology of this disorder is unclear, but is likely due to the rapid biochemical and hormonal changes associated with childbirth.

3. Severe postpartum psychotic depressive or manic illness is rare (1–2 per 1000 livebirths). Risk factors include younger age, primiparity, a family history of mental illness, and most importantly a personal history of psychotic illness. The risk of recurrence in a woman with a history of prior postpartum psychosis is 25–30%. The peak onset of psychotic symptoms is typically 10–14 days after delivery.

4. In patients with postpartum psychosis, pharmacologic therapy should be initiated as

Obstetric Clinical Algorithms, Second Edition. Errol R. Norwitz, George R. Saade, Hugh Miller and Christina M. Davidson.
© 2017 John Wiley & Sons, Ltd. Published 2017 by John Wiley & Sons, Ltd.

soon as possible and short-term hospitalization may be necessary. Electroconvulsant therapy (ECT) has been used in this setting with some success. Many of these women go on to develop life-long depressive disorders. Interestingly, suicide is uncommon during pregnancy and the year following delivery. Recurrence of postpartum psychosis is high (25–30%).

5. All psychotropic drugs are excreted in breast milk. The milk-to-plasma ratio of antidepressants ranges from 0.5 to 1.0, whereas only 40% of lithium is excreted in breast milk. In general, the amount of medication ingested by the baby is small. For this reason, the American Academy of Pediatrics (1983) has concluded that antipsychotic drugs and lithium are compatible with breastfeeding. However, the metabolism of drugs is impaired in infants due to hepatic immaturity. This is especially true for premature infants, and in this cohort it may be prudent to withhold breast milk if high doses of medication are required. An alternative recommendation has been to continue breastfeeding, but to monitor maternal and infant blood levels and discontinue feeding only if the drug levels are dangerously elevated or if the infant develops signs of toxicity.

6. Nonpsychotic postpartum depression complicates approximately 8–15% of all pregnancies, but the incidence may be as high as 30% in women with a prior history of depression and upwards of 70–85% in women with a previous episode of postpartum depression. Symptoms typically start between 2 and 3 months after delivery.

7. Prophylactic pharmacotherapy should be considered in women at high risk of postpartum depression or psychosis. Unfortunately, depressive illness is only identified in around one-third to one half of postpartum patients who meet *Diagnostic and Statistical Manual (DSM)-V* diagnostic criteria. The natural history of a postpartum depressive episode is one of gradual improvement over the 6–12 months following delivery. Supportive care and monthly follow-up for the first 3–6 months (watching for symptoms and signs of worsening depression, thoughts of infanticide or suicide, emergence of psychosis, and response to treatment) may be all that is required.

73 Sterilization[1]

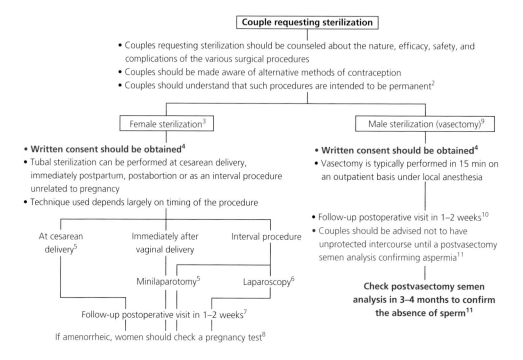

Couple requesting sterilization

- Couples requesting sterilization should be counseled about the nature, efficacy, safety, and complications of the various surgical procedures
- Couples should be made aware of alternative methods of contraception
- Couples should understand that such procedures are intended to be permanent[2]

Female sterilization[3]

- **Written consent should be obtained[4]**
- Tubal sterilization can be performed at cesarean delivery, immediately postpartum, postabortion or as an interval procedure unrelated to pregnancy
- Technique used depends largely on timing of the procedure

At cesarean delivery[5]

Immediately after vaginal delivery

Interval procedure

Minilaparotomy[5]   Laparoscopy[6]

Follow-up postoperative visit in 1–2 weeks[7]

If amenorrheic, women should check a pregnancy test[8]

Male sterilization (vasectomy)[9]

- **Written consent should be obtained[4]**
- Vasectomy is typically performed in 15 min on an outpatient basis under local anesthesia

- Follow-up postoperative visit in 1–2 weeks[10]
- Couples should be advised not to have unprotected intercourse until a postvasectomy semen analysis confirming aspermia[11]

Check postvasectomy semen analysis in 3–4 months to confirm the absence of sperm[11]

1. Sterilization refers to a surgical procedure that is aimed at permanently blocking or removing part of the female or male genital tract to prevent fertilization. It is the most common method of family planning worldwide. Over 175 million couples worldwide use surgical sterilization for contraception, 90% of whom live in developing countries. The ratio of female to male sterilization is 3:1.

2. Sterilization is designed to be permanent. That said, microsurgical tubal reanastomosis has good results if only a small segment of the tube has been damaged. Pregnancy rates following tubal reanastomosis are low with electrocoagulation (because of the large extent of the damage) and higher with clips, rings, and surgical methods. Vas deferens reanastomosis is a difficult and meticulous surgical procedure that has only a 50% success rate. The strongest indicator of future regret is young age at the time of sterilization, regardless of parity or marital status. Consider obtaining a social service consult if the patient is young or has few children.

3. Female sterilization refers to permanent surgical interruption of the fallopian tubes bilaterally. The procedure is immediately effective.

4. State laws and/or insurance regulations often require a specific interval between obtaining consent and surgical sterilization.

Obstetric Clinical Algorithms, Second Edition. Errol R. Norwitz, George R. Saade, Hugh Miller and Christina M. Davidson.
© 2017 John Wiley & Sons, Ltd. Published 2017 by John Wiley & Sons, Ltd.

5. The mini-laparotomy approach can be used in the interval, postabortion or postpartum period. Interval minilaparotomy is performed through a 2–3 cm sub-umbilical incision. The abdomen is entered, the uterus is identified, and a finger is used to elevate the fallopian tube. After the tube has been identified by its fimbriated end, the mid-portion is grasped with a Babcock clamp. Tubal occlusion is then performed. If a segment of tube is removed, it should be sent to pathology to confirm a complete cross-section of the fallopian tube. A similar procedure can be carried out following vaginal delivery (postpartum sterilization – PPS). The latter procedure is ideally performed while the uterine fundus is high in the abdomen (typically within 48 hours of delivery). Maternal and neonatal wellbeing should be confirmed prior to PPS.

6. Laparoscopic tubal ligation (LTL) is performed using one or more trocar instruments in addition to the umbilical camera site. Advantages of the laparoscopic approach over other surgical procedures include a smaller skin incision, the opportunity to inspect the abdominal and pelvic organs, and a more rapid postoperative recovery. Techniques of tubal occlusion include the following:
- *Electrocoagulation*: bipolar cautery is safer than unipolar cautery, which has the potential to cause thermal bowel injury.
- *Clips and rings*: mechanical occlusion devices, such as the silicone rubber band (Falope ring) and the spring-loaded clip (Hulka clip, Filshie clip), are less commonly used for LTL. Special applicators are necessary and each requires skill for proper application. Clips and rings destroy less oviductal tissue than electrocoagulation. Tubal adhesions or a thickened or dilated fallopian tube increase the risk of misapplication of the clip.

7. Complications of tubal ligation are rare. The mortality rate (1–2 per 100,000 procedures in the United States) is lower than that for childbirth (10 per 100,000 births). Anesthetic complication is the leading cause of death. Other potential complications include hemorrhage, infection, erroneous ligation of the round ligament, and injury to adjacent structures. Overall, when the risk of pregnancy from contraceptive failure is taken into account, sterilization is the safest of all contraceptive methods.

8. The failure rate of tubal ligation is dependent upon the specific operation performed, the skill of the surgeon, and the characteristics of the patient (age, pelvic adhesions, hydrosalpinx). When sterilization failure occurs, the resultant pregnancy is more likely to be an ectopic (tubal) pregnancy.

9. Vasectomy involves permanent surgical interruption of the vas deferens (the duct that transports sperm during ejaculation) bilaterally. Pregnancy rates following vasectomy are <1%. When compared with female tubal sterilization, vasectomy is safer, less expensive, and equally effective.

10. Postoperative complications of vasectomy include wound hematomas, infections, and rarely sperm granulomas (<3%). Putative long-term side effects (increased risk of prostate cancer, decreased libido) have never been proven.

11. Unlike tubal occlusion in women, vasectomy is not immediately effective. Spermatozoa normally mature in the vas deferens for around 70 days prior to ejaculation. For this reason, at least 3 months or 20 ejaculations are needed to deplete the vas deferens entirely of viable sperm. Postvasectomy semen analysis should be performed to determine the effectiveness of the procedure prior to unprotected intercourse.

SECTION 6
Obstetric Emergencies

Levels of evidence

The levels of evidence used in this book are those recommended by the U.S. Preventive Services Task Force, an independent panel of experts responsible for developing evidence-based recommendations for primary care and prevention, in 2007 (http://www.ahrq.gov/clinic/uspstmeth.htm):

Level I: Evidence obtained from at least one properly designed randomized controlled trial.
Level II: Evidence obtained from controlled trials without randomization or cohort / case-controlled studies that include a comparison group.
Level III: Evidence from uncontrolled descriptive studies (including case series) or opinions of respected authorities or expert committees.
Level IV: Evidence from uncontrolled descriptive studies (including case series) or opinions of respected authorities or expert committees.

74 Acute Abdomen in Pregnancy

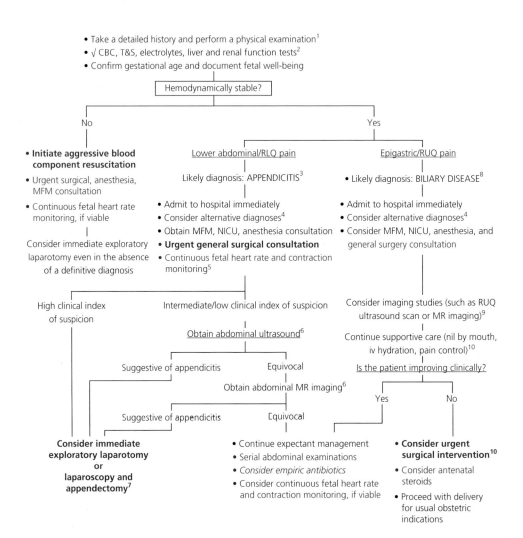

- Take a detailed history and perform a physical examination[1]
- √ CBC, T&S, electrolytes, liver and renal function tests[2]
- Confirm gestational age and document fetal well-being

Hemodynamically stable?

No

- **Initiate aggressive blood component resuscitation**
- Urgent surgical, anesthesia, MFM consultation
- Continuous fetal heart rate monitoring, if viable

Consider immediate exploratory laparotomy even in the absence of a definitive diagnosis

Yes

Lower abdominal/RLQ pain

Likely diagnosis: APPENDICITIS[3]

- Admit to hospital immediately
- Consider alternative diagnoses[4]
- Obtain MFM, NICU, anesthesia consultation
- **Urgent general surgical consultation**
- Continuous fetal heart rate and contraction monitoring[5]

High clinical index of suspicion

Intermediate/low clinical index of suspicion

Obtain abdominal ultrasound[6]

Suggestive of appendicitis

Equivocal

Obtain abdominal MR imaging[6]

Suggestive of appendicitis

Equivocal

Consider immediate exploratory laparotomy or laparoscopy and appendectomy[7]

- Continue expectant management
- Serial abdominal examinations
- *Consider empiric antibiotics*
- Consider continuous fetal heart rate and contraction monitoring, if viable

Epigastric/RUQ pain

- Likely diagnosis: BILIARY DISEASE[8]

- Admit to hospital immediately
- Consider alternative diagnoses[4]
- Consider MFM, NICU, anesthesia, and general surgery consultation

Consider imaging studies (such as RUQ ultrasound scan or MR imaging)[9]

Continue supportive care (nil by mouth, iv hydration, pain control)[10]

Is the patient improving clinically?

Yes

No

- **Consider urgent surgical intervention[10]**
- Consider antenatal steroids
- Proceed with delivery for usual obstetric indications

---

1. History taking should be brief and focused. Ask about underlying medical conditions, prior surgery, medications, and allergies. Ask about pregnancy complications including vaginal bleeding, leakage of fluid, contractions, and fetal movements. Physical examination may reveal generalized or focal tenderness, presence/absence of guarding and rebound tenderness,

---

Obstetric Clinical Algorithms, Second Edition. Errol R. Norwitz, George R. Saade, Hugh Miller and Christina M. Davidson.
© 2017 John Wiley & Sons, Ltd. Published 2017 by John Wiley & Sons, Ltd.

and increased/decreased bowel sounds. Confirm gestational age and document fetal well-being, especially if >24 weeks of gestation.

2. White blood cell count in normal pregnancy ranges from 10,000 to 14,000 cells/mm³. In labor, the white blood cell count may be as high as 20,000 to 30,000 cells/mm³. Counts that are significantly higher than that or have evidence of a left shift suggest underlying infection/inflammation.

3. Acute appendicitis is the most common general surgical problem encountered during pregnancy, complicating 1 in 1500 deliveries. Although it can occur in any trimester, there appears to be a slight predominance in the second trimester. It is not more common in pregnancy, but pregnancy is associated with a higher rate of perforation, likely due to delay in diagnosis. The clinical manifestations and diagnosis of appendicitis in pregnancy are similar to those in nonpregnant individuals. Pain in the right lower quadrant is the most common presenting symptom, regardless of gestational age. Fever and leukocytosis are less reliable indicators of appendicitis in pregnancy.

4. The differential diagnosis is extensive, including any cause of abdominal pain, such as, among others, gastroenteritis, constipation, peptic ulcer disease, small bowel obstruction, inflammatory bowel disease (Crohn's disease or ulcerative colitis), pancreatitis, ectopic pregnancy, ruptured ovarian cyst, ovarian torsion, renal colic, pyelonephritis, and (rarely) such disorders as sickle cell crisis, pneumonia, diabetic ketoacidosis, and porphyria.

5. Unruptured appendicitis is associated with a fetal loss rate of 3–5%, with little effect on maternal mortality. By contrast, the fetal loss rate in the setting of ruptured appendicitis is 20–25%. Preterm labor and birth can also occur, especially if there is peritonitis, but this is rare.

6. Abdominal ultrasonography is recommended in pregnant patients suspected of having appendicitis, although visualization of the appendix may be difficult, especially if the woman is obese and the uterus is large. If ultrasonography suggests appendicitis, surgery is indicated. If clinical findings and ultrasound are inconclusive, magnetic resonance imaging (MRI) should be considered, where available, because it avoids fetal exposure to ionizing radiation and performs well in the diagnosis of lower abdominal/pelvic disorders. The routine incorporation of MRI into the evaluation of patients with suspected appendicitis has reduced the negative laparotomy rate by half without a significant change in the perforation rate. If MRI suggests appendicitis, surgery is indicated. Computed tomography (CT) imaging can be used when MRI is not available, given its proven value in nonpregnant individuals.

7. The decision to proceed to surgery should be based on the clinical findings, diagnostic imaging results, and clinical judgment. Laboratory tests are not particularly useful other than to rule in an alternative diagnosis. Delaying intervention for more than 24 hours increases the risk of perforation. When the diagnosis is relatively certain, appendectomy can be performed through a muscle-splitting incision over the point of maximal tenderness. However, when the diagnosis is less certain or if there is a chance that a cesarean delivery may need to be performed (e.g., in the setting of early labor), it may be more prudent to approach the appendix through a lower midline vertical or paramedian incision. Laparoscopic appendectomy may be performed safely in pregnant patients and is considered by many to be the standard of care in the first half of pregnancy.

8. Acute cholecystitis is the second most common condition necessitating surgery in pregnancy, occurring in 1 in 1,600–10,000 pregnancies. Symptoms include nausea, vomiting, and colicky upper abdominal pain that radiates around to

the back. Cholecystectomy is performed in 0.01–0.08% of pregnancies. Cholelithiasis is the main cause of cholecystitis in pregnancy, accounting for >90% of cases.

9. Ultrasound remains the best initial modality to evaluate the liver and biliary system. Cholelithiasis with either positive sonographic Murphy sign or gallbladder wall thickening (>3 mm) is highly predictive of cholecystitis. Secondary findings such as pericholecystic fluid and wall hyperemia may also be helpful. However, common bile duct stones will often be missed on ultrasound. MR cholangiopancreatography (MRCP) can be used as a second-line imaging modality.

10. Surgical intervention is indicated for obstructive jaundice, acute cholecystitis unresponsive to medical management, gallstone pancreatitis, or suspected peritonitis. The initial management of symptomatic cholelithiasis includes bowel rest, intravenous hydration, narcotics, and antibiotics where appropriate. Morphine should be avoided because it can exacerbate biliary colic. Relapse of biliary colic is common.

75 Acute Asthma Exacerbation

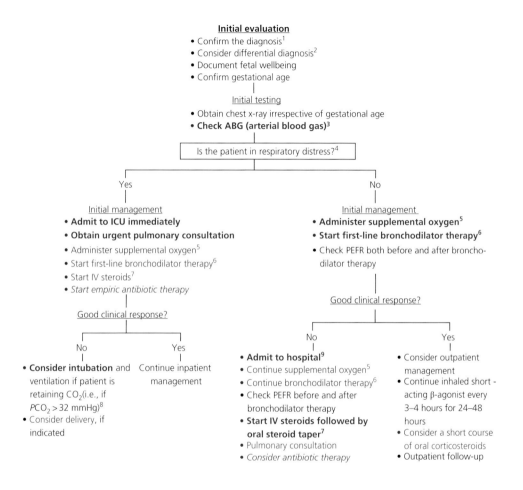

Initial evaluation
- Confirm the diagnosis[1]
- Consider differential diagnosis[2]
- Document fetal wellbeing
- Confirm gestational age

Initial testing
- Obtain chest x-ray irrespective of gestational age
- **Check ABG (arterial blood gas)[3]**

Is the patient in respiratory distress?[4]

Yes

Initial management
- **Admit to ICU immediately**
- **Obtain urgent pulmonary consultation**
- Administer supplemental oxygen[5]
- Start first-line bronchodilator therapy[6]
- Start IV steroids[7]
- *Start empiric antibiotic therapy*

Good clinical response?

No
- **Consider intubation** and ventilation if patient is retaining CO_2 (i.e., if $PCO_2 > 32$ mmHg)[8]
- Consider delivery, if indicated

Yes
Continue inpatient management

No

Initial management
- **Administer supplemental oxygen[5]**
- **Start first-line bronchodilator therapy[6]**
- Check PEFR both before and after bronchodilator therapy

Good clinical response?

No
- **Admit to hospital[9]**
- Continue supplemental oxygen[5]
- Continue bronchodilator therapy[6]
- Check PEFR before and after bronchodilator therapy
- **Start IV steroids followed by oral steroid taper[7]**
- Pulmonary consultation
- *Consider antibiotic therapy*

Yes
- Consider outpatient management
- Continue inhaled short-acting β-agonist every 3–4 hours for 24–48 hours
- Consider a short course of oral corticosteroids
- Outpatient follow-up

1. Asthma is a chronic inflammatory disorder of the airways characterized by intermittent episodes of reversible bronchospasm. The "classic" signs and symptoms of asthma are intermittent dyspnea, cough, and wheezing. To confirm the diagnosis, take a detailed history, perform a physical examination, and perform relevant pulmonary function tests, including peak expiratory flow rate (PEFR) and spirometry, which includes measurement of forced expiratory volume in one second (FEV1) and forced vital capacity (FVC) before and after administration of a bronchodilator.

2. The differential diagnosis of an acute asthma exacerbation includes pneumonia, pulmonary

Obstetric Clinical Algorithms, Second Edition. Errol R. Norwitz, George R. Saade, Hugh Miller and Christina M. Davidson.
© 2017 John Wiley & Sons, Ltd. Published 2017 by John Wiley & Sons, Ltd.

embolism, pneumothorax, congestive cardiac failure, pericarditis, pulmonary edema, and rib fracture.

3. Respiratory adaptations in pregnancy are designed to optimize maternal and fetal oxygenation, and to facilitate transfer of CO_2 waste from the fetus to the mother (see Chapter 6, Asthma). Pregnancy thus represents a state of *compensated respiratory alkalosis*.

	pH	Po_2 (mmHg)	Pco_2 (mmHg)
Non-pregnant	7.40	93–100	35–40
Pregnant	7.40	100–105	28–30

4. Symptoms and signs suggestive of a serious asthma attack and respiratory distress include marked breathlessness, inability to speak more than short phrases, use of accessory muscles, or drowsiness. A PEFR of <50% expected or of personal best (or <200 L/minute in most adults) indicates a need for urgent medical intervention.

5. Supplemental oxygen is typically administered by non-rebreather mask at 4–8 L/min to keep the O_2 saturation >95% in pregnancy (>92% in non-pregnant women).

6. As initial treatment, inhaled short-acting β-agonists should be used early and frequently. Albuterol can be given either as 4–8 puffs of a metered dose inhaler (MDI) with spacer every 20 minutes for up to four hours or by nebulizer treatment (2.5 mg repeated every 20 minutes for two or three doses or 10–15 mg given by continuous nebulization over one hour).

Consider concomitant use of ipratropium bromide for severe exacerbations given as 500 mcg by nebulization every 20 minutes for 3 doses or 8 puffs by MDI with spacer every 20 minutes as needed for up to 3 hours.

7. Start systemic glucocorticoids if there is not an immediate and marked response to the inhaled short-acting β-agonists. Recommended steroid regimens include methylprednisolone 60–125 mg IV or prednisone 40–60 mg orally; alternative regimens include dexamethazone 6–10 mg IV or hydrocortisone 150–200 mg IV. Steroids may be given IM or orally if IV access is unavailable. Steroids should be repeated at 8–12 hourly intervals. Other treatment options for asthma that is severe and unresponsive to standard therapies include terbutaline (0.25 mg by SC injection every 30 minutes for 3 doses) or epinephrine (0.2–0.5 mL of 1:1000 solution by SC injection). Give either terbutaline or epinephrine, but not both.

8. Hypercapnia (a sign of impending respiratory failure) usually only occurs if the PEFR is <25% of normal (or <100–150 L/min). In the absence of anticipated intubation difficulty, rapid sequence intubation is preferred. Nasal intubation is not recommended.

9. Patients should be admitted to hospital if they do not respond well after 4–6 hours in a setting of high surveillance and care. Frequent (every 1–2 hourly) objective clinical assessments of the response to therapy are needed once admitted until a definite and sustained improvement is documented.

76 Acute Shortness of Breath

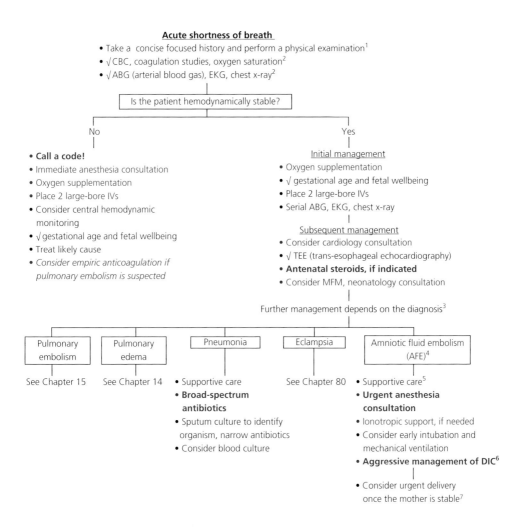

Acute shortness of breath
- Take a concise focused history and perform a physical examination[1]
- √ CBC, coagulation studies, oxygen saturation[2]
- √ ABG (arterial blood gas), EKG, chest x-ray[2]

Is the patient hemodynamically stable?

No

- **Call a code!**
- Immediate anesthesia consultation
- Oxygen supplementation
- Place 2 large-bore IVs
- Consider central hemodynamic monitoring
- √ gestational age and fetal wellbeing
- Treat likely cause
- *Consider empiric anticoagulation if pulmonary embolism is suspected*

Yes

Initial management
- Oxygen supplementation
- √ gestational age and fetal wellbeing
- Place 2 large-bore IVs
- Serial ABG, EKG, chest x-ray

Subsequent management
- Consider cardiology consultation
- √ TEE (trans-esophageal echocardiography)
- **Antenatal steroids, if indicated**
- Consider MFM, neonatology consultation

Further management depends on the diagnosis[3]

| Pulmonary embolism | Pulmonary edema | Pneumonia | Eclampsia | Amniotic fluid embolism (AFE)[4] |

Pulmonary embolism
See Chapter 15

Pulmonary edema
See Chapter 14

Pneumonia
- Supportive care
- **Broad-spectrum antibiotics**
- Sputum culture to identify organism, narrow antibiotics
- Consider blood culture

Eclampsia
See Chapter 80

Amniotic fluid embolism (AFE)[4]
- Supportive care[5]
- **Urgent anesthesia consultation**
- Ionotropic support, if needed
- Consider early intubation and mechanical ventilation
- **Aggressive management of DIC[6]**
- Consider urgent delivery once the mother is stable[7]

1. Ask about acute-onset shortness of breath (dyspnea), pleuritic chest pain, cough, and/or hemoptysis. On examination, look for low-grade fever, tachypnea, tachycardia, diminished oxygen saturation, diminished breath sounds, audible crackles, and/or evidence of pleural effusion on pulmonary examination.

2. Laboratory tests may reveal acidosis and an elevated A-a gradient on arterial blood gas

Obstetric Clinical Algorithms, Second Edition. Errol R. Norwitz, George R. Saade, Hugh Miller and Christina M. Davidson.
© 2017 John Wiley & Sons, Ltd. Published 2017 by John Wiley & Sons, Ltd.

analysis (ABG), and evidence of right-heart strain (S1Q3T3 pattern with or without right axis deviation, T wave inversion) on EKG. CXR may be normal or show evidence of multiple peripheral wedge-shaped areas of consolidation, pulmonary edema, or pleural effusion. However, if ABG reveals an arterial pO2 > 80 mm-Hg, the diagnosis of pulmonary embolism (PE) is highly unlikely. Measurement of D-dimer levels in pregnancy is generally unhelpful in making the diagnosis of PE.

3. The differential diagnosis of acute shortness of breath includes pulmonary embolism, amniotic fluid embolism (AFE), pneumonia (including aspiration pneumonitis (Mendelson's syndrome)), pneumothorax, congestive cardiac failure, pericarditis, pulmonary edema, venous air embolism (rare, associated with ruptured uterus, placenta previa, and persistent atrial septal defect), eclampsia, drug overdose/withdrawal, and rib fracture.

4. Amniotic fluid embolism (AFE) is an obstetric emergency with 80–90% maternal and perinatal mortality. It accounts for 10% of maternal deaths in the United States. AFE is seen most commonly during labor, delivery, and in the immediate postpartum period. Risk factors include cesarean delivery, chorioamnionitis, multiparity, preeclampsia, prolonged labor, fetal demise, amniotomy, intrauterine pressure catheter, intrauterine saline injection (abortion), and placental abruption. It is characterized by acute-onset dyspnea, hypotension, and hypoxemia.

Prodromal symptoms may include sudden chills, sweating, or anxiety. Physical examination may reveal acute-onset respiratory distress, cyanosis, hypotension, tachycardia, hypoxemia, neurologic manifestations (seizures, coma), and/or hemorrhage. Disseminated intravascular coagulopathy (DIC) is usually acute and severe. AFE is a clinical diagnosis. CXR and V/Q scan is of little value in the acute setting. Components of amniotic fluid (fetal squames, mucin) may be identified in the pulmonary vasculature at post-mortem, but this is not pathognemonic.

5. Therapy is primarily supportive. Cardiovascular support should be optimized. This includes maintaining O_2 saturation >90%, arterial PO_2 >60 mmHg, systolic BP >90 mmHg, and urine output >25 mL/h. Ionotropic support (dopamine) and mechanical ventilation should be considered, if needed. Treat bronchospasm (terbutaline, aminophylline, steroids) as needed. CPR and cardiopulmonary bypass may be required.

6. DIC is typically a predominant clinical feature of AFE. Serial CBC and coagulation studies should be followed, and aggressive blood product replacement initiated. Avoid heparin in established DIC.

7. The fetus is at risk of hypoxic ischemic cerebral injury and/or IUFD. Urgent delivery may be necessary regardless of gestational age. Regional anesthesia is contraindicated in the acute setting. General endotracheal anesthesia may be needed for cesarean.

77 Cord Prolapse

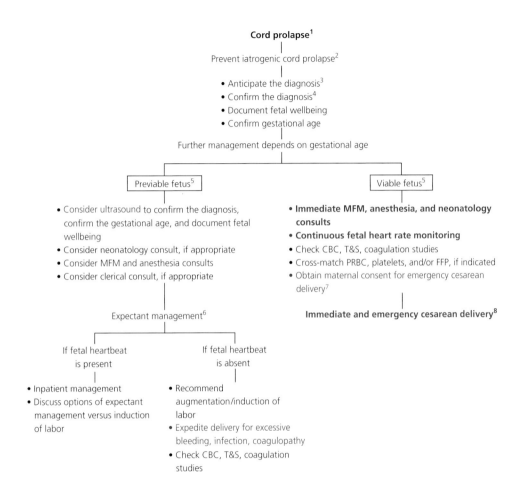

Cord prolapse[1]

Prevent iatrogenic cord prolapse[2]

- Anticipate the diagnosis[3]
- Confirm the diagnosis[4]
- Document fetal wellbeing
- Confirm gestational age

Further management depends on gestational age

Previable fetus[5]

- Consider ultrasound to confirm the diagnosis, confirm the gestational age, and document fetal wellbeing
- Consider neonatology consult, if appropriate
- Consider MFM and anesthesia consults
- Consider clerical consult, if appropriate

Viable fetus[5]

- **Immediate MFM, anesthesia, and neonatology consults**
- **Continuous fetal heart rate monitoring**
- Check CBC, T&S, coagulation studies
- Cross-match PRBC, platelets, and/or FFP, if indicated
- Obtain maternal consent for emergency cesarean delivery[7]

Immediate and emergency cesarean delivery[8]

Expectant management[6]

If fetal heartbeat is present

- Inpatient management
- Discuss options of expectant management versus induction of labor

If fetal heartbeat is absent

- Recommend augmentation/induction of labor
- Expedite delivery for excessive bleeding, infection, coagulopathy
- Check CBC, T&S, coagulation studies

1. Cord prolapse is an obstetric emergency characterized by prolapse of the umbilical cord into the vagina after rupture of the fetal membranes.

2. To prevent iatrogenic cord prolapse, perform amniotomy (artificial rupture of the membranes) only once the vertex is well applied to the cervix and always with fundal pressure.

3. The diagnosis should be anticipated in the setting of rupture of the fetal membranes if any of the following risk factors are present: (i) prematurity; (ii) a small fetus; (iii) funic (cord)

Obstetric Clinical Algorithms, Second Edition. Errol R. Norwitz, George R. Saade, Hugh Miller and Christina M. Davidson.
© 2017 John Wiley & Sons, Ltd. Published 2017 by John Wiley & Sons, Ltd.

presentation on ultrasound examination; and (iv) fetal malpresentation. (Incidence at term is 0.4% of cephalic pregnancies, 0.5% of frank breech pregnancies, 4–6% of complete breech pregnancies, 15–18% of footling breech pregnancies, and up to 25% with transverse lie.)

4. Cord prolapse is a *clinical* diagnosis made by palpation of the umbilical cord on vaginal examination with or without fetal bradycardia. In the acute setting with a viable fetus, there is no place for ultrasound to confirm the diagnosis.

5. Fetal viability is variably defined. In the United States, most obstetric care providers regard the limit of fetal viability as being between 23 and 24 weeks of gestation.

6. Given the urgency of the situation, verbal consent for emergency cesarean delivery is adequate. However, the surgeon should consider having a second provider witness and document the verbal consent and getting written consent from the patient once she has fully recovered from anesthesia. If this is done, it should be made clear that the written consent was obtained after the procedure.

7. Contraindications to emergency cesarean delivery include intrauterine fetal demise, maternal hemodynamic instability (shock), coagulopathy, and failure to secure maternal consent.

8. Once the diagnosis of cord prolapse has been made in a viable pregnancy with confirmation of a live fetus (usually by palpation of a pulsatile umbilical cord), subsequent management should include the following:
- CALL FOR HELP.
- Manual replacement of the umbilical cord into the uterus by the obstetric care provider, who should continue manual replacement until the infant is delivered.
- Place the patient in the knee–chest position.
- Establish intravenous access.
- O_2 supplementation by facemask.
- Transfer the patient immediately to the operating room.
- Notify anesthesia, neonatology, and/or high-risk obstetrics.
- Check CBC, T&S, coagulation studies.
- Continued assessment of fetal well-being (usually confirmation of a pulsatile umbilical cord is adequate).
- Emergency cesarean delivery, usually under general endotracheal anesthesia (epidural analgesia may be used only if it is already in place and has been tested).

78 Cardiopulmonary Resuscitation

CPR in pregnancy[1]

- Be aware of the physiologic changes in pregnancy which may predispose to acute cardiovascular collapse[2]
- Understand risk factors for cardiovascular collapse[3]

Confirm acute cardiovascular collapse

Initial interventions

- **Call for help. Call a code![4,5]**

- **C – Circulation** (place 2 large-bore iv, initiate fluid resuscitation, order blood products)
- **A – Airway** (turn patient on her side, ensure airway is patent, consider early intubation)
- **B – Breathing** (ensure patient is breathing; if not, perform chest compressions/CPR while preparing for intubation and ventilation)

Subsequent management

- √ CBC, liver/renal function tests, coagulation profile
- **√ EKG, arterial blood gas,** CXR, toxicology screen
- Consider differential diagnosis and manage accordingly[3]
- **Continue aggressive CPR, including early intubation and left lateral tilt**

Initial resuscitation efforts successful

- Transfer to ICU
- Confirm gestational age and fetal well-being[6]
- Search for an underlying cause

Resuscitation unsuccessful

Confirm gestational age and fetal well-being[6]

Gestational age <24 weeks and/or nonviable fetus

- **Continue aggressive CPR**
- Consider emptying the uterus within 5–10 min to facilitate CPR[7]
- Transfer to ICU once stable
- Continue to search for an underlying cause

Gestational age ≥24 weeks and a viable fetus

- **Empty the uterus within 5–10 min[7]**
- Pediatrics present at delivery
- Continue aggressive CPR
- Transfer to ICU once stable
- Continue to search for an underlying cause

Obstetric Clinical Algorithms, Second Edition. Errol R. Norwitz, George R. Saade, Hugh Miller and Christina M. Davidson.
© 2017 John Wiley & Sons, Ltd. Published 2017 by John Wiley & Sons, Ltd.

1. Cardiovascular collapse may occur in pregnancy as it does in nonpregnant women. Obstetricians should be able to anticipate, diagnose, and manage cardiac arrest in pregnancy, although it is rare (estimated to occur in <1:20,000 pregnancies).

2. Physiologic adaptations in the mother occur in response to the demands of pregnancy. Pregnancy represents a high-flow, low resistance state characterized by a high cardiac output (CO) and low systemic vascular resistance. CO increases by 50% of non-pregnant values, and the uterus receives up to 30% of CO each minute compared with 2–3% in the non-gravid patient. Hypoxia and acidosis can develop rapidly in pregnancy because of a higher basal metabolic rate, decreased functional residual capacity, and fetal oxygen requirements. Pregnancy is also associated with a dilutional anemia. All these factors limit the ability of a pregnant woman to meet the demands of acute cardiovascular collapse. Moreover, significant aortocaval compression occurs after 20 weeks of gestation due to the rapidly enlarging uterus. In the supine position, this uterine obstruction can lead to sequestration of up to 30% of circulating blood volume, decreasing venous return, causing supine hypotension, and decreasing effectiveness of thoracic compressions during CPR. Pregnant women are also at increased risk of aspiration chemical pneumonitis (Mendelson syndrome).

3. The American Heart Association (AHA) has developed a mnemonic (BEAUCHOPS) for the factors contributing to cardiac arrest in pregnancy: **B**leeding/DIC, **E**mbolism, **A**nesthetic complications, **U**terine atony, **C**ardiac disease, **H**ypertension, **O**ther, **P**lacental abruption/previa, **S**epsis. Management should be tailored to the likely cause. For example, empiric broad-spectrum antibiotics should be started immediately if septic shock is suspected. If massive blood loss is suspected, the source of the blood loss should be identified and stopped, fluid resuscitation should be started, and coagulopathy aggressively treated.

4. Immediate and effective communication is critically important during maternal cardiac arrest, because of the number of teams that must be mobilized and coordinated. All response team members should be familiar with the location of critical equipment. Protocols should be developed and systems tested in periodic multidisciplinary emergency drills. Deficiencies should be addressed. A common error is a failure to "close the loop" of communication leading to redundancy of effort and a delay in critical interventions. The use of periodic "time-outs" during CPR may help to coordinate and optimize care. During the brief time-out, the leader or timer/documenter should review the working diagnosis, the interventions that have been completed, and the goals and priorities moving forward. Chest compressions should not be interrupted.

5. Chest compressions should be started immediately to optimize maternal and fetal outcomes. Optimal compressions should be hard (achieving a depth of 5 cm), fast (100/min), and uninterrupted. The 2010 AHA guidelines now recommend C-A-B (compressions, airway, breathing) rather than A-B-C. Left uterine displacement is recommended if the uterus is palpable at or above the umbilicus in order to minimize the adverse effects of vena caval compression by the gravid uterus. The CO produced from chest compressions is optimized when the patient is placed on a firm surface (backboard). CPR should be performed while a defibrillator or automated external defibrillator (AED) is readied for use. Defibrillation should be performed as soon as possible using the same energy settings as for nonpregnant patients. Defibrillation is safe for the fetus. Fetal monitors should ideally be removed, but defibrillation should not be unnecessarily delayed as the risk of an electrical burn is minimal. In sudden cardiac arrest with ventricular

fibrillation, the earlier defibrillation occurs, the greater the chance of survival. Although many interventions have not been well studied in pregnancy, few are contraindicated when the alternative is death. These include inotrope and vasopressor medications (which may reduce uteroplacental blood flow) and thrombolytics (for the acute management of myocardial infarction and pulmonary embolism).

6. Initial efforts at maternal resuscitation should not be delayed to document fetal wellbeing. Fetal monitoring is not necessary and may distract staff or unnecessarily delay maternal CPR efforts.

7. CPR does not adequately perfuse the uterus, and fetal survival is unlikely if >10 minutes have passed since loss of maternal vital signs. Based on isolated case reports, cesarean delivery should be considered for both maternal and fetal benefit approximately 4 minutes after a woman has experienced cardiopulmonary arrest in the third trimester (so-called perimortem cesarean delivery and the "4-minute rule"). In this emergency setting, patient consent is not required. Similarly, taking the time to transport the patient to the operating room is not recommended. A vertical skin incision should be performed and the uterine contents should be evacuated immediately. If the fetus is viable, it should be passed over to the waiting pediatricians. Adequate maternal analgesia is essential, and this can be rapidly achieved though general anesthesia since the patient is typically intubated. The uterus should be rapidly closed using a single full-thickness suture. The abdomen should be left open (covered with a sterile transparent sheet) to ensure that the uterus does not fill with blood, thereby further impairing CPR. The skin can be closed at a later time. CPR should be continued throughout this procedure.

79 Diabetic Ketoacidosis[1]

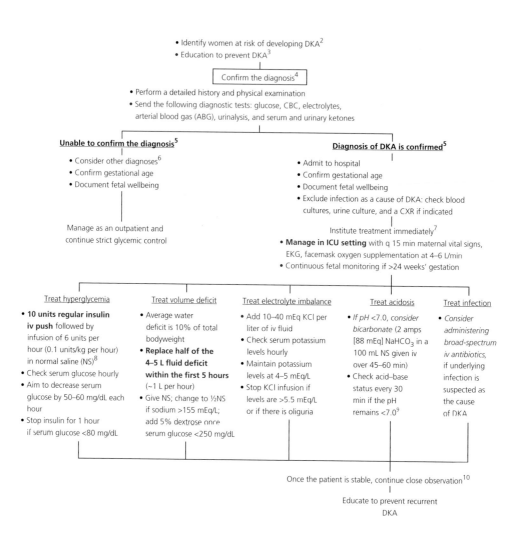

- Identify women at risk of developing DKA[2]
- Education to prevent DKA[3]

Confirm the diagnosis[4]

- Perform a detailed history and physical examination
- Send the following diagnostic tests: glucose, CBC, electrolytes,
  arterial blood gas (ABG), urinalysis, and serum and urinary ketones

Unable to confirm the diagnosis[5]

- Consider other diagnoses[6]
- Confirm gestational age
- Document fetal wellbeing

Manage as an outpatient and
continue strict glycemic control

Diagnosis of DKA is confirmed[5]

- Admit to hospital
- Confirm gestational age
- Document fetal wellbeing
- Exclude infection as a cause of DKA: check blood
  cultures, urine culture, and a CXR if indicated

Institute treatment immediately[7]
- **Manage in ICU setting** with q 15 min maternal vital signs,
  EKG, facemask oxygen supplementation at 4–6 L/min
- Continuous fetal monitoring if >24 weeks' gestation

Treat hyperglycemia	Treat volume deficit	Treat electrolyte imbalance	Treat acidosis	Treat infection
• **10 units regular insulin iv push** followed by infusion of 6 units per hour (0.1 units/kg per hour) in normal saline (NS)[8] • Check serum glucose hourly • Aim to decrease serum glucose by 50–60 mg/dL each hour • Stop insulin for 1 hour if serum glucose <80 mg/dL	• Average water deficit is 10% of total bodyweight • **Replace half of the 4–5 L fluid deficit within the first 5 hours** (~1 L per hour) • Give NS; change to ½NS if sodium >155 mEq/L; add 5% dextrose once serum glucose <250 mg/dL	• Add 10–40 mEq KCl per liter of iv fluid • Check serum potassium levels hourly • Maintain potassium levels at 4–5 mEq/L • Stop KCl infusion if levels are >5.5 mEq/L or if there is oliguria	• *If pH <7.0, consider bicarbonate* (2 amps [88 mEq] NaHCO$_3$ in a 100 mL NS given iv over 45–60 min) • Check acid–base status every 30 min if the pH remains <7.0[9]	• *Consider administering broad-spectrum iv antibiotics,* if underlying infection is suspected as the cause of DKA

Once the patient is stable, continue close observation[10]

Educate to prevent recurrent
DKA

1. Diabetic ketoacidosis (DKA) results from a relative or absolute deficiency of circulating insulin in the setting of excessive glucose counterregulatory (anti-insulin) hormones (such as catecholamines, growth hormone, cortisol, and glucagon). Insulin is an anabolic hormone that drives glucose into cells. Insulin deficiency results in a fundamental paradox: although there is an adequate supply of glucose, the body believes that it is starving and begins to make

Obstetric Clinical Algorithms, Second Edition. Errol R. Norwitz, George R. Saade, Hugh Miller and Christina M. Davidson.
© 2017 John Wiley & Sons, Ltd. Published 2017 by John Wiley & Sons, Ltd.

ketones for use by the vital organs (heart and brain). This leads to ketoacidosis in the setting of hyperglycemia.

2. Diabetic ketoacidosis develops in 2–10% of all pregnancies complicated by pregestational diabetes. It is extremely rare in gestational diabetes (<<1%), and effectively absent in nondiabetic women. Risk factors for the development of DKA include undiagnosed pregestational diabetes, pregnancy, emesis, noncompliance, infection, β-agonist therapy, and (perhaps) antepartum corticosteroid therapy.

3. Diabetic ketoacidosis can be effectively prevented by intensive diabetic education, rigorous glycemic control, and early identification and treatment of infection.

4. A high clinical index of suspicion is necessary to make the diagnosis of DKA. Any pregnant woman with pregestational diabetes who complains of nausea, vomiting, polydipsia, polyuria, abdominal pain, and/or decreased caloric intake should be evaluated to exclude ketosis. Physical examination may demonstrate dehydration, poor tissue turgor, tachycardia, hypotension, a fruity smell (acetone) on breath, and clinical evidence of acidosis (fatigue, hyperventilation, and Kussmaul breathing or coma).

5. The following five criteria are typically used for the diagnosis of DKA:
- Plasma glucose >250 mg/dL (although normal or near-normal plasma glucose levels are not sufficient to preclude DKA; indeed, up to 40% of pregnant diabetic women with DKA have plasma glucose levels on presentation of <200 mg/dL)
- pH ≤7.30
- Plasma bicarbonate ≤15 mEq/L
- Anion gap (calculated as $Na^+ - [Cl- + HCO_3-]$) >12 mEq/L

- Osmolality (calculated as 2 x $[Na^+ + K^+]$ + [glucose/18]) >280 mOsm/kg

6. The differential diagnosis of altered mental status in the setting of DKA includes hyperglycemic coma in women with pregestational diabetes, preeclampsia/eclampsia, seizure, drug overdose (especially alcohol), encephalopathy, uremia, infection, and psychosis.

7. Diabetic ketoacidosis is associated with a high maternal (5%) and perinatal mortality (35–50%). Other perinatal complications include preterm birth and newborn encephalopathy. Prognosis depends in large part on early diagnosis and rapid and effective inpatient treatment. The primary objectives of therapy include correction of volume deficit, hyperglycemia, electrolyte imbalance, acidosis, and treatment of the precipitating cause (such as infection). Fetuses die of acidosis and not high glucose levels. As such, the immediate goal of treatment is reversal of ketoacidosis, not euglycemia.

8. The half-life of IV insulin is 2–4 min. DKA can recur in the absence of exogenous insulin. Subcutaneous insulin should therefore be restarted once the patient is eating.

9. If the acidosis persists despite initial treatment, consider inadequate insulin administration, sepsis, or hypophosphatemia.

10. Once stable, it is important to: (i) follow fingerstick blood glucose hourly; (ii) check serum electrolytes and arterial blood gas (ABG) q 2–4 hourly, as indicated; (iii) check BUN/creatinine and urinary ketones q 4 hourly; (iv) catheterize patient if unconscious or not passing urine; (v) decompress stomach if unconscious; and (vi) undertake continuous fetal surveillance and delivery, if indicated.

80 Eclampsia

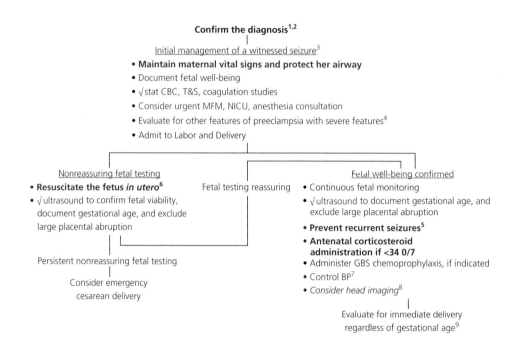

Confirm the diagnosis[1,2]
|
Initial management of a witnessed seizure[3]
- **Maintain maternal vital signs and protect her airway**
- Document fetal well-being
- √stat CBC, T&S, coagulation studies
- Consider urgent MFM, NICU, anesthesia consultation
- Evaluate for other features of preeclampsia with severe features[4]
- Admit to Labor and Delivery

Nonreassuring fetal testing
- **Resuscitate the fetus *in utero*[6]**
- √ultrasound to confirm fetal viability, document gestational age, and exclude large placental abruption

Fetal testing reassuring

Fetal well-being confirmed
- Continuous fetal monitoring
- √ultrasound to document gestational age, and exclude large placental abruption
- **Prevent recurrent seizures[5]**
- **Antenatal corticosteroid administration if <34 0/7**
- Administer GBS chemoprophylaxis, if indicated
- Control BP[7]
- *Consider head imaging[8]*

Persistent nonreassuring fetal testing
|
Consider emergency cesarean delivery

Evaluate for immediate delivery regardless of gestational age[9]

1. Eclampsia is defined as the presence of new-onset grand mal seizures in a woman with preeclampsia in the absence of other neurologic explanations. It is one manifestation of preeclampsia with severe features (see Chapter 12, Preeclampsia). Symptoms that may predict impending eclampsia include persistent occipital or frontal headaches, blurred vision, photophobia, epigastric or right upper quadrant pain, and altered mental status. Eclampsia is an obstetric emergency. Both the fetus and the mother are at immediate risk of death or lifelong neurologic disability. Major maternal complications include placental abruption (10%), HELLP syndrome (10%), DIC (5%), neurological deficits and aspiration pneumonia (5-10%), pulmonary edema (5%), cardiopulmonary arrest (1–5%), acute renal failure (1–5%), and maternal death (1%). In developed countries, the reported incidence of eclampsia ranges from 1 in 2000 to 1 in 3500 pregnancies.

2. Eclampsia can occur antepartum, intrapartum, or postpartum. The majority of cases (>90%) develop at 28 weeks of gestation or greater. Most cases of postpartum eclampsia occur within the first 48 hours of delivery; however, late postpartum eclampsia can occur up to 4 weeks after delivery.

3. The immediate management of an eclamptic seizure should include maintaining maternal

Obstetric Clinical Algorithms, Second Edition. Errol R. Norwitz, George R. Saade, Hugh Miller and Christina M. Davidson.
© 2017 John Wiley & Sons, Ltd. Published 2017 by John Wiley & Sons, Ltd.

vital functions, controlling convulsions and blood pressure, prevention of subsequent seizures, and evaluation for delivery. If witnessed, the parturient should be rolled onto her left side and a padded tongue blade placed in her mouth to maintain airway patency and prevention of aspiration, which are the first responsibilities of management. The bedside rails should be elevated and physical restraints may be needed. During the convulsive episode, hypoventilation and respiratory acidosis often occur and so it is important to administer supplemental oxygen via a face mask at 8–10 L/min.

4. Other manifestations of preeclampsia with severe features may co-exist with eclampsia, including HELLP syndrome (**H**emolysis, **E**levated **L**iver enzymes and **L**ow **P**latelets), disseminated intravascular coagulopathy (DIC), renal failure, hepatocellular injury, liver rupture, congestive cardiac failure, and pulmonary edema.

5. After maternal stabilization, the next step in the management of eclampsia is to prevent recurrent convulsions. Approximately 10% of eclamptic women will have a second convulsion in the absence of seizure prophylaxis. Magnesium sulfate is the drug of choice to prevent subsequent convulsions in women with eclampsia. It is administered as a continuous IV infusion: 4–6 g IV over 15–20 min followed by an infusion of 2 g/h. The infusion should only be given if patellar reflexes are present, respirations are >12 per min, and urine output is >100 mL in 4 hours. Serum magnesium levels only require monitoring in the presence of renal dysfunction and/or when there are absent reflexes. They can be followed every 6 hours with levels maintained at 4.8–8.4 mg/dL. Seizure prophylaxis should be continued during labor and delivery and for 24–48 hours postpartum (or 24 hours after the last convulsion). Women who do have a seizure on magnesium should be given another bolus of 2 g of magnesium sulfate IV over 3–5 min. In a woman with no IV access, magnesium sulfate can be administered intramuscularly: 10 g of

50% solution IM (5 g into each buttock). If seizures persist despite additional boluses of magnesium sulfate, another anticonvulsant agent may be given as a single dose: (i) Midazolam (Versed) 1–2 mg IV; (ii) Diazepam (Valium) 1–10 mg IV; (iii) Lorazepam (Ativan) 2–4 mg IV; or (iv) Sodium amobarbital. If these measures fail, general anesthesia may be necessary to terminate the seizure activity.

6. Transient fetal bradycardia lasting 3–5 min is a common finding after a seizure and does not necessitate immediate delivery. Resolution of maternal seizure activity is often associated with compensatory fetal tachycardia and even with transient fetal heart rate decelerations. These changes usually resolve spontaneously within 3–10 min after the termination of convulsions and the correction of maternal hypoxemia. Every attempt should be made to stabilize the mother and resuscitate the fetus *in utero* before making a decision about delivery. However, if the bradycardia or recurrent late decelerations persist beyond 10–15 min despite all resuscitative efforts, then a diagnosis of abruptio placentae should be considered.

7. The magnitude of BP elevation is predictive of cerebrovascular accident (stroke), but not eclampsia (seizures). The degree of systolic hypertension (as opposed to the level of diastolic hypertension or relative increase or rate of increase of mean arterial pressure from baseline) may be the most important predictor of cerebral injury and hemorrhagic infarction. Acute-onset severe systolic hypertension (>160 mmHg) and/or severe diastolic hypertension (>110 mmHg) should be treated with antihypertensive therapy with the aim of achieving BP of 140–150/90–100 mmHg. First line treatment for the management of acute severe hypertension includes IV labetalol, IV hydralazine, or oral nifedipine. Hydralazine is administered as 5 mg IV push followed by 5–10 mg boluses as needed every 20 min. The initial dose of labetalol is 10–20 mg IV push followed by repeated doses every

10–20 min with doubling doses not to exceed 80 mg in any single dose for a maximum total cumulative dose of 300 mg. The initial dose of nifedipine is 10 mg orally followed by 20 mg orally every 20 min, not to exceed a cumulative dose of 50 mg in one hour.

8. Eclampsia is indistinguishable clinically or by EEG from other causes of generalized tonic-clonic seizures. Not all women with eclampsia require head imaging. However, if the seizure lasts >10 min, is recurrent, occurs postpartum or on seizure prophylaxis, or if there is evidence of localizing neurologic signs, head imaging is indicated. The differential diagnosis includes cerebrovascular accident (intracerebral hemorrhage, cerebral venous thrombosis), hypertensive encephalopathy, space-occupying lesions (brain tumor, abscess), metabolic disorders (hypoglycemia, uremia, inappropriate antidiuretic hormone secretion resulting in water intoxication), infectious etiology (meningitis, encephalitis), thrombotic thrombocytopenic purpura (TTP), and idiopathic epilepsy.

9. Eclampsia is an absolute contraindication to continued expectant management of preeclampsia with severe features. Immediate delivery is indicated regardless of gestational age. However, immediate delivery does not mean cesarean. Induction of labor and attempted vaginal delivery are a reasonable option, but prolonged induction of labor should be avoided. The decision about route of delivery should be individualized based on such factors as parity, gestational age, cervical examination (Bishop score), and fetal status and presentation. Regional anesthesia is preferred for women with eclampsia so long as close attention is paid to volume expansion and anesthetic technique, and there is no thrombocytopenia. Eclampsia always resolves following delivery although this may take a few days to weeks. Diuresis (>4 L/day) is the most accurate clinical indicator of resolving preeclampsia.

81 Shoulder Dystocia[1]

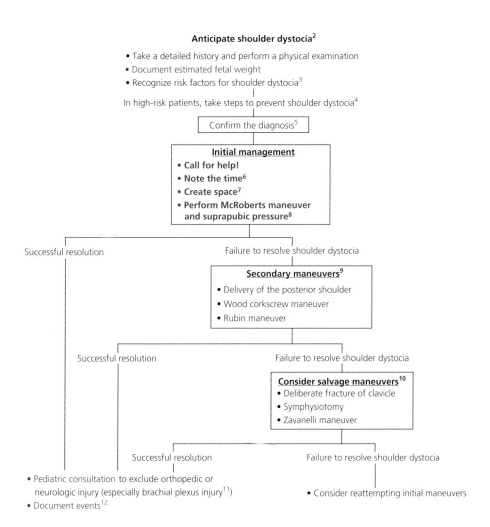

Anticipate shoulder dystocia[2]
- Take a detailed history and perform a physical examination
- Document estimated fetal weight
- Recognize risk factors for shoulder dystocia[3]

In high-risk patients, take steps to prevent shoulder dystocia[4]

Confirm the diagnosis[5]

Initial management
- **Call for help!**
- **Note the time[6]**
- **Create space[7]**
- **Perform McRoberts maneuver and suprapubic pressure[8]**

Successful resolution

Failure to resolve shoulder dystocia

Secondary maneuvers[9]
- Delivery of the posterior shoulder
- Wood corkscrew maneuver
- Rubin maneuver

Successful resolution

Failure to resolve shoulder dystocia

Consider salvage maneuvers[10]
- Deliberate fracture of clavicle
- Symphysiotomy
- Zavanelli maneuver

Successful resolution

Failure to resolve shoulder dystocia

- Pediatric consultation to exclude orthopedic or neurologic injury (especially brachial plexus injury[11])
- Document events[12]

- Consider reattempting initial maneuvers

1. Shoulder dystocia refers to impaction of the anterior shoulder of the fetus behind the pubic symphysis following delivery of the head. It is most often defined as a delivery that requires additional obstetric maneuvers following failure of gentle downward traction on the fetal head to effect delivery of the shoulders. It can also occur from impaction of the posterior fetal shoulder on the sacral promontory. It is an obstetric emergency associated with neonatal birth trauma (neurologic injuries; fractures of the humerus, skull, clavicle) in up to 40% of

Obstetric Clinical Algorithms, Second Edition. Errol R. Norwitz, George R. Saade, Hugh Miller and Christina M.Davidson.
© 2017 John Wiley & Sons, Ltd. Published 2017 by John Wiley & Sons, Ltd.

cases. Shoulder dystocia complicates 0.6–1.4% of all vaginal deliveries. Immediate identification and prompt intervention may prevent neonatal birth trauma and hypoxic ischemic encephalopathy in some cases.

2. Although several risk factors for shoulder dystocia have been identified (see below), most cases occur in women with no risk factors. As such, it is not possible to accurately predict all cases of shoulder dystocia. Obstetric care providers should be prepared to deal with shoulder dystocia at every vaginal delivery.

3. Risk factors for shoulder dystocia include a previous shoulder dystocia, fetal macrosomia, previous history of a macrosomic birth, diabetes mellitus (including gestational diabetes), obesity, multiparity, post-term pregnancy, labor induction, epidural anesthesia, and operative vaginal delivery. While risk factors for shoulder dystocia may be identified, their predictive value is not high enough to be clinically useful. The labor curve has not been found to be a useful predictor of shoulder dystocia.

4. Although the diagnosis of fetal macrosomia (estimated fetal weight >4500 gm) is imprecise, prophylactic cesarean delivery to reduce the risk of permanent brachial plexus injury may be considered for suspected fetal macrosomia with estimated fetal weights >5000 gm in non-diabetic women and >4500 gm in diabetic women. Labor induction for the sole indication of suspected macrosomia is not appropriate since it has not been shown to decrease the occurrence of shoulder dystocia or the rate of cesarean delivery. Delivery management of women at risk of shoulder dystocia should be individualized. It may be prudent to have one or more experienced clinicians on hand. Forceps delivery should be avoided for midpelvic arrest of the fetus with suspected macrosomia.

5. Failure of the shoulders to deliver after delivery of the head should be noted immediately, especially if the head retracts into the birth canal ("turtle sign").

6. Delivery of the fetus within approximately 10 min minimizes the risk of hypoxic ischemic injury. Following delivery of the fetal head, compression of the umbilical cord in the birth canal occurs with concomitant inability of the fetus to spontaneously breathe, with a resultant drop in pH of 0.04 units per minute following delivery of the head.

7. If not already done, remove the bottom of the bed, empty the patient's bladder, and consider performing a generous episiotomy (to provide more room for posterior manipulation).

8. The *McRoberts maneuver* refers to hyperflexion of the patient's thighs onto her abdomen. This maneuver does not increase the dimensions of the pelvis, but the cephalad rotation of the symphysis pubis leads to a decrease in the angle of pelvic inclination, which frees the impacted anterior shoulder. Simultaneous oblique suprapubic (not fundal) pressure may be applied at a 45 degree angle to assist in dislodging the impacted shoulder. These are the primary maneuvers recommended when shoulder dystocia is recognized. Together, they are successful in 24–62% of cases.

9. If the combination of the McRoberts maneuver and suprapubic pressure is unsuccessful, a number of other maneuvers have been described. These maneuvers include: (i) the *Wood corkscrew maneuver* which is aimed at progressively rotating the posterior shoulder 180° in a corkscrew fashion to dislodge the anterior shoulder; (ii) the *Rubin maneuver* in which pressure is applied laterally to the most accessible shoulder towards the anterior chest of the fetus with a view to decreasing the bisacromial (shoulder-to-shoulder) diameter and freeing the impacted shoulder; and (iii) *delivery of the posterior shoulder* which consists of sweeping the posterior arm of the fetus across the chest, flexing

the elbow manually, and delivering the posterior arm by traction on the wrist. This maneuver can result in fracture of the humerus, although humeral fractures usually heal without complication. When the posterior arm cannot be reached (for example, if the arm is fully extended or if the fetus is lying on its posterior arm), a modified technique has been reported. It involves delivering the posterior shoulder before delivering the posterior arm by placing the two middle fingers into the posterior axilla and applying traction outward and downward on the posterior shoulder following the curve of the sacrum. Once the shoulder has emerged from the pelvis, the posterior arm is delivered. At other times, the shoulder may not actually be delivered first but instead is brought down low enough in the pelvis that the posterior arm can be grasped and brought out. Recent evidence suggests that delivery of the posterior shoulder has the highest overall rate of success (84%) when compared with all other maneuvers, and thus should be the first maneuver considered when McRoberts and suprapubic pressure fail to deliver the anterior shoulder. None of the maneuvers demonstrated a loss of efficacy and both McRoberts and suprapubic pressure became more effective the later they were used. Thus, at no point in the acute management of shoulder dystocia should any maneuver be completely abandoned.

10. If secondary maneuvers are unsuccessful, "salvage" maneuvers can be attempted. These include: (i) *deliberate fracture of the anterior clavicle* which is performed manually by pushing the clavicle outwards against the ramus of the maternal pubis. The clavicle should not be fractured by pushing inwards towards the fetal chest since this can result in fetal pneumothorax, subclavian vascular injury or brachial plexus injury. In the absence of neurologic injury, the fracture will heal rapidly without incident; (ii) *symphysiotomy* consisting of surgical separation of the maternal pubic rami by transecting the cartilaginous symphysis pubis. It is very effective in expediting delivery, but is technically challenging and should not be attempted by inexperienced practitioners. It is associated with long-term nonunion and chronic severe pain to the mother. As such, it is rarely performed; (iii) the *Zavanelli maneuver*, which involves manual flexion and replacement of the fetal head back into the uterus followed by cesarean delivery. Reported success rates vary considerably; (iv) *abdominal rescue* may be considered if the Zavanelli maneuver is unsuccessful. A low transverse hysterotomy is performed to assist the fetal shoulder below the symphysis pubis, followed by vaginal delivery of the infant.

11. Brachial plexus injury complicates 11.8–16.8% of shoulder dystocia cases. It reportedly results from "excessive" lateral traction on the head and neck at delivery with resultant injury to the brachial plexus, usually to cervical nerve roots C5/C6 (Erb/Duchenne palsy). On examination, the arm hangs limply at the side of the body with the forearm extended and internally rotated, the classic "waiter's tip" deformity. The function of the fingers is usually retained. The lower brachial plexus (C8/T1) may also be involved, resulting in paralysis of the hand, but isolated lower plexus injuries (Klumpke palsy) are rare. Fewer than 10% of all cases of shoulder dystocia result in persistent brachial plexus injury. Most cases recover within the first 6 months and most of those that will resolve do so by 18 months. Elective cesarean delivery will prevent most (but not all) brachial plexus injuries. However, given the difficulty of predicting and preventing shoulder dystocia, cesarean delivery cannot be recommended for all women with identifiable risk factors.

12. The American College of Obstetricians and Gynecologists Patient Safety Checklist on Documenting Shoulder Dystocia can be used to guide the documentation of the delivery.

82 Thyroid Storm

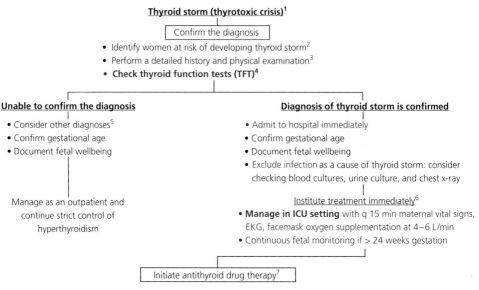

Thyroid storm (thyrotoxic crisis)[1]

Confirm the diagnosis

- Identify women at risk of developing thyroid storm[2]
- Perform a detailed history and physical examination[3]
- **Check thyroid function tests (TFT)[4]**

Unable to confirm the diagnosis

- Consider other diagnoses[5]
- Confirm gestational age
- Document fetal wellbeing

Manage as an outpatient and continue strict control of hyperthyroidism

Diagnosis of thyroid storm is confirmed

- Admit to hospital immediately
- Confirm gestational age
- Document fetal wellbeing
- Exclude infection as a cause of thyroid storm: consider checking blood cultures, urine culture, and chest x-ray

Institute treatment immediately[6]

- **Manage in ICU setting** with q 15 min maternal vital signs, EKG, facemask oxygen supplementation at 4–6 L/min
- Continuous fetal monitoring if > 24 weeks gestation

Initiate antithyroid drug therapy[7]

- **Propylthiouracil (PTU)** 600–800 mg orally stat, then 150–200 mg orally every 4–6 hours. If oral administration is not possible, use methimazole rectal suppositories
- Starting 1–2 hours after PTU, administer **saturated solution of potassium iodide (SSKI)** 2–5 drops orally every 8 hours. Alternative sources of iodine may include sodium iodide (0.5–1.0 g iv every 8 hours) or Lugol solution (8 drops every 6 hours) or lithium carbonate (300 mg orally every 6 hours)
- **Dexamethasone** 2 mg iv or im every 6 hours for four doses
- **Propranolol** 20–80 mg orally every 4–6 hours or 1–2 mg iv every 5 minutes for a total of 6 mg, then 1–10 mg iv every 4 hours. If the patient has a history of severe bronchospasm, consider reserpine (1–5 mg im every 4–6 hours) or guanethidine (1 mg/kg orally every 12 hours) or diltiazem (60 mg orally every 6–8 hours)
- Phenobarbital 30–60 mg orally every 6–8 hours as needed for extreme restlessness

Once the patient is stable, continue close observation[8]

1. Thyroid storm (thyrotoxic crisis) is a medical emergency characterized by a severe acute exacerbation of the signs and symptoms of hyperthyroidism. It is a rare complication, occurring in approximately 1% of pregnant patients with hyperthyroidism, but is associated with significant maternal and perinatal mortality and morbidity.

Obstetric Clinical Algorithms, Second Edition. Errol R. Norwitz, George R. Saade, Hugh Miller and Christina M. Davidson. © 2017 John Wiley & Sons, Ltd. Published 2017 by John Wiley & Sons, Ltd.

2. The vast majority of women presenting with thyroid storm have a history of hyperthyroidism. Hyperthyroidism refers to the clinical state resulting from an excess production of and exposure to thyroid hormone. The most common cause is Graves' disease, which accounts for 95% of all cases of hyperthyroidism in pregnancy and is caused by circulating thyroid-stimulating autoantibodies. Ophthalmopathy (exophthalmos, lid lag, lid retraction) and dermopathy (pretibial edema) are clinical signs that are specific to Graves' disease. Other causes of hyperthyroidism in pregnancy include inflammation (thyroiditis), toxic multinodular goiter, solitary toxic thyroid nodule, hyperemesis gravidarum/gestational trophoblastic neoplasia, ingestion of exogenous thyroid hormone, and a TSH-secreting pituitary adenoma. In order to minimize complications (including thyroid storm), hyperthyroidism is best diagnosed and treated prior to pregnancy. An inciting event (such as infection, hypoglycemia, diabetic ketoacidosis, venous thromboembolism, surgery, and/or labor and delivery) can be identified in many instances of thyroid storm.

3. Thyroid storm is diagnosed by a combination of symptoms and signs in patients with thyrotoxicosis, including fever, tachycardia out of proportion to the fever >140–160 bpm, altered mental status (such as restlessness, nervousness, confusion or seizures), diarrhea, vomiting, and cardiac arrhythmia. However, the diagnosis can be difficult to make clinically.

4. If thyroid storm is suspected, serum thyroid function tests (TFTs) should be sent immediately. Biochemical findings supportive of the diagnosis include suppressed levels of thyroid-binding globulin (<0.05 mU/mL) and increased free levothyroxine (T_4) and L-triiodithyronine (T_3) in the maternal circulation. Although most women with Graves' disease will have circulating anti-TSH receptor, antimicrosomal, and/or antithyroid peroxidase autoantibodies, measurement of such antibodies is neither required nor recommended to establish the diagnosis. Moreover, antibody levels do not correlate well with either maternal or perinatal outcome.

5. The differential diagnosis of thyroid storm includes anxiety disorders, drug intoxication and/or withdrawal, and pheochromocytoma.

6. Thyroid storm is associated with significant maternal and perinatal mortality and morbidity, including shock, stupor, coma, and death. If the clinical index of suspicion for thyroid storm is high, treatment should be initiated immediately and should not be withheld pending the results of the biochemical tests.

7. The goals of treatment of thyroid storm are: (i) to reduce the synthesis and release of hormone from the thyroid gland using thioamides (such as propylthiouracil (PTU) or methimazole), supplemental iodide, and/or glucocorticoids; (ii) to block the peripheral actions of thyroid hormones using glucocorticoids, PTU, and/or β-blockers; (iii) to treat complications and support physiologic functions (manage in an ICU setting, acetaminophen, cooling blankets, supplemental oxygen, fluid and caloric replacement); and (iv) to identify and treat precipitating events (such as hypoglycemia, thromboembolic events, and diabetic ketoacidosis). As with other acute maternal illnesses, fetal well-being should be appropriately evaluated and consideration given to delivery, if appropriate. Fetal tachycardia (>160 bpm) is a sensitive index of fetal hyperthyroidism. Only 1–5% of neonates born to women with poorly controlled thyrotoxicosis will develop transient hyperthyroidism or neonatal Graves' disease caused by the transplacental passage of maternal antithyroid antibodies.

8. Once stable, it is important: (i) to follow serum electrolytes (especially potassium) and arterial blood gas q 2–4 hourly, as indicated;

(ii) to catheterize the patient if unconscious or not passing urine; (iii) to decompress the stomach if unconscious; and (iv) to continue fetal surveillance. For women who fail to respond to initial medical therapy, options are limited.

Radioactive iodine (^{131}I) administration to ablate the thyroid gland is absolutely contraindicated in pregnancy, because it will permanently damage the fetal thyroid. Surgery is best avoided, but may be required.

Recommended Reading

1 Abnormal Pap Smear in Pregnancy

American College of Obstetricians and Gynecologists. ACOG Practice Bulletin No. 131: Screening for cervical cancer. *Obstetrics & Gynecology* 2012;**120** (5):1222–1238.

American College of Obstetricians and Gynecologists. ACOG Practice Bulletin No. 140: Management of abnormal cervical cancer screening test results and cervical cancer precursors. *Obstetrics & Gynecology* 2013;**122**(5):1338–1367.

Massad, L. Stewart,; Einstein, Mark H., Huh, Warnerer K, *et al*. 2012 Updated consensus guidelines for the management of abnormal cervical cancer screening tests and cancer precursors. *Obstetrics & Gynecology* 2012;**121**(4):829–846.

Moyer VA. Screening for cervical cancer: U.S. Preventive Services Task Force recommendation statement. U.S. Preventive Services Task Force. *Annals of International Medicine* 2012;**156**:880–891.

Saslow D, Solomon D, Lawson HW, Killackey M, Kulasingam SL, Cain J, *et al*. American Cancer Society, American Society for Colposcopy and Cervical Pathology, and American Society for Clinical Pathology screening guidelines for the prevention and early detection of cervical cancer. *CA: A Cancer Journal for Clinicians* 2012;**62**:147–172.

2 Immunization

American College of Obstetricians and Gynecologists. ACOG Committee Opinion #608, Influenza vaccination during pregnancy. September 2014 Prevention and control of seasonal influenza with vaccines. Recommendations of the Advisory Committee on Immunization Practices—United States, 2013–2014. Centers for Disease Control and Prevention (CDC) [published erratum appears in MMWR, Morbidity and Mortality Weekly Report 2013;62:906]. MMWR Recommendation Report 2013;**62**(RR-7):1–43.

American College of Obstetricians and Gynecologists. ACOG Committee Opinion No. 566, Update on immunization and pregnancy: tetanus, diphtheria, and pertussis vaccination. June 2013.

3 Preconception Care

American Academy of Pediatrics and American College of Obstetricians and Gynecologists. *Obstetrics & Gynecology*. 6th edition, Washington, DC; American Academy of Pediatrics and American College of Obstetricians and Gynecologists, 2007.

American College of Obstetricians and Gynecologists. ACOG Committee Opinion No. 313. The importance of preconception care in the continuum of women's health care. *Obstetrics & Gynecology* 2005;**106**:665–666.

Coonrod DV, Jack BW, Boggess KA, *et al*. The clinical content of preconception care: immunizations as part of preconception care. *Obstetrics & Gynecology* 2008;**199**:S290–295.

Coonrod DV, Jack BW, Stubblefield PG, *et al*. The clinical content of preconception care: infectious diseases in preconception care. *Obstetrics & Gynecology* 2008;**199**:S296–309.

4 Prenatal Care

American Academy of Pediatrics and American College of Obstetricians and Gynecologists. *Guidelines for Perinatal Care*, 6th edition. American Academy of Pediatrics and American College of Obstetricians and Gynecologists, Washington, DC, 2007.

American Academy of Pediatrics and the American College of Obstetricians and Gynecologists. *Guidelines for Perinatal Care*, 7th edition. Elk Grove Village, Illinois: AAP; Washington, DC: ACOG, 2012.

American College of Obstetricians and Gynecologists. ACOG Committee Opinion No. 511. Health care for pregnant and postpartum incarcerated women and adolescent females. *Obstetrics & Gynecology* 2011; **118**(5):1198–1202.

De-Regil LM, Fernández-Gaxiola AC, Dowswell T, Peña-Rosas JP. Effects and safety of periconceptional folate supplementation for preventing birth defects. *Obstetrics & Gynecology* 2010;(**10**):CD007950.

Visintin C, Mugglestone MA, James D, Kilby MD; *Guideline Development Group. Antenatal care for twin and triplet pregnancies: summary of NICE guidance.* *Obstetrics & Gynecology* 2011;**343**:d5714.

Obstetric Clinical Algorithms, Second Edition. Errol R. Norwitz, George R. Saade, Hugh Miller and Christina M. Davidson.
© 2017 John Wiley & Sons, Ltd. Published 2017 by John Wiley & Sons, Ltd.

5 Antiphospholipid Antibody Syndrome

American College of Obstetricians and Gynecologists. ACOG Practice Bulletin No. 118. Antiphospholipid syndrome. *Obstetrics & Gynecology* 2011;**117**(1):192–199.

Erkan D, Aguiar CL, Andrade D, *et al*. 14th International Congress on Antiphospholipid Antibodies Task Force Report on antiphospholipid syndrome treatment trends. *Obstetrics & Gynecology* 2014;**13**(6):685–696.

Lim W, Crowther MA, Eikelboom JW. Management of antiphospholipid antibody syndrome: a systematic review. *Obstetrics & Gynecology* 2006;**295**(9):1050–1057.

Lockshin MD. Anticoagulation in management of antiphospholipid antibody syndrome in pregnancy. *Obstetrics & Gynecology* 2013;**33**(2):367–376.

7 Cholestasis of Pregnancy

Chappell LC, Gurung V, Seed PT, *et al*. Ursodeoxycholic acid versus placebo, and early term delivery versus expectant management, in women with intrahepatic cholestasis of pregnancy: semifactorial randomised clinical trial. *Obstetrics & Gynecology* 2012;**344**:e3799.

Williamson C, Geenes G. Clinical expert series: intrahepatic cholestasis of pregnancy. *Obstetrics & Gynecology* 2014;**124**:120–133.

8 Chronic Hypertension

American College of Obstetricians and Gynecologists. Task Force on Hypertension in Pregnancy. hyper-tension in pregnancy. American College of Obstetricians and Gynecologists Washington, DC, 2013.

American College of Obstetricians and Gynecologists. ACOG Committee Opinion, No. 560. Medically indicated late-preterm and early-term deliveries. ACOG, Washington, DC. 2013.

American College of Obstetricians and Gynecologists Committee Opinion No. 623. Emergent therapy for acute-onset, severe hypertension during pregnancy and the postpartum period. *Obstetrics & Gynecology* 2015;**125**(2):521–525.

9 Deep Vein Thrombosis

American College of Chest Physicians Evidence-Based Clinical Practice Guidelines. *Obstetrics & Gynecology* 2012;**141**(2 Suppl):e691S-736S. DOI: 10.1378/chest.11-2300.

American College of Obstetricians and Gynecologists. Practice Bulletin No. 123. Thromboembolism in pregnancy. *Obstetrics & Gynecology* 2011;**118**(3):718–729.

Bates SM, Greer IA, Middeldorp S, *et al*. *VTE, Thrombophilia, Antithrombotic Therapy, and Pregnancy: Antithrombotic Therapy and Prevention of Thrombosis*, 9th edition. American College of Chest Physicians, Washington, DC.

Duhl AJ, Paidas MJ, Ural SH, *et al*.; Pregnancy and Thrombosis Working Group. Antithrombotic therapy and pregnancy: consensus report and recommendations for prevention and treatment of venous thromboembolism and adverse pregnancy outcomes. *Obstetrics & Gynecology*. 2007;**197**(5):457.e1–21.

Horlocker TT, Wedel DJ, Rowlingson JC, Enneking FK. American Society of Regional Anesthesia and Pain Medicine Evidence-Based Guideline. Executive summary: regional anesthesia in the patient receiving antithrombotic or thrombolytic therapy: 3rd edition. *Obstetrics & Gynecology* 2010;**35**:102–105.

Marik PE, Plante LA. Venous thromboembolic disease and pregnancy. *Obstetrics & Gynecology*. 2008;**359**(19):2025–2033.

11 Gestational Hypertension

American College of Obstetricians and Gynecologists. Task Force on Hypertension in Pregnancy. *Obstetrics & Gynecology*. American College of Obstetricians and Gynecologists, Washington, DC, 2013.

Barton JR, O'Brien JM, Bergauer RN, Jacques DL, Sibai BM. *Mild gestational hypertension remote from term: progression and outcome Obstetrics & Gynecology* 2001;**184**:979–983.

Buchbinder A, Sibai BM, Caritis S, *et al*. Adverse perinatal outcomes are significantly higher in severe gestational hypertension than in mild preeclampsia. National Institute of Child Health and Human Development Network of Maternal-Fetal Medicine Units. *Obstetrics & Gynecology* 2002;**186**:66–71.

Sibai B. Diagnosis, prevention, and management of eclampsia. *Obstetrics & Gynecology* 2005;**105**:402–410.

Sibai BM, Stella CL. Diagnosis and management of atypical preeclampsia-eclampsia. *Obstetrics & Gynecology* 2009;**200**:481.e1-481.e7.

12 Preeclampsia

American College of Obstetricians and Gynecologists. Committee Opinion No. 623: Emergent therapy for acute-onset, severe hypertension during pregnancy and the postpartum period. *Obstetrics & Gynecology* 2015;**125**(2):521–525.

American College of Obstetricians and Gynecologists. Task Force on Hypertension in Pregnancy. *Hypertension in Pregnancy*. Task Force on Hypertension in Pregnancy, editor. American College of Obstetricians and Gynecologists, Washington, DC, 2013.

Martin JN Jr, Thigpen BD, Moore RC, Rose CH, Cushman J, May W. Stroke and severe preeclampsia and eclampsia: a paradigm shift focusing on systolic blood pressure. *Obstetrics & Gynecology* 2005;**105**:246–254.

14 Pulmonary Edema

American College of Obstetricians and Gynecologists. ACOG Practice Bulletin No. 100. Critical care in pregnancy. *Obstetrics & Gynecology* 2009;**113**(2): 443–450.

American College of Obstetricians and Gynecologists, Task Force on Hypertension in Pregnancy. Hypertension in pregnancy. Report of the American College of Obstetricians and Gynecologists' Task Force on Hypertension in Pregnancy. *Obstetrics & Gynecology* 2013;**122**:1122.

Mighty HE. Acute respiratory failure in pregnancy. *Obstetrics & Gynecology* 2010;**53**:360.

Pollock W, Rose L, Dennis CL. Pregnant and postpartum admissions to the intensive care unit: a systematic review. *Obstetrics & Gynecology* 2010;**36**:1465.

Thornton CE, von Dadelszen P, Makris A, *et al*. Acute pulmonary oedema as a complication of hypertension during pregnancy. *Obstetrics & Gynecology* 2011;**30**:169.

15 Pulmonary Embolism

American College of Obstetricians and Gynecologists. Practice Bulletin No. 123. Thromboembolism in pregnancy. *Obstetrics & Gynecology* 2011;**118**(3): 718–729.

Bates SM, Greer IA, Middeldorp S, *et al*. American College of Chest Physicians. *VTE, Thrombophilia, Antithrombotic Therapy, and Pregnancy: Antithrombotic Therapy and Prevention of Thrombosis*, 9th edition. American College of Chest Physicians Evidence-Based Clinical Practice Guidelines. Chest. 2012 Feb;**141**(2 Suppl):e691S–736S. doi: 10.1378/chest.11-2300.

Cahill AG, Stout MJ, Macones GA, *et al*. Diagnosing pulmonary embolism in pregnancy using computed-tomographic angiography or ventilation–perfusion. *Obstetrics & Gynecology* 2009;**114**:124–129.

Duhl AJ, Paidas MJ, Ural SH, *et al*. Pregnancy and Thrombosis Working Group. Antithrombotic therapy and pregnancy: consensus report and recommendations for prevention and treatment of venous thromboembolism and adverse pregnancy outcomes. *Obstetrics & Gynecology* 2007;**197**(5): 457.e1-21.

Horlocker TT, Wedel DJ, Rowlingson JC, Enneking FK. Executive summary: regional anesthesia in the patient receiving antithrombotic or thrombolytic therapy: American Society of Regional Anesthesia and Pain Medicine Evidence-Based Guideline. 3rd ed. *Regional Anesthesia and Pain Medicine* 2010;**35**:102–105.

Leung AN, Bull TM, Jaeschke R, *et al*; ATS/STR Committee on Pulmonary Embolism in Pregnancy. American Thoracic Society documents: an official American Thoracic Society/Society of Thoracic Radiology Clinical Practice Guideline. Evaluation of suspected pulmonary embolism in pregnancy. *Radiology* 2012;**262**(2):635–646.

Marik PE, Plante LA. Venous thromboembolic disease and pregnancy. *New England Journal of Medicine* 2008;6;**359**(19):2025–2033.

16 Renal Disease

Lindheimer MD, Kanter D. *Clinical expert series. interpreting abnormal proteinuria in pregnancy: the need for a more pathophysiological approach. Obstetrics & Gynecology* 2010;**115**:365–375.

Morris RK, Riley RD, Doug M, *et al*. Diagnostic accuracy of spot urinary protein and albumin to creatinine ratios for detection of significant proteinuria or adverse pregnancy outcome in patients with suspected pre-eclampsia: systematic review and meta-analysis. *Obstetrics & Gynecology* 2012; **345**:e4342.

Nevis IF, Reitsma A, Dominic A, *et al*. Pregnancy outcomes in women with chronic kidney disease: a systematic review. *Obstetrics & Gynecology* 2011;**6**:2587.

17 Seizure Disorder

Borthen I, Eide MG, Daltveit AK, Gilhus NE. Obstetric outcome in women with epilepsy: a hospital-based, retrospective study. *Obstetrics & Gynecology* 2011;**118**:956.

Bromley R, Weston J, Adab N, *et al*. Treatment for epilepsy in pregnancy: neurodevelopmental outcomes in the child. *Cochrane Database of Systematic Reviews* 2014 Oct **30**;10.

Harden CL, Hopp J, Ting TY, *et al*. Practice parameter update: management issues for women with epilepsy: focus on pregnancy (an evidence-based review): obstetrical complications and change in seizure frequency: report of the Quality Standards Subcommittee and Therapeutics and Technology Assessment Subcommittee of the American Academy of Neurology and American Epilepsy Society. *Obstetrics & Gynecology* 2009;**73**:126.

Meador KJ, Baker GA, Browning N, *et al.* Cognitive function at 3 years of age after fetal exposure to antiepileptic drugs. *Obstetrics & Gynecology* 2009;**360**:1597.

Mølgaard-Nielsen D, Hviid A. Newer-generation antiepileptic drugs and the risk of major birth defects. *Obstetrics & Gynecology* 2011;**305**:1996.

18 Systemic Lupus Erythematosus (SLE)

Izmirly PM, Costedoat-Chalumeau N, Pisoni CN, *et al.* Maternal use of hydroxychloroquine is associated with a reduced risk of recurrent anti-SSA/Ro-antibody-associated cardiac manifestations of neonatal lupus. *Obstetrics & Gynecology* 2012;**126**:76.

Landy, H, Powell, M, Hill, D, *et al.* Belimumab Pregnancy Registry: prospective cohort study of pregnancy outcomes. *Obstetrics & Gynecology.* 2014; **123**:62S.

Silver, RM, Parker, CB, Reddy, UM *et al.* Antiphospholipid antibodies in stillbirth. *Obstetrics & Gynecology*2013; **122**(3):641–657.

Tsokos GC. Mechanisms of disease: systemic lupus erythematosus. *New England Journal of Medicine* 2011;**365**:2110–2121.

19 Thrombocytopenia

Adams TM, Allaf MB, Vintzileos AM. Maternal thrombocytopenia in pregnancy: diagnosis and management. *Obstetrics & Gynecology* 2013;**33**(2): 327–341.

American College of Obstetricians and Gynecologists. ACOG Practice Bulletin No. 6.Thrombocytopenia in pregnancy. *Obstetrics & Gynecology* 1999;**67**(2): 117–128.

Espinoza JP, Caradeux J, Norwitz ER, Illanes SE. Fetal and neonatal alloimmune thrombocytopenia. *Obstetrics & Gynecology* 2013;**6**(1):e15–21.

Martí-Carvajal AJ, Peña-Martí GE, Comunián-Carrasco G. Medical treatments for idiopathic thrombocytopenic purpura during pregnancy. *Obstetrics & Gynecology* 2009;(**4**):CD007722.

20 Thyroid Dysfunction

American College of Obstetricians and Gynecologists. ACOG Practice Bulletin No. 148. Thyroid disease in pregnancy. *Obstetrics & Gynecology* 2015;**125**: 996–1005.

Casey B, Leveno K. Thyroid disease in pregnancy. *Obstetrics & Gynecology* 2006;**108**:1283–1292.

25 Hepatitis B

American College of Obstetricians and Gynecologists. ACOG Practice Bulletin No. 86. Viral hepatitis in pregnancy. *Obstetrics & Gynecology* 2007;**110**(4): 941–956.

Dunkelberg JC, Berkley EM, Thiel KW, Leslie KK. Hepatitis B and C in pregnancy: a review and recommendations for care. *Obstetrics & Gynecology* 2014;**34**(12):882–891.

Kubo A, Shlager L, Marks AR, *et al.* Prevention of vertical transmission of hepatitis B: an observational study. *Obstetrics & Gynecology* 2014;**160**:828.

Shi Z, Yang Y, Ma L, *et al.* Lamivudine in late pregnancy to interrupt in utero transmission of hepatitis B virus: a systematic review and meta-analysis. *Obstetrics & Gynecology* 2010;**116**:147.

26 Herpes Simplex Virus (HSV)

American College of Obstetricians and Gynecologists. ACOG Practice Bulletin No 82. Management of herpes in pregnancy. *Obstetrics & Gynecology* 2007;**109**(6): 1489–1498.

Delaney S, Gardella C, Saracino M, *et al.* Seroprevalence of herpes simplex virus type 1 and 2 among pregnant women, 1989–2010. *Obstetrics & Gynecology* 2014;**312**:746.

Linthavong, OR, Franasiak J, Ivester T. Febrile illness in pregnancy: disseminated herpes simplex virus. *Obstetrics & Gynecology.* 2013;**121**(3):675–681.

Westhoff GL, Little SE, Caughey AB, Herpes simplex virus and pregnancy: a review of the management of antenatal and peripartum herpes infections. *Obstetrics & Gynecology* 2011;**66**:629.

27 Human Immunodeficiency Virus (HIV)

American College of Obstetricians and Gynecologists. ACOG Committee Opinion No. 596. Routine human immunodeficiency virus screening. *Obstetrics & Gynecology* 2014;**123**:1137.

Centers for Disease Control and Prevention (CDC). Laboratory testing for the diagnosis of hiv infection: updated recommendations. http://www.cdc.gov/hiv/pdf/HIVtestingAlgorithmRecommendation-Final.pdf. (accessed July 7, 2014).

Nielsen-Saines K, Watts DH, Veloso VG, *et al.* Three postpartum antiretroviral regimens to prevent intrapartum HIV infection. *Obstetrics & Gynecology* 2012;**366**:2368.

Panel on Treatment of HIV-Infected Pregnant Women and Prevention of Perinatal Transmission. Recommendations for Use of Antiretroviral Drugs in Pregnant HIV-1-Infected Women for Maternal Health and Interventions to Reduce Perinatal HIV Transmission in the United States. http://aidsinfo. nih.gov/guidelines/html/3/perinatal-guidelines/0/ (accessed March 28, 2014).

28 Parvovirus B19

De Jong EP, Lindenburg IT, van Klink JM, *et al.* Intrauterine transfusion for parvovirus B19 infection: long-term neurodevelopmental outcome. *Obstetrics & Gynecology* 2012;**206**:204.e1.

Lassen J, Jensen AK, Bager P, *et al.* Parvovirus B19 infection in the first trimester of pregnancy and risk of fetal loss: a population-based case-control study. *Obstetrics & Gynecology* 2012; **176**:803.

Puccetti C, Contoli M, Bonvicini F, *et al.* Parvovirus B19 in pregnancy: possible consequences of vertical transmission. *Prenatal Diagnosis* 2012; **32**:897.

29 Syphilis

Centers for Disease Control and Prevention (CDC). Syphilis testing algorithms using treponemal tests for initial screening—four laboratories, New York City, 2005–2006. *Obstetrics & Gynecology* 2008;**57**: 872–875.

U.S. Preventive Services Task Force. Screening for syphilis infection in pregnancy: U.S. Preventive Services Task Force reaffirmation recommendation statement. *Obstetrics & Gynecology* 2009;**150**: 705–709.

Wendel GD Jr, Sheffield JS, Hollier LM, *et al.* Treatment of syphilis in pregnancy and prevention of congenital syphilis. *Obstetrics & Gynecology* 2002;**35**: S200–209.

Workowski KA, Berman SM. Centers for Disease Control and Prevention Sexually Transmitted Disease Treatment Guidelines. *Obstetrics & Gynecology* 2011;**53**(3):S59–63.

30 Tuberculosis (TB)

Lighter-Fisher J, Surette AM. Performance of an interferon-gamma release assay to diagnose latent tuberculosis infection during pregnancy. *Obstetrics & Gynecology* 2012;**119**:1088.

Worjoloh A, Kato-Maeda M, Osmond D, *et al.* Interferon gamma release assay compared with the tuberculin skin test for latent tuberculosis detection in pregnancy. *Obstetrics & Gynecology* 2011;**118**:1363.

Wright A, Zignol M, Van Deun A, *et al.* Epidemiology of anti-tuberculosis drug resistance 2002-07: an updated analysis of the Global Project on Anti-Tuberculosis Drug Resistance Surveillance. *Lancet* 2009; **373**:1861.

31 Chorioamnionitis (Intraamniotic Infection)

Black, LP, Hinson, L Duff, P. Limited course of antibiotic treatment for chorioamnionitis. *Obstetrics & Gynecology* 2012;**119**(6):1102–1105.

Combs CA, Gravett M, Garite TJ, *et al.* Amniotic fluid infection, inflammation, and colonization in preterm labor with intact membranes. *Obstetrics & Gynecology* 2014;**210**:125.e1.

Goodnight W, Newman R, Society of Maternal-Fetal Medicine. *Optimal nutrition for improved twin pregnancy outcome. Obstetrics & Gynecology* 2009;**114**:1121.

Shatrov JG, Birch SC, Lam LT, *et al.* Chorioamnionitis and cerebral palsy: a meta-analysis. *Obstetrics & Gynecology* 2010; **116**:387.

34 Breast Lesions

Chen L, Zhou WB, Zhao Y, *et al.* Bloody nipple discharge is a predictor of breast cancer risk: a meta-analysis. *Obstetrics & Gynecology* 2012;**132**:9.

Griffin JL, Pearlman MD. Clinical expert series: breast cancer screening in women at average risk and high risk. *Obstetrics & Gynecology* 2010;**116**(6):1410–1421.

Pearlman MD, Griffin JL. Clinical expert series: benign breast disease. *Obstetrics & Gynecology* 2010;**116**(3): 747–758.

Satenn RJ, Mansel R. Benign breast disorders. *Obstetrics & Gynecology* 2005;**353**:275.

US Preventive Services Task Force. Screening for Breast Cancer: United States Preventive Services Task Force recommendation statement. *Obstetrics & Gynecology* 2009;**151**:716–726.

36 First Trimester Vaginal Bleeding

Doubilet PM, Benson CB, Bourne T, Blaivas M; Society of Radiologists in Ultrasound Multispecialty Panel on Early First Trimester Diagnosis of Miscarriage and Exclusion of a Viable Intrauterine Pregnancy, Barnhart KT *et al.* Diagnostic criteria for nonviable pregnancy early in the first trimester. *Obstetrics & Gynecology* 2013;**369**(15):1443–1451.

Lane BF, Wong-You-Cheong JJ, Javitt MC, *et al.* American College of Radiology. ACR appropriateness Criteria® first trimester bleeding. *Obstetrics & Gynecology* 2013; **9**(2):91–96.

Lykke JA, Dideriksen KL, Lidegaard O, Langhoff-Roos J. First-trimester vaginal bleeding and complications later in pregnancy. *Obstetrics & Gynecology* 2010;**115**:935–944.

Nanda K, Lopez LM, Grimes DA, *et al.* Expectant care versus surgical treatment for miscarriage. *Obstetrics & Gynecology* 2012;(**3**):CD003518.

37 Higher-Order Multifetal Pregnancy

American College of Obstetricians and Gynecologists. ACOG Committee Opinion No. 455. Magnesium sulfate before anticipated preterm birth for neuroprotection. *Obstetrics & Gynecology* 2010;**115**: 669–671.

American College of Obstetricians and Gynecologists. ACOG Committee Opinion No. 553. Multifetal pregnancy reduction. *Obstetrics & Gynecology* 2013; **121**:405–410.

American College of Obstetricians and Gynecologists. ACOG Practice Bulletin No. 144: Multifetal gestations: twin, triplet, and higher-order multifetal pregnancies. *Obstetrics & Gynecology.* 2014; **123**(5):1118.

Goodnight W, Newman R, Society of Maternal-Fetal Medicine. *Optimal nutrition for improved twin pregnancy outcome. Obstetrics & Gynecology* 2009; **114**:1121.

38 Hyperemesis Gravidarum (HEG)

American College of Obstetricians and Gynecologists. ACOG Practice Bulletin No. 52. Nausea and vomiting of pregnancy. *Obstetrics & Gynecology* 2004;**103**: 803–814.

Magee LA, Mazzotta P, Koren G. Evidence-based view of safety and effectiveness of pharmacologic therapy for nausea and vomiting of pregnancy (NVP). *Obstetrics & Gynecology* 2002;**186**:S256–261.

Matthews A, Haas DM, O'Mathúna DP, Dowswell T, Doyle M. Interventions for nausea and vomiting in early pregnancy. *Obstetrics & Gynecology* 2014; (**3**):CD007575.

39 Intrauterine Fetal Demise (IUFD)

American College Obstetricians and Gynecologists. ACOG Practice Bulletin No. 102. Management of stillbirth. *Obstetrics & Gynecology* 2009;**113**:748–761.

American College Obstetricians and Gynecologists. ACOG Committee Opinion No. 383. Evaluation of stillbirths and neonatal deaths. *Obstetrics & Gynecology* 2007;**110**:963–966.

Silver RM, Heuser CC. Stillbirth workup and delivery management. *Obstetrics & Gynecology* 2010; **53**(3):681–690.

Silver RM, Varner MW, Reddy U, *et al. Obstetrics & Gynecology* 2007;**196**(5):433–444.

40 Fetal Growth Restriction (FGR)

American College of Obstetricians and Gynecologists. ACOG Committee Opinion, No. 560. Fetal Growth Restriction. Washington, DC: ACOG, 2013.

American College of Obstetricians and Gynecologists. ACOG Practice Bulletin, No. 134. Fetal Growth Restriction. Washington, DC, May 2013.

Garite TJ, Clark R, Thorp JA: Intrauterine growth restriction increases morbidity and mortality among premature neonates. *Obstetrics & Gynecology* 2004;**191**:481.

Low JA, Handley-Derry MH, Burke SO, *et al.* Association of intrauterine fetal growth retardation and learning deficits at age 9 to 11 years. *Obstetrics & Gynecology* 1992;**167**:1499.

Pilliod RA, Cheng YW, Snowden JM, *et al.* The risk of intrauterine fetal death in the small-for-gestational-age fetus. *Obstetrics & Gynecology* 2012;**207**:318.e1-6.

Society for Maternal-Fetal Medicine Publications Committee, Berkley E, Chauhan SP, Abuhamad A. Doppler assessment of the fetus with intrauterine growth restriction. *Obstetrics & Gynecology.* 2012;**206**: 300–308.

Unterscheider J, Daly S, Geary MP, *et al.* Optimizing the definition of intrauterine growth restriction: the multicenter prospective PORTO trial. *Obstetrics & Gynecology.* 2013;**208**:280–290.e1-6.

41 Isoimmunization

American College of Obstetricians and Gynecologists. Management of alloimmunization during pregnancy. *Obstetrics & Gynecology* 2006;**108**(2):457–464.

Mari GI, Deter RL, Carpenter RL, Rahman F, Zimmerman R, Moise KJ Jr, *et al.* Noninvasive diagnosis by Doppler ultrasonography of fetal anemia due to maternal red-cell alloimmunization. *Obstetrics & Gynecology* 2000;**342**(1):9–14.

Society for Maternal-Fetal Medicine, Norton ME, Chauhan SP, Dashe JS. SMFM Clinical Guideline No. 7. Nonimmune hydrops fetalis. *Obstetrics & Gynecology* 2015; **212**(2):127–139.

42 Macrosomia

American College of Obstetricians and Gynecologists. ACOG Technical Bulletin No. 159. Fetal macrosomia. *Obstetrics & Gynecology* 1992;**39**(4):341–345.

American College of Obstetricians and Gynecologists. ACOG Practice Bulletin No. 58. Ultrasonography in pregnancy. *Obstetrics & Gynecology* 2004;**104**(6): 1449–1458.

Irion O, Boulvain M. Induction of labour for suspected fetal macrosomia. *Obstetrics & Gynecology* 2000; (2):CD000938.

Poolsup N, Suksomboon N, Amin M. Effect of treatment of gestational diabetes mellitus: a systematic review and meta-analysis. *Obstetrics & Gynecology* 2014;**9**(3):e92485.

43 Medically-Indicated Late Preterm and Early Term Delivery

American College of Obstetricians and Gynecologists. ACOG Practice Bulletin No. 107. *Induction of labor Obstetrics & Gynecology* 2009;**114**:386–397.

American College of Obstetricians and Gynecologists. ACOG Committee Opinion No. 560Medically indicated late-preterm and early-term deliveries. *Obstetrics & Gynecology* 2013;**121**:908–910.

American College of Obstetricians and Gynecologists. ACOG Committee Opinion No. 561. Nonmedically indicated early-term deliveries. *Obstetrics & Gynecology* 2013; **121**:911–915.

Holland MG, Refuerzo JS, Ramin SM, Saade GR, Blackwell SC. Late preterm birth: how often is it avoidable? *Obstetrics & Gynecology* 2009;**201**(4):404.e1–4.

Spong CY, Mercer BM, D'Alton M, *et al.* Timing of indicated late-preterm and early-term birth. *Obstetrics & Gynecology* 2011;**118**:323–333.

44 Obesity

American College of Obstetricians and Gynecologists. ACOG Committee Opinion Number 549. Obesity in pregnancy. *Obstetrics & Gynecology* 2013;**121**(1):213–217.

American College of Obstetricians and Gynecologists. ACOG Committee Opinion Number 319. The role of the obstetrician-gynecologist in the assessment and management of obesity. *Obstetrics & Gynecology* 2005;**106**:895–899.

Catalano PM. Management of obesity in pregnancy. *Obstetrics & Gynecology* 2007;**109**:419–433.

Institute of Medicine. Nutritional status and weight gain. In: *Nutrition during Pregnancy*. Washington, DC: National Academies Press, 1990. pp. 227–233.

Yu CK, Teoh TG, Robinson S. Obesity in pregnancy. *Obstetrics & Gynecology* 2006;**113**:1117–1125.

45 Oligohydramnios

American College of Obstetricians and Gynecologists. ACOG Practice Bulletin No. 9. Antepartum fetal surveillance *Obstetrics & Gynecology* 2000;**68**(2): 175–185.

American College of Obstetricians and Gynecologists. ACOG Practice Bulletin No. 101. Ultrasonography in pregnancy. *Obstetrics & Gynecology* 2009;**113**(2): 451–461.

Nabhan AF, Abdelmoula YA. Amniotic fluid index versus single deepest vertical pocket as a screening test for preventing adverse pregnancy outcome. *Obstetrics & Gynecology* 2008;(**3**):CD006593.

Rossi AC, Prefumo F. Perinatal outcomes of isolated oligohydramnios at term and post-term pregnancy: a systematic review of literature with meta-analysis. *Obstetrics & Gynecology* 2013;**169**(2):149–154.

46 Recurrent Pregnancy Loss (RPL)

American College Obstetricians and Gynecologists. ACOG Practice Bulletin No. 24. Management of recurrent pregnancy loss. *International Journal of Gynaecology and Obstetrics* 2002;**78**:179–190.

American College Obstetricians and Gynecologists. ACOG Practice Bulletin No. 118. Antiphospholipid antibody syndrome. *Obstetrics & Gynecology* 2011;**117**:192–199.

Hyde KJ, Schust DJ. Genetic considerations in recurrent pregnancy loss. *Cold Spring Harbor Perspectives in Medicine* 2015;**5**(3):a023119.

47 Placenta Accreta

American College of Obstetricians and Gynecologists. ACOG Committee Opinion. Placenta accreta. Washington, DC: ACOG, July 2012.

American College of Obstetricians and Gynecologists. ACOG Committee Opinion, No. 560. Medically indicated late-preterm and early-term deliveries Washington, DC: ACOG, 2013.

Belfort MA. Indicated preterm birth for placenta accreta. *Seminars in Perinatology* 2011;**35**(5): 252–256.

Oyelese Y, Smulian J. Placenta previa, placenta accreta, and vasa previa. *Obstetrics & Gynecology* 2006;**107**: 927–941.

Society for Maternal-Fetal Medicine. Placenta accreta. *Obstetrics & Gynecology* 2010;**203**:430–439.

Usta I, Hobeika E, Musa A, Gabriel G, Nassar A. Placenta pevia-accreta: risk factors and complications. *Obstetrics & Gynecology* 2005;**193**:1045–1049.

48 Placenta Previa

Oyelese Y, Smulian J. Placenta previa, placenta accreta, and vasa previa. *Obstetrics & Gynecology* 2006;**107**:927--941.

Rao KP, Belogolovkin V, Yankowitz J, Spinnato JA 2nd. Abnormal placentation: evidence-based diagnosis and management of placenta previa, placenta accreta, and vasa previa. *Obstetrics & Gynecology Survey* 2012; **67**(8):503–519.

Silver RM Abnormal placentation: placenta previa, vasa previa, and placenta accreta. *Obstetrics & Gynecology*. 2015;**126**(3):654–668.

49 Placental Abruption

Ananth CV, Berkowitz GS, Savitz DA, *et al*. Placental abruption and adverse perinatal outcomes. *Journal of the American Medical Association* 1999;**282**:1646–1651.

Cunningham FG, Leveno KJ, Bloom SL, *et al.*, eds. Obstetrical haemorrhage. In: Cunningham FG, Leveno KJ, Bloom SL, et al, eds. *Williams Obstetrics*. 24th ed. McGraw-Hill, New York, NY, 2014, pp. 780–828.

Glantz C, Purnell L. Clinical utility of sonography in the diagnosis and treatment of placental abruption. *Journal of Ultrasound Medicine*. 2002.**21**:837–840.

Hurd WW, Miodovnik M, Hertzberg V, *et al*. Selective management of abruption placentae: a prospective study. *Obstetrics & Gynecology* 1983;**61**:467–479.

Stafford I, Belfort MS, Dildy III GA. Etiology and management of haemorrhage. In: Belfort M, Saade G, Foley M, Phelan J, Dildy G, eds. *Critical Care Obstetrics*. 5th ed. Wiley-Blackwell, Chichester, 2010:308–326.

50 Polyhydramnios

American College of Obstetricians and Gynecologists. ACOG Practice Bulletin No. 9. Antepartum fetal surveillance. *Obstetrics & Gynecology* 2000;**68**(2): 175–185.

American College of Obstetricians and Gynecologists. ACOG Practice Bulletin No. 101. Ultrasonography in pregnancy. *Obstetrics & Gynecology* 2009;**113**(2): 451–461.

Moore TR. The role of amniotic fluid assessment in evaluating fetal well-being. *Obstetrics & Gynecology* 2011;**38**(1):33–46.

51 Post-Term Pregnancy

American College of Obstetricians and Gynecologists. ACOG Practice Bulletin No. 55. Management of postterm pregnancy. *Obstetrics & Gynecology* 2004;**104**(3):639–646.

Clinical Practice Obstetrics Committee; Maternal Fetal Medicine Committee, Delaney M, Roggensack A, Leduc DC, Ballermann C, *et al*. Guidelines for the management of pregnancy at 41+0 to 42+0 weeks. *Obstetrics & Gynecology* 2008;**30**(9):800–823.

Crowley P. Interventions for preventing or improving the outcome of delivery at or beyond term. *Obstetrics & Gynecology* 2000;(**2**):CD000170.

Gülmezoglu AM, Crowther CA, Middleton P, Heatley E. Induction of labour for improving birth outcomes for women at or beyond term. *Obstetrics & Gynecology* 2012;(**6**):CD004945.

Hannah ME, Hannah WJ, Hellmann J, *et al*. Induction of labor as compared with serial antenatal monitoring in post-term pregnancy. A randomized controlled trial. The Canadian Multicenter Post-term Pregnancy Trial Group. *Obstetrics & Gynecology* 1992; **326**(24):1587–1592.

The National Institute of Child Health and Human Development Network of Maternal-Fetal Medicine Units A clinical trial of induction of labor versus expectant management in postterm pregnancy.. *Obstetrics & Gynecology* 1994;**170**(3):716–723.

52 Pregnancy Termination

ACOG Practice Bulletin No. 135: Second-trimester abortion. *Obstetrics & Gynecology*. 2013;**121**(6):1394.

ACOG Practice Bulletin No. 143: Medical Management of First-Trimester Abortion. *Obstetrics & Gynecology*. 2014;**123**(3):676.

Raymond EG, Grimes DA. The comparative safety of legal induced abortion and childbirth in the United States. *Obstetrics & Gynecology* 2012;**119**:215.

53 Prenatal Diagnosis

American College of Obstetricians and Gynecologists. ACOG Practice Bulletin No. 77. Screening for fetal chromosomal abnormalities. *Obstetrics & Gynecology* 2007; **109**(1):217–227.

American College of Obstetricians and Gynecologists. ACOG Practice Bulletin No. 78.Hemoglobinopathies in pregnancy. *Obstetrics & Gynecology* 2007; **109**(1):229–237.

American College of Obstetricians and Gynecologists. ACOG Practice Bulletin No. 88. Invasive prenatal testing for aneuploidy. *Obstetrics & Gynecology* 2007;**110**(6):1459–1467.

American College of Obstetricians and Gynecologists. ACOG Practice Bulletin No. 58. OUltrasonography in pregnancy. *bstetrics & Gynecology* 2004;**104**(6): 1449–1458.

Norwitz ER, Levy B. Noninvasive prenatal testing: the future is now. *Obstetrics & Gynecology* 2013;**6**(2):48–62.

54 Preterm Labor

American College of Obstetricians and Gynecologists. ACOG Practice Bulletin No. 38. Perinatal care at the threshold of viability. *Obstetrics & Gynecology* 2002;**79**(2):181–188.

American College of Obstetricians and Gynecologists. ACOG Committee Opinion No. 475. Antenatal corticosteroid therapy for fetal maturation. *Obstetrics & Gynecology* 2011; **17**(2):422–424.

American College of Obstetricians and Gynecologists. ACOG Practice Bulletin No. 127. Management of preterm labor. *Obstetrics & Gynecology* 2012;**119**(6): 1308–1317.

Dodd JM, Jones L, Flenady V, Cincotta R, Crowther CA. Prenatal administration of progesterone for preventing preterm birth in women considered to be at risk of preterm birth. *Obstetrics & Gynecology* 2013;(**7**):CD004947.

Flenady V, Hawley G, Stock OM, Kenyon S, Badawi N. Prophylactic antibiotics for inhibiting preterm labour with intact membranes. *Obstetrics & Gynecology* 2013;(**12**):CD000246.

Haas DM, Caldwell DM, Kirkpatrick P, McIntosh JJ, Welton NJ. Tocolytic therapy for preterm delivery: systematic review and network meta-analysis. *Obstetrics & Gynecology* 2012 **345**:e6226.

Norwitz ER, Robinson JN, Challis JR. The control of labor. *Obstetrics & Gynecology* 1999; **341**(9):660–666.

55 Screening for Preterm Birth

American College of Obstetricians and Gynecologists. ACOG Practice Bulletin No. 130. Prediction and prevention of preterm birth. *Obstetrics & Gynecology* 2012;**120**(4):964–973.

American College of Obstetricians and Gynecologists. ACOG Committee Opinion No. 560. Medically indicated late-preterm and early-term deliveries. *Obstetrics & Gynecology* 2013; **121**(4):908–10.

Deshpande SN, van Asselt AD, Tomini F, *et al*. Rapid fetal fibronectin testing to predict preterm birth in women with symptoms of premature labour: a systematic review and cost analysis. *Obstetrics & Gynecology* 2013;**17**(40):131–138.

Iams JD, Goldenberg RL, Meis PJ, *et al*. The length of the cervix and the risk of spontaneous premature delivery. National Institute of Child Health and Human Development Maternal Fetal Medicine Unit Network. *Obstetrics & Gynecology* 1996;**334**(9): 567–572.

Iams JD, Romero R, Culhane JF, Goldenberg RL. Primary, secondary, and tertiary interventions to reduce the morbidity and mortality of preterm birth. *Obstetrics & Gynecology* 2008; **371**:164–175.

Lim K, Butt K, Crane JM. SOGC Clinical Practice Guideline. Ultrasonographic cervical length assessment in predicting preterm birth in singleton pregnancies. *Obstetrics & Gynecology* 2011;**33**(5):486–499.

Society for Maternal-Fetal Medicine Publications Committee. Progesterone and preterm birth prevention: translating clinical trials data into clinical practice. *Obstetrics & Gynecology* 2012;**206**:376–386.

Sosa C, Althabe F, Belizán J, Bergel E. Bed rest in singleton pregnancies for preventing preterm birth. *Obstetrics & Gynecology* 2004;(**1**):CD003581.

56 Preterm Premature Rupture of the Membranes

American College of Obstetricians and Gynecologists Committee on Obstetric Practice. ACOG Committee Opinion No. 485. Prevention of early-onset group B streptococcal disease in newborns *Obstetrics & Gynecology* 2011;**117**(4):1019–1027.

American College of Obstetricians and Gynecologists Practice Bulletin No. 139. Premature rupture of membranes *Obstetrics & Gynecology* 2013;**122**(4): 918–930.

Gyamfi-Bannerman C, Son M. Preterm premature rupture of membranes and the rate of neonatal sepsis after two courses of antenatal corticosteroids. *Obstetrics & Gynecology* 2014;**124**:999–1003.

Pierson RC, Gordon SS, Haas DH. A retrospective comparison of antibiotic regimens for preterm premature rupture of membranes. *Obstetrics & Gynecology* 2014;**124**:515–519.

Waters TP, Mercer BM. The management of preterm premature rupture of the membranes near the limit of fetal viability. *American Journal of Obstetrics & Gynecology* 2009;**201**:230–240.

57 Vaginal Birth After Cesarean (VBAC)

American College of Obstetricians and Gynecologists. ACOG Committee Opinion No. 342. Induction of labor for vaginal birth after cesarean delivery. *Obstetrics & Gynecology* 2006;**108**:465–468.

American College of Obstetricians and Gynecologists. Vaginal birth after cesarean delivery. *Obstetrics & Gynecology* 2010;**116**:450–463.

Cheng YW, Eden KB, Marshall N, et al. Delivery after prior cesarean: maternal morbidity and mortality. *Clinics in Perinatology* 2011;**38**(2):297–309.

Spong CY, Landon MB, Gilbert S, *et al.*; National Institute of Child Health and Human Development (NICHD) Maternal-Fetal Medicine Units (MFMU) Network. *Obstetrics & Gynecology* 2007;**110**(4): 801–807.

58 Teratology

Adam MP, Polifka JE, Friedman JM. Evolving knowledge of the teratogenicity of medications in human pregnancy. *Medical Genetics Part C* 2011;**157C**:175.

Buhimschi CS, Weiner CP. Clinical expert series: medications in pregnancy and lactation. Part 1. Teratology. *Obstetrics & Gynecology* 2009;**113**:166–188.

Buhimschi CS, Weiner CP. Clinical expert series: medications in pregnancy and lactation. Part 2. Drugs with minimal or unknown human teratogenic Effect. *Obstetrics & Gynecology* 2009;**113**:417–432.

Department of Health and Human Services. Food and Drug Administration 21 CFR Part 201 [Docket No. FDA-2006-N-0515 (formerly Docket No. 2006 N-0467).

59 Term Premature Rupture of the Membranes

American College of Obstetricians and Gynecologists. Committee on Obstetric Practice. ACOG Committee Opinion No. 485: Prevention of early-onset group B streptococcal disease in newborns. *Obstetrics & Gynecology*. 2011;**117**(4):1019–1027.

American College of Obstetricians and Gynecologists. Practice Bulletin No. 139. Premature rupture of membranes. *Obstetrics & Gynecology*. 2013;**122**(4): 918–930.

60 Twin Pregnancy

American College of Obstetricians and Gynecologists. ACOG Committee Opinion No. 455. Magnesium sulfate before anticipated preterm birth for neuroprotection. *Obstetrics & Gynecology* 2010;**115**:669–671.

American College of Obstetricians and Gynecologists. ACOG Practice Bulletin No. 144: Multifetal gestations: twin, triplet, and higher-order multifetal pregnancies. *Obstetrics & Gynecology*. 2014;**123**(5):1118.

Goodnight W, Newman R, Society of Maternal-Fetal Medicine. *Optimal nutrition for improved twin pregnancy outcome. Obstetrics & Gynecology* 2009; **114**:1121.

Higgins JR, Dornan J, Morrison JJ, *et al.*; Perinatal Ireland Research Consortium. Definition of intertwin birth weight discordance. *Obstetrics & Gynecology* 2011;**118**(1):94–103.

61 Breech Presentation

Alarab M, Regan C, O'Connell M, *et al.* Singleton vaginal breech delivery at term: still a safe Option. *Obstetrics & Gynecology* 2004;**103**:407–412.

American College of Obstetricians and Gynecologists. ACOG Committee Opinion Number 340. Mode of term singleton breech delivery. July 2006.

American College of Obstetricians and Gynecologists. ACOG Practice Bulletin Number 13. External Cehalic Version. February 2000.

American College of Obstetricians and Gynecologists. ACOG; SMFM. Safe prevention of the primary cesarean delivery. *Obstetrics & Gynecology* 2014; **123**(3):693–711.

Gilstrap LC, Cunningham FG, VanDorsten JP, eds, Breech delivery. In: *Operative Obstetrics*. 2nd ed. McGraw-Hill, New York, NY, 2002, pp. 89–122.

Su M, McLeod L, Ross S, Willan A, *et al.* Term Breech Trial Collaborative Group. Factors associated with adverse perinatal outcome in the Term Breech Trial. *Obstetrics & Gynecology* 2003;**189**(3):740–745.

62 Intrapartum Fetal Testing

Alfirevic Z, Devane D, Gyte GM. Continuous cardiotocography (CTG) as a form of electronic fetal monitoring (EFM) for fetal assessment during labour. *Cochrane Database of Systematic Reviews* 2013; **5**:CD006066.

American College Obstetricians and Gynecologists. ACOG Practice Bulletin. Neonatal encephalopathy and cerebral palsy: executive summary. *Obstetrics & Gynecology* 2004;**103**(4):780–781.

American College Obstetricians and Gynecologists. Umbilical cord blood gas and acid-base analysis. *Obstetrics & Gynecology* 2006;**108**(5):1319–1322.

Macones GA, Hankins GD, Spong CY, Hauth J, Moore T. The 2008 National Institute of Child Health and Human Development workshop report on electronic fetal monitoring: update on definitions, interpretation, and research guidelines. *Obstetrics & Gynecology* 2008;**112**(3):661–666.

63 Cesarean Delivery

American College of Obstetricians and Gynecologists. ACOG Practice Bulletin No. 115.Vaginal birth after cesarean delivery. *Obstetrics & Gynecology* 2010;**116**: 450–463.

American College of Obstetricians and Gynecologists. ACOG Committee Opinion No. 559. Cesarean delivery on maternal request. *Obstetrics & Gynecology* 2013;**121**(4):904–907.

Mackeen AD, Packard RE, Ota E, Berghella V, Baxter JK. Timing of intravenous prophylactic antibiotics for preventing postpartum infectious morbidity in women undergoing cesarean delivery. *Cochrane Database of Systematic Reviews* 2014;**5**:12:CD009516.

64 Operative Vaginal Delivery

American College of Obstetricians and Gynecologists. ACOG Practice Bulletin No. 154. Operative vaginal delivery. November 2015.

American College of Obstetricians and Gynecologists. ACOG; SMFM. Safe prevention of the primary cesarean delivery. *Obstetrics & Gynecology* 2014;**123**(3):693–711.

Gilstrap LC, Cunningham FG, VanDorsten JP, eds. Forceps. In *Operative Obstetrics*. 2nd ed. McGraw-Hill: New York, NY, 2002, pp. 89–122.

Gilstrap LC, Cunningham FG, Van Dorsten JP, eds. Operative delivery by vacuum. In: *Operative Obstetrics*. 2nd ed. McGraw-Hill, NY, 2002, pp. 123–143.

Yeomans E. Operative vaginal delivery. *Obstetrics & Gynecology* 2010;**115**:645–653.

65 Severe Perineal Lacerations

Boggs EW, Berger H, Urquia M, McDermott CD. Recurrence of obstetric third-degree and fourth-degree anal sphincter injuries. *Obstetrics & Gynecology*. 2014;**124**(6):1128–1134.

Farrell S, Flowerdew G, Gilmour D. Overlapping compared with end-to-end repair of complete third-degree or fourth-degree obstetric tears: three-year follow-up of a randomized controlled trial. *Obstetrics & Gynecology* 2012;**120**:803–808.

Fernando R, Sultan A, Kettle C, et al*et al*. Repair techniques for obstetric anal sphincter injuries: a randomized controlled trial. *Obstetrics & Gynecology* 2006;**107**:1261–1268.

Gilstrap LC, Cunningham FG, Van Dorsten JP, eds. Episiotomy In: *Operative Obstetrics*. 2nd ed. McGraw-Hill, New York, NY, 2002, pp. 63–88.

Hale R, Ling F. *Episiotomy: Procedure and Repair Techniques*. American College of Obstetricians and Gynecologists, Washington, DC, 2007.

Landy HJ, Laughon SK, Bailit JL, *et al*; Consortium on Safe Labor. Characteristics associated with severe perineal and cervical lacerations during vaginal delivery. *Obstetrics & Gynecology*. 2011;**117**(3):627–635.

Lewicky-Gaupp C, Leader-Cramer A, Johnson L, *et al*. Wound complications after obstetric anal sphincter injuries. *Obstetrics & Gynecology* 2015;**125**:1088–1093.

Stock L, Basham E, Gossett DR, *et al*. Factors associated with wound complications in women with obstetric anal sphincter injuries (OASIS). *Obstetrics & Gynecology* 2013;**208**:327.e1-6.

66 Intrapartum Mangement of Twin Pregnancy

American College of Obstetricians and Gynecologists. ACOG Practice Bulletin No. 144: Multifetal gestations: twin, triplet, and higher-order multifetal pregnancies. *Obstetrics & Gynecology*. 2014; **123**(5):1118.

Barrett JF, Hannah ME, Hutton EK, *et al*. A randomized trial of planned cesarean or vaginal delivery for twin pregnancy. Twin Birth Study Collaborative Group. *Obstetrics & Gynecology*2013;**369**:1295–1305.

Higgins JR, Dornan J, Morrison JJ, *et al*. Perinatal Ireland Research Consortium. Definition of inter-twin birth weight discordance. *Obstetrics & Gynecology* 2011;**118**(1):94–103.

67 Postpartum Hemorrhage

American College of Obstetricians and Gynecologists. ACOG Practice Bulletin No. 76. Postpartum hemorrhage. *Obstetrics & Gynecology* 2006;**108**:1039–1047.

Brown H. Trauma in pregnancy. *Obstetrics & Gynecology* 2009;**114**:147–160.

Lyndon A, Lagrew D, Shields L, Main E, Cape V. Improving Health Care Response to Obstetric Hemorrhage. (California Maternal Quality Care Collaborative Toolkit to Transform Maternity Care) Developed under contract #11-10006 with the California Department of Public Health; Maternal, Child and Adolescent Health Division; Published by the California Maternal Quality Care Collaborative, 3/17/15.

Lyndon A, Lagrew D, Shields L, Melsop K, Bingham D, Main E. ACOG Practice Bulletin No. 76. Patient Safety Checklist 2. Postpartum hemorrhage. *Obstetrics & Gynecology* 2013;**121**(5):1151–1152.

68 Retained Placenta

American College of Obstetricians and Gynecologists. ACOG Practice Bulletin No. 120: Use of prophylactic antibiotics in labor and delivery. *Obstetrics & Gynecology*. 2011;**117**(6):1472–1483.

Duffy J, Mylan S, Showell M, *et al*. Pharmacologic intervention for retained placenta: a systematic review and meta-analysis. *Obstetrics & Gynecology* 2015;**125**:711–718.

Weeks AD. The retained placenta. *Best Practice & Research Clinical Obstetrics & Gynaecology* 2008;**22**(6):1103–1117.

69 Postpartum Endomyometritis

American College of Obstetricians and Gynecologists. Prophylactic antibiotic in labor and delivery. *Obstetrics & Gynecology* 2004;**84**(3):300–307.

American College of Obstetricians and Gynecologists. ACOG Practice Bulletin No. 120. Use of prophylactic antibiotics in labor and delivery. *Obstetrics & Gynecology* 2011;**117**(6):1472–1483.

Baaqeel H, Baaqeel R. Timing of administration of prophylactic antibiotics for caesarean section: a systematic review and meta-analysis. *Obstetrics & Gynecology* 2013;**120**(6):661–669.

Conroy K, Koenig AF, Yu YH, Courtney A, Lee HJ, Norwitz ER. Infectious morbidity after cesarean delivery: 10 strategies to reduce risk. *Obstetrics & Gynecology* 2012;**5**(2):69–77.

Tita AT, Rouse DJ, Blackwell S, *et al*. Emerging concepts in antibiotic prophylaxis for cesarean delivery: a systematic review. *Obstetrics & Gynecology* 2009;**113**:675–682.

70 Mastitis

Committee on Health Care for Underserved Women, American College of Obstetricians and Gynecologists. ACOG Committee Opinion No. 361: Breastfeeding: maternal and infant aspects. *Obstetrics & Gynecology* 2007;**109**:479.

Schoenfeld EM, McKay MP. Mastitis and methicillin-resistant Staphylococcus aureus (MRSA): the calm before the storm? *Journal of Emergency Medicine* 2010;**38**:e31.

Stafford I, Hernandez J, Laibl V, *et al*. Community-acquired methicillin-resistant Staphylococcus aureus among patients with puerperal mastitis requiring hospitalization. *Obstetrics & Gynecology* 2008;**112**:533.

Trop I, Dugas A, David J, El Khoury M, *et al*. Breast abscesses: evidence-based algorithms for diagnosis, management, and follow-up. *Radiographics*. 2011; **31**(6):1683–1699.

71 Vasa Previa

Bronsteen R, Whitten A, Balasubramanian M, *et al*. Vasa previa: clinical presentations, outcomes, and implications for management. *Obstetrics & Gynecology* 2013;**122**(2):352–357.

Gagnon R, Morin L, Bly S, Butt K, *et al*. Diagnostic Imaging Committee; Maternal Fetal Medicine Committee. SOGC Clinical Practice GuidelinE: guidelines for the management of vasa previa. *Obstetrics & Gynecology* 2010;**108**(1):85–89.

Rebarber A, Dolin C, Fox NS, Klauser CK, Saltzman DH, Roman AS. Natural history of vasa previa across gestation using a screening protocol. *Obstetrics & Gynecology* 2014;**33**(1):141–147.

72 Postpartum Psychiatric Disorders

American College of Obstetricians and Gynecologists. ACOG Practice Bulletin No. 92. Use of psychiatric medications during pregnancy and lactation. *Obstetrics & Gynecology* 2008;**111**(4):1001–1020.

Dennis CL, Dowswell T. Psychosocial and psychological interventions for preventing postpartum depression. *Obstetrics & Gynecology* 2013;(**2**):CD001134.

Haran C, van Driel M, Mitchell BL, Brodribb WE. Clinical guidelines for postpartum women and infants in primary care-a systematic review. *Obstetrics & Gynecology* 2014;**14**:51.

Yonkers KA, Wisner KL, Stewart DE, et al. The management of depression during pregnancy: a report from the American Psychiatric Association and the American College of Obstetricians and Gynecologists. *Obstetrics & Gynecology* 2009;**114**(3):703–713.

73 Sterilization

American College of Obstetricians and Gynecologists. ACOG Practice Bulletin No. 133. Benefits and risks of sterilization. *Obstetrics & Gynecology* 2013;**121**(2):392–404.

ESHRE Capri Workshop Group, Crosignani PG, Glasier A. Family planning 2011: better use of existing methods, new strategies and more informed choices for female contraception. *Obstetrics & Gynecology* 2012;**18**(6):670–681.

Lawrie TA, Nardin JM, Kulier R, Boulvain M. Techniques for the interruption of tubal patency for female sterilisation. *Obstetrics & Gynecology* 2011; (**2**):CD003034.

Zite N, Borrero S. Female sterilisation in the United States. *Obstetrics & Gynecology* 2011;**16**(5):336–340.

74 Acute Abdomen in Pregnancy

Khandelwal A, Fasih N, Kielar A. Imaging of acute abdomen in pregnancy. *Radiology Clinics of North America.* 2013;**51**:1005–1022.

Korndorffer JR, Fellinger E, Reed W. SAGES guideline for laparoscopic appendectomy. *Surgical Endoscopy* 2010;**24**(4):757–761.

Lu EJ, Curet MJ, El-Sayed YY, Kirkwood KS. Medical versus surgical management of biliary tract disease in pregnancy. *Surgery* 2004;**188**(6):755–759.

Mourad J, Elliott JP, Erickson L, Lisboa L. Appendicitis in pregnancy: new information that contradicts long-held clinical beliefs. *Obstetrics & Gynecology* 2000;**182**(5):1027–1029.

Tamir IL, Bongard FS, Klein SR. Acute appendicitis in the pregnant patient. *Surgery* 1990;**160**(6):571.

76 Acute Shortness of Breath

American College of Obstetricians and Gynecologists. ACOG Practice Bulletin No. 123. Thromboembolism in pregnancy. *Obstetrics & Gynecology* 2011;**118**:718–729.

Clark SL. Amniotic fluid embolism. *Obstetrics & Gynecology* 2014;**123**:337–348.

77 Cord Prolapse

American College of Obstetricians and Gynecologists. ACOG Committee Opinion No. 104. Anesthesia for emergency deliveries. *Obstetrics & Gynecology* 1992;**39**(2):148.

Holbrook BD, Phelan ST. Umbilical cord prolapse. *Obstetrics & Gynecology* 2013;**40**(1):1–14.

Uygur D, Kiş S, Tuncer R, Ozcan FS, Erkaya S. Risk factors and infant outcomes associated with umbilical cord prolapse. *Obstetrics & Gynecology* 2002;**78**(2):127–130.

78 Cardiopulmonary Resuscitation

American College of Obstetricians and Gynecologists. ACOG Practice Bulletin No. 100: Critical care in pregnancy. *Obstetrics & Gynecology* 2009;**113**:443–450.

Lipman S, Cohen S, Einav S. The Society for Obstetric Anesthesia and Perinatology Consensus Statement on the Management of Cardiac Arrest in Pregnancy. *Anesthesia Analgesics* 2014;**118**:1003–1016.

Vanden Hoek TL, Morrison LJ, Shuster M, *et al.* Part 12: Cardiac arrest in special situations: 2010. American Heart Association Guidelines for Cardiopulmonary Resuscitation and Emergency Cardiovascular Care. *Circulation* 2010;**122**:S829–861.

80 Eclampsia

American College of Obstetricians and Gynecologists. Task Force on Hypertension in Pregnancy. *Hypertension in Pregnancy.* Task Force on Hypertension in Pregnancy, editor. American College of Obstetricians and Gynecologists, Washington, DC, 2013.

American College of Obstetricians and Gynecologists. ACOG Committee Opinion No. 623. Emergent therapy for acute-onset, severe hypertension during pregnancy and the postpartum period. *Obstetrics & Gynecology* 2015;**125**(2):521–525.

Duley L, Gulmezoglu AM, Henderson-Smart DJ, Chou D. Magnesium sulphate and other anticonvulsants for women with pre-eclampsia. *Cochrane Database of Systematic Reviews* 2010, Issue 11.

Duley L, Henderson-Smart DJ, Walker GJ, Chou D. Magnesium sulphate versus diazepam for eclampsia. *Cochrane Database of Systematic Reviews* 2010, Issue 12.

Mattar F, Sibai BM. Eclampsia: VIII. *Risk factors for maternal morbidity. Obstetrics & Gynecology* 2000;**182**:307.

Sibai BM. Diagnosis, prevention, and management of eclampsia. *Obstetrics & Gynecology* 2005;**105**:402–410.

81 Shoulder Dystocia

American College of Obstetricians and Gynecologists. ACOG Practice Bulletin No. 22. Fetal Macrosomia. *Obstetrics & Gynecology* 2000.

American College of Obstetricians and Gynecologists. ACOG Practice Bulletin No. 40. Shoulder Dystocia *Obstetrics & Gynecology* 2002;**100**:1045–1050.

American College of Obstetricians and Gynecologists. Patient Safety Checklist No. 6: Documenting Shoulder Dystocia. *Obstetrics & Gynecology* 2012; **120**(2), Part 1:430–431.

Hoffman MK, Bailit JL, Branch W, *et al.* for the Consortium on Safe Labor A Comparison of Obstetric Maneuvers for the Acute Management of Shoulder Dystocia. *Obstetrics & Gynecology* 2011;**117**:1272–1278.

Menticoglou SM. A modified technique to deliver the posterior arm in severe shoulder dystocia. *Obstetrics & Gynecology* 2006;**108**:755–757.

Wood C, Ng KH, Dounslow D, Benning H. Time-an important variable in normal delivery. *Journal of Obstetrics of the British Commonwealth* 1973;**80**:295.

82 Thyroid Storm

Abalovich M, Amino N, Barbour LA, *et al.* Management of thyroid dysfunction during pregnancy and postpartum: an Endocrine Society Clinical Practice Guideline. *Obstetrics & Gynecology* 2007;**92**:S1–47.

American College of Obstetricians and Gynecologists. ACOG Technical Bulletin No. 181. Thyroid disease in pregnancy. *Obstetrics & Gynecology* 1993;**43** (1):82–88.

Bahn Chair RS, Burch HB, Cooper DS, *et al.* Hyperthyroidism and other causes of thyrotoxicosis: management guidelines of the American Thyroid Association and American Association of Clinical Endocrinologists. *Obstetrics & Gynecology* 2011; **21**(6):593–646.

Khoo CM, Lee KO. Endocrine emergencies in pregnancy. *Obstetrics & Gynecology* 2013;**27**(6): 885–891.

Stagnaro-Green A, Abalovich M, Alexander E, *et al.* Guidelines of the American Thyroid Association for the diagnosis and management of thyroid disease during pregnancy and postpartum. *Obstetrics & Gynecology* 2011;**21**:1081–1125.

Index

Obstetric Clinical Algorithms, Second Edition. Errol R. Norwitz, George R. Saade, Hugh Miller and Christina M. Davidson.
© 2017 John Wiley & Sons, Ltd. Published 2017 by John Wiley & Sons, Ltd.